Medical Memories and Experie
in Postwar East Germany

This book draws on the example of the major cities of Leipzig and Dresden to illustrate continuity and change in public health in the German Democratic Republic. Based on archival work, it will demonstrate how members of the medical profession successfully manipulated their pre-1945 past in order to continue practising, leading to persistence in the social conception of medicine and disease after Communism took hold. This was particularly evident in attitudes towards and treatment of sexually transmitted diseases and the pathology of deviant behaviour among young people.

Markus Wahl is a Research Fellow at the Institute for the History of Medicine at the Robert Bosch Stiftung in Stuttgart, Germany. In his current project, he investigates the experiences of patients with diabetes, sexually transmitted diseases, and alcohol addiction in the socialist healthcare system of East Germany. In 2017, he received his PhD from the University of Kent. His most recent publication is 'The Workhouse Dresden-Leuben After 1945: A Microstudy of Local Continuities in Postwar East Germany', *Journal of Contemporary History* (Online First: published 26 July 2018). In general, his research interests include Modern German History, Social History of Medicine, Socialist History, Memory and Addiction Studies as well as broader studies of sexual health in the past and around the world.

Routledge Studies in the History of Science, Technology and Medicine

Closing the Door on Globalization
Internationalism, Nationalism, Culture and Science in the Nineteenth and Twentieth Centuries
Fernando Clara and Cláudia Ninhos

Johann Friedrich Blumenbach
Race and Natural History, 1750–1850
Edited by Nicolaas Rupke and Gerhard Lauer

Health Policies in Transnational Perspective
Europe in the Interwar Years
Josep-Lluís Barona-Vilar

Urban Histories of Science
Making Knowledge in the City, 1820–1940
Edited by Oliver Hochadel and Agustí Nieto-Galan

Pioneering Health in London, 1935–2000
The Peckham Experiment
David Kuchenbuch

Soviet Science and Engineering in the Shadow of the Cold War
Hiroshi Ichikawa

Cold Science
Environmental Knowledge in the North American Arctic During the Cold War
Stephen Bocking and Daniel Heidt

Medical Memories and Experiences in Postwar East Germany
Treatments of the Past
Markus Wahl

For the full list of titles in the series, please visit: www.routledge.com/Routledge-Studies-in-the-History-of-Science-Technology-and-Medicine/book-series/HISTSCI

Medical Memories and Experiences in Postwar East Germany

Treatments of the Past

Markus Wahl

Routledge
Taylor & Francis Group

LONDON AND NEW YORK

First published 2019
by Routledge
2 Park Square, Milton Park, Abingdon, Oxon OX14 4RN

and by Routledge
605 Third Avenue, New York, NY 10017

First issued in paperback 2021

Routledge is an imprint of the Taylor & Francis Group, an informa business

British Library Cataloguing-in-Publication Data
A catalogue record for this book is available from the British Library

Library of Congress Cataloging-in-Publication Data
A catalog record for this book has been requested

ISBN 13: 978-0-367-78619-9 (pbk)
ISBN 13: 978-0-367-13870-7 (hbk)

Typeset in Times
by Apex CoVantage, LLC

Gewidmet meinem Großvater

Max Joachim Wahl (*1925–†2012)

Contents

Figures

Tables

Acknowledgements

Even if a book project and the PhD journey sometimes feel like a lonely endeavour, I had the privilege to enjoy great input and support from many people all over the world. This book would not have been finished or even possible without them, and I am very grateful for this.

First of all, I would like to express my sincere gratitude to my two advisors at the University of Kent, UK, Ulf Schmidt and Stefan Goebel, for leading me to this topic and supporting me in my academic career. I am also really grateful for an engaging viva with Juliette Pattinson and Patrick Major, which helped me to re-shape my dissertation into this book.

After my PhD in the UK, I found a new home at the Institute for the History of Medicine at the Robert Bosch Stiftung in Stuttgart, and I want to thank Robert Jütte, Martin Dinges, and the rest of my colleagues for allowing me to finish this book while working on new projects. Moreover, the input and support of Francesca Weil, Erika Dyck, Kateřina Lišková, and Heather Wolffram were always highly appreciated and helped me to broaden my horizons on that topic.

As I have often been quite relentless in my inquiries to the archives and collections relevant to my topic, I am very grateful for the patience and legwork of Maria Fiebrandt, my archivist at the Archive of the former State Security Service of East Germany, and Marion Schneider from the German Hygiene Museum, as well as all other staff members of the consulted city and federal archives, which helped me to uncover many new and important files for my research.

As a non-native speaker, however, I sometimes struggle to express my ideas as clearly as possible in the English language. Therefore, I am particularly grateful for the help of my proofreaders and friends, who were happy to sacrifice some time and sweat to look over my abstract ideas, above all Stuart Palmer and Grant Goszik.

For the daily coffee infusions, philosophical discussions, and emotional support I would like to thank in particular my friends Aske Brock, Julius Günther, Sebastian Beese, and Anja Lubosch. I would not have been able to push through such a stressful endeavour without them.

Last but not least, I would like to thank my family, who has been a great emotional but also financial support and without whom I could not have reached the stage in which I am now. Therefore, my sincere gratitude goes to my parents Uwe Kersten Wahl and Kerstin Wahl, who made my life as a historian possible.

However, the deepest gratitude for whom and where I am now goes to my grandfather, Max Joachim Wahl. He had a major influence on me and encouraged my interest in history and historical inquiry. For this crucial contribution to my life, I want to dedicate my first book to him and hope that he is proud of me. Rest in peace, Opa Achim.

Abbreviations

Abbreviation	Original name	English translation
Aufn.-Nr.	*Aufnahmenummer*	Number of the Picture
BArch	*Bundesarchiv*	Federal Archive of Germany
BDC	*Berlin Document Centre*	Berlin Document Centre
BDM	*Bund Deutscher Mädel*	German Girls' League
Bl.	*Blatt*	Page
BStU	*Der Bundesbeauftragte für die Unterlagen des Staatssicherheitsdienstes der ehemaligen Deutschen Demokratischen Republik*	The Federal Commissioner for the Files of the State Security Service of the former German Democratic Republic
BV	*Bezirksverwaltung*	Regional Administration of the MfS
CDU	*Christlich-Demokratische Union Deutschlands*	Christian Democratic Union of Germany
DAF	*Deutsche Arbeitsfront*	German Labour Front
DFD	*Demokratischer Frauenbund Deutschlands*	Democratic Women Association of Germany
DHDM	*Deutsches Hygiene Museum Dresden*	German Hygiene Museum in Dresden
DJV	*Deutsches Jungvolk*	German Youth Folk
DM	*Deutsche Mark*	German Mark
DRK	*Deutsches Rotes Kreuz*	German Red Cross
DSF	*Gesellschaft für Deutsch–Sowjetische Freundschaft*	German–Soviet Friendship Association
DVJ	*Deutsche Vereinigung für Jugendpsychiatrie*	German Association for Youth Psychiatry
DZVGW	*Deutsche Zentralverwaltung für Gesundheitswesen*	German Central Administration of Healthcare
DZVJ	*Deutsche Zentralverwaltung der Justiz [DJV]*	German Central Administration of Justice
FDGB	*Freier Deutscher Gewerkschaftsbund*	Free German Trade Union
FDJ	*Freie Deutsche Jugend*	Free German Youth
FRG	*Bundesrepublik Deutschland [BRD]*	Federal Republic of Germany
GDR	*Deutsche Demokratische Republik [DDR]*	German Democratic Republic

Abbreviation	Original name	English translation
HA IX/11	*Hauptabteilung IX/11 des MfS*	Head Department IX/11 of the MfS; responsible for discovering Nazi and war-crimes
HA XX	*Hauptabteilung XX des MfS*	Head Department XX of the MfS; responsible for the areas of medicine, culture, education, post, church, party organisations, and the general state apparatus
HJ	*Hitlerjugend*	Hitler Youth
HSA DD	*Hauptstaatsarchiv Dresden*	Main (Saxon) State Archive Dresden
hwG	*häufig wechselnden Geschlecht-sverkehr/-partner*	frequent promiscuous behaviour
IM	*Inoffizieller Mitarbeiter des MfS*	Unofficial collaborator of the MfS
KPD	*Kommunistische Partei Deutschlands*	Communist Party of Germany
LDPD	*Liberal-Demokratische Partei Deutschlands*	Liberal Democratic Party of Germany
MfG	*Ministerium für Gesundheitswesen*	Ministry of Healthcare
MfS	*Ministerium für Staatssicherheit [Stasi]*	Ministry of State Security
MVD	*Министерство внутренних дел*	Soviet Interior Ministry
NDPD	*National-Demokratische Partei Deutschlands*	National Democratic Party of Germany
NSÄB	*Nationalsozialistischer Ärztebund*	National Socialist Doctors' Association
NSDAP	*Nationalsozialistische Deutsche Arbeiterpartei*	National Socialist German Workers' Party
NSFK	*Nationalsozialistisches Fliegerkorps*	National Socialist Flyers Corps
NSV	*Nationalsozialistische Volkswohlfahrt*	National Socialist People's Welfare
NVA	*Nationale Volksarmee*	National People's Army
POW	*Kriegsgefangener*	Prisoner of War
PTSD	*Posttraumatische Belastungsstörung*	Post-Traumatic Stress Disorder
RHE	*Rechtshilfeersuchen*	Rogatory Letter
SA	*Sturmabteilung*	Storm Unit
SAJ	*Sozialistische Arbeiter-Jugend*	Socialist Workers' Youth
SBZ	*Sowjetische Besatzungszone*	Soviet Occupied Zone of Germany
SED	*Sozialistische Einheitspartei Deutschlands*	Socialist Unity Party of Germany
SLUB	*Sächsische Landesbibliothek, Staats- und Universitätsbibliothek Dresden*	Saxon State's Library, National and University Library Dresden
SMAD	*Sowjetische Militäradministration in Deutschland*	Soviet Military Administration in Germany

Abbreviation	Original name	English translation
SMAS	*Sowjetische Militäradministration in Sachsen*	Soviet Military Administration in Saxony
SS	*Schutzstaffel*	Protection Squadron
StA DD	*Stadtarchiv Dresden*	City Archive Dresden
StA Lpz	*Stadtarchiv Leipzig*	City Archive Leipzig
STD	*Geschlechtskrankheit*	Sexually transmitted disease
SU	*Sowjetunion*	Soviet Union
Tbc	*Tuberkulosis*	Tuberculosis
UFJ	*Untersuchungsausschuss Freiheitlicher Juristen*	Inquiry Committee of Liberal Jurists
UK	*Vereinigtes Königreich*	United Kingdom
USA	*Vereinigte Staaten von Amerika*	United States of America
VP	*Volkspolizei*	People's Police
ZAIG	*Zentrale Auswertungs- und Informationsgruppe*	Central Analysis and Information Group of the MfS

Translation note

Unless otherwise noted or cited, all translations from German in this book are my own.

Disclaimer

Terms and phrases in inverted commas indicate the author's awareness of their ambiguous or ideological character, their political incorrectness, or their colloquial nature. However, it was important to use contemporary language to capture the voices and mentalities of the people. Direct citations are always in double quotation marks.

Introduction

Medical memories and experiences

It was almost midnight, the day before Christmas Eve in 1959. A car of the *Ministerium für Staatssicherheit* [Ministry of State Security – MfS] of the *Deutsche Demokratische Republik* [German Democratic Republic – GDR] came to a halt outside house number 25 on Goethe-Allee in Dresden. Shortly afterwards, the MfS officers handcuffed and accompanied a man to their car, interrupting his holiday season and leaving his wife ignorant to the reason for his arrest. Back at the District Headquarters, the MfS officers interrogated him from 1 am to 8 am in the morning, after which he was taken into custody for several months to await trial. In a nine-page report, the responsible MfS officer, Frank Becker, explained the reasons for these proceedings: he had been informed about a double life of the arrested man that had started immediately at the end of the Second World War.[1]

In 1945, a man with the name Alfredo "Fred" Ceccetti appeared and offered his services to the local Soviet command in Dresden. He pretended to be of Italian origin with fluent Russian, so the *Sowjetische Militäradministration in Sachsen* [Soviet Military Administration in Saxony – SMAS] decided to employ him as an interpreter. However, as archival sources suggest, he evidently used this position and his connections to the West for illegal trade. The latter might be one of the reasons why he and his wife suddenly disappeared in 1950. Becker's report from 1960, which described these circumstances, continued that, not long after his disappearance, a man at a doctors' ball in Dresden created many rumours among the participants. The *Inoffizielle Mitarbeiter* [unofficial collaborator – IM] with the codename "Vogel" had informed the MfS about the following conversation during the ball:

> "I know this guy that is Fred Cichetti[sic]". [. . .] Hereupon another doctor answered: "You must have been mistaken, this is not Fred Cichetti[sic], this is Dr Korinek" "Why Dr Korinek?" – "Yes, he is a doctor [. . .] in orthopaedics. He is an excellent physician".[2]

In his report, Becker seemed very excited that he might have exposed that Ceccetti and Korinek were the same person – one man with a double life. However, the MfS files reveal that the state security service had arrested both Ceccetti, whose real name was Czeck, and Korinek already by the time the author wrote this report in February 1960. According to the investigation reports, the MfS officers were unable to find out why Siegfried Czeck (*1922) had in 1945 changed his name to Alfredo Ceccetti and assumed an Italian origin through a lengthy biography. One reason, they presumed, could be that he was part of a *Schutzstaffel* [SS] unit during the Second World War.[3]

Nevertheless, rumours could have consequences for an individual, and in Becker's report not everything was false; Walter Korinek (*1914) represents an exceptional case of the abuse of the chaotic situation of the postwar years. After 1945, he was able to conceal that he had never finished his medical studies and thus had no specialisation; yet, through excuses and his opportunistic behaviour he had persuaded authorities to employ him. The medical experiences and skills he had obtained while working as a medical assistant in a military hospital during the Second World War enabled him to continue working as a doctor without raising much suspicion. He even became the senior consultant of orthopaedics at a Dresden hospital until his arrest during Christmas 1959.[4]

The life of Walter Korinek is probably the most striking case that I have found during my archival research. Many fraud doctors operated during the postwar years, benefitting from the chaotic surroundings. However, as far as I can judge, Korinek's cunningness and his remarkable luck throughout his career were unique. If one reads the sources against the grain, his case simultaneously reveals the blatant issues in the early years of East Germany, which proclaimed a new era under the banner of Socialism. If someone without a medical licence could fall through the institutional nets, it is easy to imagine how many doctors with a Nazi past managed to get through the de-Nazification procedures unharmed.

The smooth transition of most doctors, nurses, and other medical personnel from the Third Reich into the GDR ultimately meant a continued existence of medical concepts, clichés, stigmatisations, and prejudices that formed part of their individual medical memories. Moreover, these persistent mentalities and professional views – manifested in a doctor's person – had a direct impact on the treatment, doctor–patient relationship, and consequent medical experience of people within health clinics across the GDR. For the state, this was an important fact, as the healthcare system was crucial to East Germany's legitimacy. Ludwig Mecklinger even stated in his position as Health Minister at a conference in 1981 that "[i]n the encounter with the health, and social, care system, Socialism has a name, face, and address for the citizen".[5] Health provision thus became a tool with which to implement the new vision of society, to demarcate itself from Western systems, and to support its claim to superiority in the Cold War. Accordingly, the GDR wanted to ensure that all interactions in a doctor's examination room adhered to socialist doctrines. Such an ideal, however, never reflected the reality.

The subtitle of this book, *Treatments of the Past*, captures the impact of the past on people's present in three particular contexts. Firstly, it reveals the strategies taken by doctors, such as Walter Korinek, to *treat their past* and adapt to a new system after 1945. Furthermore, it shows the opportunistic behaviour that enabled them professionally and personally to avoid any disruptions throughout the postwar period. This endeavour was often tolerated by the state, sometimes to the extent that doctors were given support by authorities in 'sanitising' their past. Secondly, this study explores how the resulting continuity of medical personnel influenced medical and social treatments of patients who suffered from sexually transmitted diseases [STDs]. Despite medical advances and new curative, less harmful drugs, many patients, mainly women, would receive out-dated treatments – *treatments from the past* – which were applied to educate the stigmatised STD sufferer. Thirdly, the book shows that the same was true for the 'war children' who had been psychologically and physically affected by the Second World War and its aftermath. However, their medical past in the form of disease, loss, malnutrition, and violence was hardly addressed; there was no *treatment for their past*. Instead, these medical memories and experiences were incorporated into the state narrative in order to justify the road to Socialism.

The analysis of how medical memories had an impact on the medical experiences of patients in postwar East Germany concludes with a case study of the *Fürsorgeheim Leuben* [Care Home Leuben] in Dresden. Here, all three examined strands – incriminated doctors, stigmatised, syphilitic women, and 'socially deviant' children – are drawn together. This institution exemplifies that the state narrative and claims were often curtailed, interpreted, and implemented in line with local needs. Moreover, it is more an example of a continued tradition than of a new beginning in the postwar era, and thus we see the persistence of the workhouse as a concept carried over from previous decades – *institutionalised treatments of the past*.

Consequently, patients' medical experiences differed according to their locality, officials in charge, doctors, and the mentality of the general public. Therefore, while these two cities capture the war and postwar experiences of other bombed metropolises within Germany, the focus on Leipzig and in particular Dresden creates a microcosm exposing details that a nationwide approach would fail to encompass.[6]

The book makes a twofold contribution to the historiography. Firstly, it argues that postwar East Germany was not a monolithic, Soviet-dominated construct. Instead, it reveals the agency that people had, even as a care home inmate. Therefore, the East German postwar narrative was not solely dictated by the state, but twisted and adapted according to medical memories and experiences at the local level.

Secondly, 1945 does not represent a decisive rupture in the perceptions of 'deviance' by local health and social authorities, nor in the methods utilised by doctors to treat diseases, in the experiences of patients in medical institutions, or in the ideas concerning morality within the population. Therefore, this study investigates the postwar years, roughly from 1945 to 1961, yet avoids relying on historically determined watersheds so as to reveal developments beyond these fixed periods.[7]

For investigating this period, it should be clarified that for East Germany the term 'state' is misleading for the postwar context. Until the foundation of the GDR in 1949, East Germany was not a traditional state construct. Instead, it became the *Sowjetische Besatzungszone* [Soviet Occupied Zone of Germany – SBZ] and thus had no sovereignty. Under the leadership of the *Sowjetische Militäradministration in Deutschland* [Soviet Military Administration in Germany – SMAD], occupation authorities established several central administrations for governmental tasks such as health and justice. For ease of understanding, this study addresses both the central administrations and the subsequent GDR ministries as the state level.

This book uses the concept of medical memories and experiences to demonstrate that mentalities and morals concerning social constructions of diagnoses and medical concepts had a persistence that led to unexpected continuities at the local level. Despite political changes and ideological claims at the state level, the denunciation and stigmatisation of people with STDs remained a common medical experience in cities like Dresden and Leipzig in postwar East Germany.[8] Therefore, the combination of medical history and memory studies is an innovative step to establish a new perspective on this part of history.

Medical memories and experiences

Walter Korinek had a decisive advantage over many other fraud doctors after the Second World War: he actually studied medicine for five years in Prague between 1935 and 1940. However, he never finished his degree after failing some of his exams. Following this, he had to return to Dresden because his parents were unable to continue supporting him financially. At that time, the Second World War was in full swing, and any person with medical knowledge was urgently needed, a situation that was clearly favourable to Korinek. Already during the term breaks of his medical studies in Prague, he had assisted a doctor in a Dresden hospital. In April 1941, this doctor called upon Korinek to become his assistant in orthopaedics. Simultaneously, due to the emergency regulation [*Notdienstverordnung*] of the Third Reich and the granting of temporary medical approbations, Dresden officials asked him to take over a vacant doctor's surgery.[9] He worked in this position until 1943, when he was drafted and deployed in various military hospitals. During this period, he obtained comprehensive medical skills. Moreover, he was able to build a reputation as a doctor among patients in Dresden and in his field.[10] Both facts were decisive in his successful postwar masquerade, which was based on his and other people's medical memories and experiences.

In many ways, Korinek's case is a perfect introduction to the concept of medical memories and experiences, which is at the heart of the methodological approach of this book. The following paragraphs provide a brief conceptual overview of underlying theories that have been used and applied in this study. It argues that medical memories in the form of the state narrative, the medical profession's perception of diseases, the layout and equipment of institutions, and the attitudes and skills of individual doctors all had an effect on the medical experiences of patients in the everyday life of postwar East Germany.

In recent decades, the field of memory studies has flourished, producing a diverse, often contradictory, terminology.[11] The works of Aleida Assmann and Jay Winter are central to the theoretical concept of this book. Their conception is split into four overlapping, mutually dependent, but still separable levels: individual memory, mnemonic community, institutional memory, and the state narrative.[12] The following three chapters address all these categories, while the final chapter applies this framework to a case study and the epilogue illustrates avenues for future research.

Every individual has memories that shape his or her identity, and thus are indispensable for her or his social activity.[13] However, Maurice Halbwachs suggested that within memories "the past is not preserved but is reconstructed on the basis of the present", not least due to its cognitive psychological characteristics.[14] Events leave behind memory traces in the brain, which are recalled in certain contexts, such as a smell, a surrounding, and similar triggers. However, these traces never reproduce a precise copy of the actual past event. They are overwritten, reinterpreted, and manipulated throughout a person's life.[15] According to Peter A. Levin, the outcome of reconstructing memories is that they lose accuracy while gaining relevance for the current context and for possible future situations.[16] Therefore, memories are always subjective, and, as Halbwachs concluded, "[t]here is hence no memory without perception".[17]

His statement complies with Assmann's classification of four interrelated individual memory characteristics. Firstly, every person creates his own ideology and identity, derived from his perceptual reality that distinguishes him from others. Secondly, individual memory cannot exist without social activity and therefore is always linked to other people's past.[18] Assmann's last two characteristics are the biological limitations in the comprehensiveness of memories, and their fragility when facing adaptation, fading, or even erasure; both are important features that any historical investigation needs to address.[19]

For this book, the category of individual medical memories is assembled through the individual medical histories, as well as medicine-related experiences inside and outside of medical institutions, either as a patient or as medical personnel. The concept follows the outlined theoretical background by assuming that everyone has a personal medical history and potentially experienced injuries, diseases, and mental illnesses, especially during and after the war.[20] Moreover, the study analyses subsequent experiences of patients with the healthcare system and its personnel. These encounters included the availability or unavailability of medical care and treatment, the implementation of coercive measures such as forced sterilisation or hospitalisation, as well as the individual's public exposure, abuse, and other violations of ethical principles and personal integrity. All these experiences determined how patients viewed their doctor after the war and thus capture the impact of medical memories and experiences on the doctor–patient relationship.

As shown for Korinck's case, the medical practice of a doctor was shaped by numerous factors such as the acquired skills and continued existence of health concepts in the form of medical memories, or the experience of the limited availability of facilities or equipment and the ability or inability to help people during and after the war. Additionally, the involvement – direct or indirect – of physicians in medical crimes and unethical experiments in the Third Reich brought the potential of their subsequent prosecution and loss of position, something which influenced their individual identity formation. These examples are taken from a great variety of experiences that potentially formed the self-perception of people and their adaptation strategies that allowed them to confront their past and create a selective life-narrative during the postwar era.

In 1963, Korinek retrospectively explained and defended his masquerade to the head of a Dresden hospital in the following terms:

> I just found myself caught up in this situation; I earned money, stood on my own feet [was independent, M.W.]. [. . .] After the war, everything was built new. Much was destroyed. I had a secure existence and in the meantime had married and two kids; but now I did not have the courage anymore to find to the truth and to myself in time.[21]

In this way, he constructed an image of himself that fitted into the medical memories of the Dresden population and his needs at the time. He invented a new life-narrative, and if asked for his medical licence and certificates he always came up with new excuses: "I had gained a certain circle of patients before the collapse [of the Third Reich, M.W.], was known as a doctor in Dresden and thus had no difficulties in this field also after 1945".[22] In this process, Dr. med. Walter Korinek was born.

Korinek's description of the interdependency between the individual and other people's perceptions leads to the second level of medical memories and experiences: mnemonic communities. As Hannah Arendt observed, "[e]very man is born into a community with pre-existing laws which he 'obeys' first of all because there is no other way for him to enter the great game of life".[23] These associations are the Halbwachsian 'frameworks' in which the memories of a person are embedded and form part of their social remembrance.[24] Therefore, mnemonic communities, in the form of families, local communities, or professional networks, are, as Francesca Cappelletto notes, shaped through selected traditions, experiences, and remembrances that are preserved and shared among its members.

Nevertheless, the social bond of a community could also be based on a traumatic event. Cappelletto uses an example of a massacre in an Italian village during the Second World War as a case study, demonstrating how a mnemonic community could appear as a homogenous group that pursues interests common to all its members. However, Cappelletto clarifies that "they are not understood [. . .] as corporate groups, as politically and ideologically unified wholes" because every individual is still part of other frameworks, such as the family and the local community. The combination of these frameworks shapes people's specific and distinctive personalities.[25] In general, a mnemonic community can be local, national, or international in its scope. Yet, for Assmann, the term is only applicable to a group, institution, or association if they "produce strong ties of loyalty accompanied by a strong unified We-identity".[26] Consequently, the principal characteristic of remembrance activities of mnemonic communities is their conscious creation for an unlimited period and their narrow content selection.[27]

For the concept of medical memories and experiences, the medical profession itself is an example of a mnemonic community that created an overarching narrative of their professionalisation history and involvement in the Third Reich. Therefore, by following the outlined theoretical background, this study identifies both the persistence of medical concepts in the form of individuals and the conscious selection, silencing, and enforcing of medical memories by mnemonic communities. It also describes how, for example, after 1945 the medical profession applied their medical memories as a defence for the use of old medicine as a deterrence for suspected 'promiscuous' people despite the availability of new, more effective, less harmful drugs. Subsequently, their established narrative influences the individual memories of their members and potentially reconfigures their identity, which ultimately causes their integration into a social remembrance framework. Moreover, doctors legitimise medical practices, such as the use of sterilisation during the Third Reich, from this narrative and the political strategies of the medical profession, creating a sizeable impact on the medical experiences of patients.

Nevertheless, alongside people, social organisations, professions, and states, institutions also carry 'memories'. Besides the use of symbols, as Alon Confino shows for traditional *Heimat* [place of birth, belonging, or identity] illustrations in the GDR, monuments and buildings together with their equipment and furniture can represent a break or continuity with the past.[28] For the private sphere, Paul Betts has provided a pioneering work by exploring the changes in the interior design of the living room – a place for relics of the past, memories, deviance, and the new system – during the existence of the East German state.[29] For the public sphere, the *lieux de mémoire*, as described by Pierre Nora, reveal remembrance culture and how the urban landscape is shaped in line with political, ideological, cultural, and local perceptions.[30] One example is the politically motivated renaming of streets following political changes, a way in which selected famous people or oppositional members of former political systems are manifestly remembered. East German cities are a striking case of this fact as their streets were renamed four times during the twentieth century: after 1918, 1933, 1945, and 1989.[31]

Therefore, in the same way as individual or mnemonic community narratives, architecture is used as a 'carrier of remembrance', serving as a reference point that always carries a political message for contemporaries.[32] By contrast, the destruction and erasure of chosen parts of a city's architectural amalgam support a desired silence or even obliteration of certain aspects of the past.[33] Both the physical construction and demolition of artefacts are tools for use in the remembrance activities of groups or the state when looking to legitimise the present or future via a selected history.

This study proposes two forms of institutional memory. Firstly, a building is designed according to contemporary knowledge and opinions – such as the effect of environment upon healing[34] – which means a 'building in' of memories. Later, the building might be changed and extended, like the urban landscape, reconfiguring not only its composition but also its memories. This process is similar to the human brain, which can never reproduce the exact copy of an event. However, structural changes are also limited by memories represented by existing layout and architecture. The demolishing of a building, however, signifies the erasure of spatial memory. In this study, the medical memories of an institution include its layout, interior, and used medical devices and equipment that influence the medical experiences of patients and medical personnel within that institution.[35]

The second characteristic of institutional memory is the range of concepts and memories projected on a building by the state, local officials, communities, or individuals. For example, even in an institution whose name habitually changes throughout its existence, the memories in the form of its past, location, and address evoke associations among the people according to their experiences with, and knowledge about, this place. Moreover, spaces, like the Care Home Leuben, always provide a purpose for the local government and the state. Therefore, authorities incorporate this institution into their narratives to justify its existence and the confinement of 'socially deviant' people, which the last level of the concept of medical memories and experiences, the state narrative, addresses.

The nineteenth-century nation-state theorist Ernest Renan declared that "[t]he forgetting – I would almost say: the historical aberration – plays in the creation of a nation an important role, and therefore the progress of the historical sciences is often a threat to the nation".[36] This quotation has been true for states ever since. Governments often attempt to establish a 'master narrative' and remembrance practices that reinforce power relations and stabilise the current political system; in doing so, they aim to create a 'collective identity' for their citizens. However, the term 'collective' homogenises individual experience and memories, which has led to the critique and often the outright refutation of a Halbwachsian 'collective memory' in recent literature.[37]

The state narrative, which is based on individual memories, as well as the family, generational, and mnemonic community frameworks, contains highly differentiated remembrance practices and interpretations. Winter identifies this area as the "civil society" that is influenced, but far from dominated, by either the authoritarian or democratic state.[38] Instead, this level contains a continuous struggle of various, but often unequally powerful, agents, such as stakeholders, communities, professional associations, or the state, over the subject and form of commemoration practices.

In his book *Secret Science*, Ulf Schmidt refers to these often state-dominated agents who determine forms of commemoration. His chapter on the 'politics of medical memories' for the cases of the Porton Down veterans exposes the biased nature of the United Kingdom [UK] 'master narrative'. The state consciously excluded the victims of their chemical and biological warfare experiments as they had no place in the broader commemoration of the 'heroic' twentieth-century world wars.[39] However, Stefan Goebel's comparison of the negotiation between different agents, not limited to the state, over commemoration practices with the market system is valuable as these stakeholders interfere with each other in a 'supply and demand relationship' within civil society.[40] Therefore, this level describes a heterogeneous state narrative or commemoration practices that are greatly influenced by all other levels of the concept of medical memories.[41]

For a state, this complex edifice of commemoration is both the guard of, and challenger to, 'social norm' and 'behaviour'. Such a conceptualisation is a bridge to the sociological studies of Erving Goffman, with whom this study critically engages. Memories in the form of traditions and societal expectations – described by Goffman as the required social conduct when publicly encountering other people, or the respect of hierarchical and social organisations – are decisive in creating a common identity. However, this socially constructed order also defines and condemns 'abnormal behaviour' and 'social deviance' to protect social occasions from disturbances. As such, the sociological studies of Goffman are integral to the following analysis.[42]

One example of an enforced social order is the practice of silence, explored in this study by the biased 'postwar silence and narratives'. On the one hand, as Konrad H. Jarausch and Dorothee Wierling note, hunger, rape, bombing, fleeing, and even rebuilding were predominantly remembered in the first decades after the war, since they were experiences shared by a majority of the German population.[43] On the other hand, however, the Holocaust, the exclusion and deportation of minorities, and other crimes against humanity had no role in postwar commemoration. One reason for disregarding the Third Reich's victims was that, as Henry Rousso emphasises, the state of war continued for many beyond 8 May 1945; with the loss of housing and relatives, for example, continuing to determine the narrative of people's lives for a period longer than the duration of the conflict.[44]

Alongside personal affection, the 'political or strategic silences' discussed by Winter help to explain this bias in the remembrance of the Second World War. According to Winter, political or strategic silences are creations of a group, a state, or the international community to suppress tensions in society over facets of the past and secure 'social order' – a fact that can equally be identified within East Germany.[45] The state provided a socially constructed framework of silence for its population as postwar guidance to adapt their lives to, and thus a space to integrate into, the new political system – not least by serving the widespread 'willingness to forget' the Third Reich and Second World War.[46] Selective commemoration was supposed to gain the required legitimacy among the population for both East and West Germany after their formation in 1949, but the desired 'master narrative' by the state was unachievable.[47] According to Jarausch, the postwar consumer culture, demonstrated in "the exciting purchase of the first car, whether VW beetle or Trabi", rather than the political transformations became the predominant subject of individual commemoration.[48] Consequently, the proposed concept of medical memories and experiences is not a strictly top-down model but consists of a continuous exchange between all other levels that shape and replace the memories and remembrance practices.[49]

This book follows the theories of Assmann and Winter in defining the state narrative for the concept of medical memories and experiences as fragile: a constantly contested field of remembrance practices. For the GDR's state narrative the socialist healthcare system offered political legitimisation and an opportunity to demarcate itself from the West German private healthcare system.[50] The free, universally accessible, state-run health clinics were viewed as Socialism's most significant achievement and were thus emphasised throughout the existence of East Germany.[51] Therefore, the study analyses the state's emphasis on, and selection of, a medical narrative, which, for example, justified strict laws against prostitution or 'promiscuous behaviour', originally introduced by previous political systems. Through discussions of this 'master narrative', it exposes how state policies, shaped by medical memories and experiences of people in charge, were altered and limited by memories of mnemonic communities and individuals at the local level. Local authorities and doctors influenced laws that dispute the assumption of a strictly centralised state construct and the unhindered transmission of SED claims into society's reality.

In short, medical memories and experiences are broadly defined as the relationship of the medical past with the medical experiences of the present and perception of the future. This dependency often meant that persistence of medical treatments, mentalities, and terminologies at the local level could be recognised; oftentimes these were asynchronical with medical and political advances of the time. In order to ground this abstract definition in the interactions between a doctor and a patient for the particular context of the book, the concept uses the microcosmic study of Dresden and Leipzig, embedding this into the macrocosm of the state narrative and broader, longer-term developments of postwar East Germany and Europe.

Historiography

Korinek's life offers a starting point for defining the place of this book within the existing literature and historiographical landscape. As discussed earlier for memory studies, the book's aim is to investigate individual life and state narratives, medical case histories, and the social and medical treatment of patients in the East German context with the cultural, political, and social developments that followed the Second World War. To accomplish this endeavour, it proposes the combination of memory studies with the history of medicine in order to establish the outlined concept of medical memories and experiences.

Therefore, individuals like Korinek play a crucial role in this study. At first glance, his case of an adapted life-narrative could support the notion of the *Stunde Null* [Zero Hour or Year Zero] for the year 1945; for him, the end of the war meant the beginning of his masquerade and a new life story.[52] Defining historical caesura as watersheds in terms of political and societal affairs has a long tradition. However, especially recent studies about postwar eras and the First World War, linked with an increased interest in commemorative culture and the relationship of war and memory within social, cultural, and psychological contexts,[53] question these assumptions.[54] In this way, Korinek's case reveals continuity instead of a new beginning: he accomplished the transition from the old into the new political system, also transferring his political and medical views into the 'new' healthcare system. Therefore, this study refutes the definition of a caesura like 1945 as misleading in a similar way to historians like Ralph Jessen who have instead emphasised traditional features in societies that survived upheavals, wars, and other radical events.[55]

For the SBZ, and later the GDR, the postwar years were decisive for the future of the socialist state. Since its dissolution in 1989 and 1990, historians have attached a vital role to the years 1945 to 1949, and 1949 up until the construction of the Berlin Wall in 1961, for the establishment and stability of the East German state. However, the explanations for this development differ greatly among historians. In particular the disputed re-appearance of totalitarian theories used to analyse the GDR from a macrocosmic perspective divided the historiographical landscape in Germany during the 1990s.[56] Emotional debates produced mutual accusations between proponents or enemies of the totalitarian theorem: the latter were seen as exonerating the dictatorship, whereas the others were seen as Cold War warriors, leading to a typical black–white dispute.

Furthermore, the 1990s were marked by the attempt of many established historians to define a label for the GDR. They developed terms and their underlying concepts such as *durchherrschte Gesellschaft* [thoroughly ruled society],[57] modern dictatorship,[58] *konstitutiv-widersprüchliche Gesellschaft* [constitutively contradictory society],[59] and *Fürsorgediktatur* [welfare dictatorship][60] to create theoretical approaches into the microcosm of East Germany and a social and cultural history that captures the GDR's nature as a system and society. However, a single term, theory, or concept is incapable of sufficiently explaining the entire lifespan of the GDR.[61] Linda Fuller criticises the search for a specific terminology of former socialist East and Central European states as a common fallacy, suggesting that it simply "glazes over a great deal of social difference with a frosting of homogeneity".[62] Therefore, as Patrick Major concludes, the totalitarian, social, and cultural historians of the GDR "have been equally guilty of fetishising elite power fantasies, while ignoring their realizability".[63]

Major's recent book *Behind the Berlin Wall* is an example of combining the strengths of different approaches and theories into a sophisticated and multi-faceted basis for a study.[64] He categorises the GDR as a 'welfare', as well as a 'didactic', dictatorship, a terminology that captures the SED's perception that its people were too immature for Socialism. However, he also adds the social analytical tools of Alf Lüdtke's *Eigensinn*,[65] describing people's self-interest or directedness, and of Thomas Lindenberger's *Alltagsgeschichte*,[66] which recognises the visible and invisible boundaries of everyday life.[67] The latter two concepts lead to the theory of *Zweckrationalität* [purposive rationality] that Detlef Pollack establishes for individuals' behaviour with which they pursue their goals by adapting to prevailing rules in order to avoid sanctions by the system.[68] Major develops Pollack's interpretation further and describes the 'hidden transcripts' of human behaviour, asserting that people comply only on the surface and hide their criticisms and struggles to maintain some autonomous space behind the mask of 'doublespeak'.[69] This study follows Major's claim that this socio-cultural approach is "bringing ordinary people more firmly back to the centre stage" and captures the complexity of social performance.[70]

To this end, Mary Fulbrook's work offers another valuable analytical tool to the GDR's socio-cultural history.[71] In her studies, Fulbrook analyses societal developments and their origins by establishing a generational perspective.[72] By exploring the different experiences and 'life stories' of multiple generations, she explains, for example, that the '1929ers' (Fulbrook's constructed affiliation of people born around the late 1920s) were highly distinctive to those 'born into the GDR'.[73] Despite the criticisms that Fulbrook has faced, in particular for her 'normalisation' concept for the 1960s and 1970s, her 'bottom-up' approach is a crucial template for this book.[74] Exploring generations and their differentiated medical experiences and memories is an important tool, especially for analysing the life-narratives and adaptation strategies of doctors after 1945.[75]

In summary, the book follows Betts and Jarausch's suggestion that East German historiography in general should embed the GDR in broader nineteenth- and twentieth-century developments.[76] This proposition is particularly true for the specific focus of its medical history. The rapid medical advancement throughout the long-nineteenth century and the transformative developments following the two world wars, with their inventions of radiography, the tuberculin test, and Penicillin, revolutionised the medical treatment of tuberculosis [Tbc] and STDs.[77] However, medical concepts and socially constructed diagnoses did not alter at a similar pace. As such, the terminology, mentality, and treatments used in postwar East Germany were derived from previous political systems, with the emphasis on the legacy of the Weimar Republic being particularly prominent.

In locating the GDR within longer-standing developments and traditions, this study expands the works of Anna-Sabine Ernst and Gabriele Moser. Ernst focuses on the medical profession's past and outlines its often antagonistic relationship to the state between 1945 and 1961.[78] Her findings offer an important comparison to this study's analysis of doctors who became part of the socialist state along with their medical memories after 1945, bringing with them their medical skills, preconception of diseases, and potential past involvement in medical crimes.

While Ernst's study focuses on change in the East German healthcare system after the Second World War, Moser illustrates continuity by exploring the institutional development from the Weimar Republic into the GDR. She analyses the concept of social hygiene and identifies the paradigms and traditions from the 1920s that were used to establish the socialist healthcare system in East Germany after 1945.[79] Moser's term 'medicalised social hygiene' illustrates the synthesis between the medical legacy of the Weimar Republic and ideas of the 'social hygiene' movement. For the GDR, she argues that this merging point was the cornerstone of the new socialist healthcare system. To Moser, this concept indicates that postwar East Germany emphasised medical knowledge and expertise within its social hygiene policies, neglecting the notions of positive *Bevölkerungspolitik* [demographic policies] that dominated the debates during the Weimar Republic. This study differs from Moser's interpretation by showing that the *Bevölkerungspolitik* still played a major role in curbing strategies against STDs, as well as in the treatment of the 'asocial' after 1945.

Aside from this limitation, the book revisits Moser's argument to show that German socialists and health officials, rather than Soviet authorities, shaped the postwar healthcare system. The agency of different state and local actors in the forms of doctors and even patients in East Germany after 1945 is one of the main hypotheses that this study proposes and is part of each chapter's analysis. Nevertheless, the occupation power relied on selected German socialists or local physicians to implement their commands while at the same time reserving its right to intervene and punish any deviance from the socialist aims with harsh sanctions.

This postwar relationship between the occupation power, re-emigrated socialists, and occupied people is elucidated in the studies of special cases of Tbc and heart diseases by Donna Harsch and Jeannette Madarász-Lebenhagen. They discuss the East German strategies of containment and prophylaxis in the international context, as well as the persistence of old methods and the slow transitions towards innovations. They identify that resistance to progress also had an impact on the microcosms of the doctor–patient relationship, offering valuable insights for this study.[80] Moreover, Harsch builds upon Moser's findings and concept of a 'medicalised social hygiene'. She applies this concept to the tuberculosis policies in the GDR, but with the emphasis on the postwar era and its Tbc epidemic. However, some of her claims are limited by the fact that Harsch used only the Federal Archive for her research, which, in some instances, diminishes the validity of her arguments.[81]

Melanie Arndt's exploration of divided Berlin from 1948 to 1961 provides a more recent account of postwar health policies.[82] She shows the benefits and issues arising from two competing ideologies within one city, with both healthcare systems serving as "*Schaufenster* [show case or shop window] of the respective underlying political order".[83] This particular case study provides an important insight into the struggle to win over doctors and patients for the new socialist healthcare system. However, there was a significant difference between Berlin and the rest of the GDR, or even Germany, as also illuminated by Jessica Reinisch's study on the postwar health situation.[84] By focussing on Dresden and Leipzig, this book closes a gap in the historiography that commonly concentrates on the situation in Berlin, across all or one of the occupation zones.

Three decades after the reunification of Germany and the end of the Cold War, the historiography of postwar East Germany and the GDR remains politically motivated and partly burdened with emotional rhetoric, especially within Germany. However, this book situates itself in the new trend among early-career scholars of *Alltagsgeschichte*: using microstudies for the post-Second World War historiography to expose the complex processes at the local level of society. Therefore, this study is part of Andrew Beattie's postulate, summarised by Anne Krüger as the "*Aufarbeitung der Aufarbeitung* [coming to terms with the coming to terms]" of the GDR, lasting from the 1990s until today.[85] The aim is to establish a differentiated approach to people's actions in East Germany.

Sources and structure

After conducting research in multiple archives in Germany, it became evident that the existing historical literature about East Germany's healthcare system far from encompasses the full potential that this field has to offer. By examining a broad scope of primary sources that allow insight into the mechanics of East German society using the concept of medical memories and experiences, this book closes some of the gaps in GDR historiography identified earlier.

At the state level, the *Bundesarchiv* [Federal Archive of Germany – BArch] offers the archival sources illuminating the work of the SBZ central administrations and GDR ministries and their interactions with the local level. The local and community level is examined with the files of the *Stadtarchiv Dresden* [City Archive Dresden – StA DD], the *Hauptstaatsarchiv Dresden* [Main (Saxon) State Archive Dresden – HSA DD], and *Stadtarchiv Leipzig* [City Archive Leipzig – StA Lpz]. All four archives both provide and limit the insights available to researchers due to the restrictive access and privacy policies in place at each of them. In particular the City Archive Dresden denied the use of individual patient files that could have proved valuable to analysing individual memories and medical pasts of, for example, inmates of the Care Home Dresden.

The available archival files are also historically restricted themselves: often representing the opinion of the author, state narrative, or political motivation of mnemonic communities. Therefore, the insight given into East German society through these sources is biased *a priori*, and as such needs to be cautiously analysed and contextualised to avoid invalid conclusions concerning people's daily life.

A similar issue occurs when using the archive of *Der Bundesbeauftragte für die Unterlagen des Staatssicherheitsdienstes der ehemaligen Deutschen Demokratischen Republik* [The Agency of the Federal Commissioner for the Records of the State Security Service of the former German Democratic Republic – BStU]. Despite the historiographical importance of the fact that after 1989 and 1990 the files of East Germany's intelligence service became accessible to academics and the general public, in order to protect the privacy and identity of people who are still alive the archive remains highly restrictive regarding sensitive data. In order to avoid inaccuracies or grey-areas in the materials used to establish medical memories and experiences, the study combines a great number of different archival files with the collection of the *Deutsches Hygiene Museum Dresden* [German Hygiene Museum Dresden – DHMD] and published contemporary literature, newspaper articles, pictures, policies, and statistics.

The book's subtitle, *Treatments of the Past*, alludes to its discussion of a variety of perspectives surrounding postwar East German medical and social reality. The first chapter investigates the biographies of doctors who adapted differently to the new political system after Germany's defeat and *treated their past*. The establishment and use of generations is problematic as they are always historical constructions with the danger of homogenising memories and generalising experiences of highly heterogeneous age cohorts. However, in line with Fulbrook's work, the generational approach still reveals significant variances in the life strategies of, for example, doctors born in the nineteenth century and those who spent their youth during the Weimar Republic.

By using case studies for each age cohort, the study embeds the postwar era into the personal development of selected doctors and proves the hypothesis that, more often than not, 1945 meant continuity rather than a break in lives and careers. This development was possible as both the East German state and the Soviet occupation power were driven by the predicament of the epidemic diseases and thus employed pragmatism towards the urgently needed medical profession. Subsequently, doctors' medical memories and experiences, in the form of their socialisation and medical education, as well as their involvement in the Third Reich and medical crimes, were 'treated': they were altered and often sanitised to their ends, not least with the help of state authorities and the MfS.

The book argues that the continuity of local doctors and authorities resulted in the persistence of medical concepts and out-dated treatments, faced by patients inside and outside of a doctor's examination room – *treatments from the past*. As the second chapter reveals for the specialised health clinics of STDs, medicine was often used as a deterrence to teach abstinence to supposedly 'promiscuous' women. Moreover, outside of these buildings, the survival of a denunciation system propagated under previous political systems can be observed supporting East Germany's health policies and efforts to curb STDs. However, the assessment of 'promiscuous' people relied on gossip, rumours, and personal sympathy or antipathy that often led to false accusations or, on occasions, to the individual experience of a far-reaching system of medical and social control. Consequently, the chapter investigates not only medical but also social treatments of the past that patients who suffered from STDs faced in the postwar era.

To illustrate the argument of a simultaneously employed strategy of education and stigmatisation, the analysis focusses on the health clinics, categories for 'sexually deviant' people, raids, and public campaigns and exhibitions to identify medical memories in the form of mentalities, medical concepts, stigmatisations, and clichés that became the medical experiences of the targeted groups. Not least, this chapter proves the hypothesis that claims made by the state were limited at the local level of society, as Saxony often implemented an even stricter STD control system than demanded by state authorities, overstepping legal boundaries by depriving personal rights.

Treatments of the past in the form of medical memories and experiences also refer to the process of how states, mnemonic communities, or individuals altered their past to their needs. This book identifies the process of omitting and rewriting the life-narratives of doctors and also of the 'war youth' by the East German state. Therefore, the third chapter analyses the war experiences of children. This study does not diagnose 'trauma' retrospectively but establishes an overview of the complexity of children's war experiences that a single term like 'trauma' is incapable of expressing. From this basis, the chapter investigates the response by the state to a perceived 'depraved' youth and its subsequent narration. It argues that the authorities targeted youth behaviour without acknowledging the causes of their social conduct, which often had their origins in children's war experiences – there was no *treatment for their past*.

Instead, the state developed a narrative that included the 'war children' as the hope and future of the nation, a characterisation that in turn pathologised any 'socially deviant behaviour' and contributed to the pervasive East German perception of 'deviant behaviour' as a disease that required treatment. Consequently, adolescents whom the state classified as 'asocial' were often caught up in a social hygienic cycle, in which they were sent from one institution to the next without receiving the support and treatment a potentially traumatic past event necessitated. Furthermore, this chapter questions the 'para-medicalised' terminology, such as 'trauma', that was used to explain political and social phenomena. The study formulates that this transfer served as a narrative, justifying the interventions into the families and communities by the East German state in the postwar era and the interests of the proclaimed 'forgotten or traumatised generation' today.

The final chapter draws together the different strands of the study looking at various social groups – the incriminated doctors, 'promiscuous' women, and delinquent children – by investigating *institutionalised treatments of the past* within the care home in Dresden as a case study. This case study is inspired by the theoretical works of Goffman and David J. Rothman, who both studied and criticised asylums and identified the medical concepts inscribed into the institutional layout and perceptions of the supervisors and population. The final chapter questions how the state advocated the continuation of the workhouse after the war – the vision – and exposes the institutional memories that determined medical experiences of those within its premises – the reality. Furthermore, it examines discussions between mnemonic communities about the purpose and utilisation of the institution, and, finally, investigates the medical memories and experiences of the patients and staff. In this final section, the analysis systematically follows the proposed key concept of medical memories and experiences to reveal the theoretical framework and provides practical examples.

This book contributes both to memory studies and to the postwar, medical, and socio-cultural histories of the GDR. It employs an intentionally interdisciplinary approach, chosen to avoid the homogenisation of social interactions with a limited terminology or theory. Instead, the study seeks out the complex, unpredictable, and often selfish human behaviour within the broader medical realm that challenges fixed historical caesuras such as 1945.

In this way, the fraud doctor Korinek accompanies the study as a red-thread because he was not only an extraordinary case, but also the embodiment of continuity, local agency, and difficulties encountered in the postwar era in East Germany. For example, one of the reasons why Korinek did not receive his approbation was because he failed in the exams of gynaecology in 1940. Despite this fact, Korinek carried out around 15 abortions between 1950 and 1959, which were forbidden at this time in the GDR. His female costumers came to him via 'word-of-mouth' and paid him 100 to 300 Mark.[86] After his arrest Korinek stated during the interrogation after being asked why he carried out illegal abortions the following:

> In my activities, I was mainly guided by my mentality. I disagreed with the law of the German Democratic Republic regarding abortions because in my opinion, it does not take into account the social situation of pregnant women. [. . .] When then these women came to me, I simply did not "have the heart" [*konnte ich es einfach nicht "übers Herz bringen"*] to not "help" them and because of these reasons I carried out the abortions.[87]

On the one hand, Korinek's statement shows his narrative and self-defence strategy that explained his defiance towards state law because, in his opinion, abortions should be possible under certain social circumstances that affected pregnant women. On the other hand, the illegal abortions were just one more legal transgression and a welcome source of income for Korinek, who at the time had debts amounting to around 15,000 Mark.[88] Furthermore, given that he carried out the procedures in private, and that he was never a fully qualified doctor – and his medical skills cannot be judged retrospectively – his actions also likely endangered the lives of the women involved here. Therefore, his case illustrates that it is both the state health policies and, perhaps more importantly, the medical personnel on site who determine the medical experiences of their patients with their skills and mentality as well as their medical memories: the main theme of this book.

Notes

1 See BStU, MfS, BV Dresden, AU 43/60.
2 'Betr.: Bericht über die Angelegenheit Cichetti und Korinek, 12. Februar 1960': BStU, MfS, BV Dresden, AU 43/60, Bl. 42–4, here 43–4.
3 'Betr.: Bericht über die Angelegenheit Cichetti und Korinek, 12. Februar 1960': BStU, MfS, BV Dresden, AU 43/60, Bl. 44.
4 'Einschätzung zu Operativ-Vorgang "Spinne", 15. Dezember 1959': BStU, MfS, BV Dresden, AU 43/60, Bl. 17.
5 Ludwig Mecklinger, 'Der politische Auftrag des Gesundheitswesens: Aus der Rede des Ministers für Gesundheitswesen, OMR Prof. Dr. sc. med. Ludwig Mecklinger, auf der Kreisärztekonferenz', *humanitas*, 24 (1981), 1–3.
6 Jay Winter comes to the same conclusion that cities were sites of dense experience of total war. Jay Winter, 'Conclusion: Metropolitan History and National History in the Age of Total War', in *Cities into Battlefields: Metropolitan Scenarios, Experiences, and Commemorations of Total War*, ed. by Stefan Goebel and Derek Keene (Farnham: Ashgate, 2011), pp. 219–23.
7 As Henry Rousso emphasises, the war did not end for everyone on 8 May 1945. The effects of loss, for example, shaped people's lives much longer than the actual war and thus prolonged, and individualised, the duration of the postwar period. Henry Rousso, 'A New Perspective on the War', in *Experience and Memory: The Second World War in Europe*, ed. by Jörg Echternkamp and Stefan Martens (New York: Berghahn Books, 2010), pp. 1–9.
8 Monica Black, for example, reveals continuities and mentalities of burial and mourning rituals in Berlin from the Weimar Republic until the division of Germany. Monica Black, *Death in Berlin: From Weimar to Divided Germany* (Cambridge: Cambridge University Press, 2010).
9 'Brief, 08.04.1941': BArch, DQ 1/12052, unpaginated.
10 'Vernehmungsprotokoll, 24. Dezember 1959': BStU, MfS, BV DD, AU 43/60, Bl. 117–18.
11 Stefan Goebel notes that "communication in academia about memory has become increasingly difficult because the central term has different meanings to different authors". Stefan Goebel, *The Great War and Medieval Memory: War, Remembrance, and Medievalism in Britain and Germany, 1914–1940* (Cambridge: Cambridge University Press, 2007), p. 14. The problem is complicated due to the fact that 'memory' has also different connotations in different languages and cultures. Jay Winter and Emmanuel Sivan, 'Setting the Framework', in *War and Remembrance in the Twentieth Century*, ed. by Jay Winter and Emmanuel Sivan (Cambridge: Cambridge University

Press, 1999), pp. 6–39. The studies from this field's appointed founders, Maurice Halbwachs and Pierre Nora, were also too dependent on particular conditions or nations to
offer universal tools and terms for memory concepts. Maurice Halbwachs, *On Collective Memory*, trans. by Lewis A. Coser (Chicago: University of Chicago Press, 1992);
Rethinking France: Les Lieux De Mémoire: Volume 4: Histories and Memories, ed. by
Pierre Nora (Chicago: University of Chicago Press, 2010). Winter, however, refutes
the assumptions and findings of Pierre Nora. Winter and Sivan, pp. 1–3; Jay Winter, 'Thinking About Silence', in *Shadows of War: A Social History of Silence in the
Twentieth Century*, ed. by Efrat Ben-Ze'ev, Ruth Ginio, and Jay Winter (Cambridge:
Cambridge University Press, 2010), pp. 3–31.

12   This separation is based on the suggestions of Aleida Assmann, *Der lange Schatten
der Vergangenheit: Erinnerungskultur und Geschichtspolitik* (Munich: Beck, 2006),
pp. 24–61.

13   Assmann, *Der lange Schatten der Vergangenheit*, p. 24.

14   Halbwachs, p. 39.

15   Winter and Sivan, pp. 11–13.

16   Peter A. Levine, *Trauma and Memory: Brain and Body in a Search for the Living Past:
A Practical Guide for Understanding and Working with Traumatic Memory* (Berkeley: North Atlantic Books, 2015), p. 141. As Puleng Segalo explains, "[m]emory is
an active process of creating meaning from past events". Puleng Segalo, 'Trauma and
Gender', *Social and Personality Psychology Compass*, 9 (2015), 447–54.

17   Halbwachs, p. 169.

18   Assmann, *Der lange Schatten der Vergangenheit*, p. 24. Halbwachs also indicated that
"no memory is possible outside [social] frameworks". Halbwachs, pp. 40–3, here 43.

19   Assmann, *Der lange Schatten der Vergangenheit*, pp. 24–5; Winter, 'Conclusion',
pp. 219–20.

20   Assmann, *Der lange Schatten der Vergangenheit*, pp. 93–4; Winter and Sivan,
pp. 15–16.

21   'Stellungnahme zu dem mir am 2.8.1963 durch Herrn Chefarzt Dr. med. [. . .] und
Herrn [. . .] eröffneten Beschluß': BArch, DQ 1/12052, unpaginated.

22   'Vernehmungsprotokoll, 24. Dezember 1959': BStU, MfS, BV DD, AU 43/60, Bl. 117.

23   Hannah Arendt, *On Violence* (New York: Harcourt Brace, 1970), p. 97.

24   Halbwachs, p. 61.

25   Francesca Cappelletto, 'Introduction', in *Memory and World War II: An Ethnographic
Approach*, ed. by Francesca Cappelletto (Oxford: Berg, 2005), pp. 4–5, here 4; Wulf
Kansteiner, 'Finding a Meaning in Memory: A Methodological Critique of Collective
Memory Studies', *History and Theory*, 1 (2002), 179–97.

26   Assmann, *Der lange Schatten der Vergangenheit*, p. 36.

27   Assmann, *Der lange Schatten der Vergangenheit*, pp. 36–7.

28   Alon Confino, *Germany as a Culture of Remembrance: Promises and Limits of Writing
History* (Chapel Hill, NC: University of North Carolina Press, 2006), pp. 93–113.

29   Paul Betts, *Within Walls: Private Life in the German Democratic Republic* (Oxford:
Oxford University Press, 2010), pp. 6, 119–47.

30   Pierre Nora, 'Introduction', in *Rethinking France. Les Lieux De Mémoire: Volume 4:
Histories and Memories*, ed. by Pierre Nora (Chicago: University of Chicago Press,
2010), pp. VII–XIV.

31   For a contemporary documentary about the street-renaming in Dresden in 1991 after
the reunification of Germany, see the short film of Daniel Glaser, *Dresden '91: Ein
Beitrag zur Dialektik* (Filminitiative Dresden, 1991). My thanks go to the producer and
artist Daniel Glaser, who kindly sent me a copy of this film.

32   Aleida Assmann, *Geschichte im Gedächtnis: Von der individuellen Erfahrung zur
öffentlichen Inszenierung* (Munich: Beck, 2007), p. 96.

33   Winter, 'Thinking About Silence', p. 21.

34   For the medical concept of environmentalism and its reflection in asylum architecture,
see David J. Rothman, *The Discovery of the Asylum: Social Order and Disorder in the*

New Republic (Boston: Little, Brown & Company, 1971); Carla Yanni, *The Architecture of Madness: Insane Asylums in the United States* (Minneapolis, MN: University of Minnesota Press, 2007).

35 For a comparison regarding the interior of the private space and the interactions with the people who live there, see Betts, pp. 119–47.

36 Ernst Renan, 'Was ist eine Nation? Vortrag, gehalten an der Sorbonne am 11. März 1882', in *Was ist eine Nation? Und andere politische Schriften*, ed. & trans. by Henning Ritter and Walter Euchner (Wien: Folio, 1995), pp. 41–58.

37 Winter and Sivan, pp. 6, 9; Jay Winter, *Remembering War: The Great War Between Memory and History in the Twentieth Century* (New Haven: Yale University Press, 2006), p. 276; Cappelletto, pp. 8–9; Goebel, p. 17; Dorothee Wierling, 'The War in Postwar Society: The Role of the Second World War in Public and Private Spheres in the Soviet Occupation Zone and Early GDR', in *Experience and Memory: The Second World War in Europe*, ed. by Jörg Echternkamp and Stefan Martens (New York: Berghahn Books, 2010), pp. 214–28.

38 Winter and Sivan, pp. 28–33; Winter, *Remembering War*, p. 276.

39 Ulf Schmidt, *Secret Science: A Century of Poison Warfare and Human Experiments* (Oxford: Oxford University Press, 2015), pp. 408–63.

40 Goebel, pp. 17–18.

41 Winter and Sivan, pp. 27–8; Winter, *Remembering War*, p. 287.

42 Erving Goffman, *Behavior in Public Places: Notes on the Social Organization of Gatherings* (New York: The Free Press, 1985); Erving Goffman, *The Presentation of Self in Everyday Life* (New York: Anchor, 1959); Erving Goffman, *Frame Analysis: An Essay on the Organization of Experience* (Harmondsworth: Penguin Books, 1975).

43 Konrad H. Jarausch, 'Living with Broken Memories: Some Narratological Comments', in *The Divided Past: Rewriting Post-War German History*, ed. by Christoph Klessmann (Oxford: Berg, 2001), pp. 171–98; Wierling, p. 216.

44 Rousso, pp. 5–8.

45 Winter, 'Thinking About Silence', p. 5; Konrad H. Jarausch, *After Hitler: Recivilizing Germans, 1945–1995*, trans. by Brandon Hunziker (New York: Oxford University Press, 2008), p. 270.

46 An important insight of this notion is offered by Annette Weinke, *Die Verfolgung von NS-Tätern im geteilten Deutschland: Vergangenheitsbewältigung 1949–1969, oder: Eine deutsch-deutsche Beziehungsgeschichte im Kalten Krieg* (Paderborn: Schöningh, 2002), p. 333. For further information on that issue see the fundamental study of Alexander Mitscherlich and Margarete Mitscherlich, *The Inability to Mourn: Principles of Collective Behavior* (New York: Grove Press, 1975).

47 For example, the study of Alon Confino shows the conscious use of *Heimat* symbols and pictures by the GDR as continuity from the past to achieve legitimacy and integration of the population. Confino, pp. 92–113.

48 Jarausch, 'Living with Broken Memories', p. 181.

49 Winter and Sivan describe collective remembrance, or the state narrative, as the "end product of that exchange relationship". Winter and Sivan, p. 27.

50 Anna-Sabine Ernst, *'Die beste Prophylaxe ist der Sozialismus': Ärzte und Hochschullehrer in der SBZ/DDR 1945–1961* (Münster: Waxmann, 1996), p. 25; Annette F. Timm, 'The Legacy of Bevölkerungspolitik: Veneral Disease Control and Marriage Counselling in Post-WW II Berlin', *Canadian Journal of History/Annales Canadienes d'histoire*, 2 (1998), 173–214.

51 Mecklinger, p. 1.

52 For the persistence of the concept *Stunde Null* as caesura, see *Deutsche Umbrüche im 20. Jahrhundert*, ed. by Wolfgang Schieder and Dietrich Papenfuß (Cologne: Böhlau, 2000); *Die lange Stunde Null: Gelenkter sozialer Wandel in Westdeutschland nach 1945*, ed. by Everhard Holtmann, Uta Gerhardt, and Hans Braun (Baden-Baden: Nomos, 2007); Siegried Meuschel, *Legitimation und Parteiherrschaft: Zum Paradox von Stabilität und Revolution in der DDR* (Frankfurt a.M.: Suhrkamp, 1992).

53 Goebel; Winter, *Remembering War*; Nancy Wood, *Vectors of Memory: Legacies of Trauma in Postwar Europe* (Oxford: Berg, 1999).

54 *Experience and Memory: The Second World War in Europe*, ed. by Jörg Echternkamp and Stefan Martens (New York: Berghahn Books, 2010); Richard Bessel, 'Hatred After War: Emotion and the Postwar History of East Germany', *History & Memory*, 17 (2005), 195–216; Wierling; *Three Postwar Eras in Comparison: Western Europe 1918–1945–1989*, ed. by Carl Levy and Mark Roseman (Basingstoke: Palgrave, 2002).

55 Ralph Jessen, 'Die Gesellschaft im Staatssozialismus: Probleme einer Sozialgeschichte der DDR', *Geschichte und Gesellschaft*, 21 (1995), 96–110. For more recent accounts, see Rousso, pp. 1–8; Richard Bessel, *Germany 1945: From War to Peace* (London: Simon & Schuster, 2009).

56 For the origins of the totalitarian concept, see Hannah Arendt, *The Origins of Totalitarianism* (London: Allen and Unwin, 1967). For the use of this theory to explain the GDR state, see Peter Grieder, *The East German Leadership, 1946–1973: Conflict and Crisis* (Manchester: Manchester University Press, 1999), pp. 1, 5–6, Endnote 1; Klaus Schroeder, *Der SED-Staat: Geschichte und Strukturen der DDR* (Munich: Bayrische Landeszentrale für politische Bildungsarbeit, 1998), p. 633; Klaus Schroeder, *Die veränderte Republik: Deutschland nach der Wiedervereinigung* (Munich: Bayrische Landeszentrale für politische Bildungsarbeit, 2006), p. 348; Klaus Schroeder and Monika Deutz-Schroeder, *Soziales Paradies oder Stasi-Staat? Das DDR-Bild von Schülern – ein Ost-West-Vergleich* (Stamsried: Vögel, 2008), p. 92. For its critics, see Andrew I. Port, 'The Banalities of East German Historiography', in *Becoming East German: Socialist Structures and Sensibilities After Hitler*, ed. by Mary Fulbrook and Andrew I. Port (New York: Berghahn Books, 2013), pp. 1–30; Andrew H. Beattie, 'The Politics of Remembering the GDR: Official and State-Mandated Memory Since 1990', in *Remembering the German Democratic Republic: Divided Memory in a United Germany*, ed. by David Clarke and Ute Wölfel (Harmondsworth: Palgrave Macmillan, 2011), pp. 23–34; Andrew H. Beattie, *Playing Politics with History: The Bundestag Inquiries into East Germany* (New York: Berghahn Books, 2008).

57 Jürgen Kocka, 'Eine durchherrschte Gesellschaft', in *Sozialgeschichte der DDR*, ed. by Hartmut Kaelble, Jürgen Kocka, and Hartmut Zwahr (Stuttgart: Klett-Cotta, 1994), pp. 547–53.

58 Jürgen Kocka, 'The GDR: A Special Kind of Modern Dictatorship', in *Dictatorship as Experience: Towards a Socio-Cultural History of the GDR*, ed. by Konrad H. Jarausch (New York: Berghahn Books, 1999), pp. 17–26. For critics of Kocka's concept, see Christoph Kleßmann, 'Rethinking the Second German Dictatorship', in *Dictatorship as Experience: Towards a Socio-Cultural History of the GDR*, ed. by Konrad H. Jarausch (New York: Berghahn Books, 1999), pp. 363–78; Konrad H. Jarausch, 'Care and Coercion: The GDR as Welfare Dictatorship', in *Dictatorship as Experience: Towards a Socio-Cultural History of the GDR*, ed. by Konrad H. Jarausch (New York: Berghahn Books, 1999), pp. 47–69.

59 Detlef Pollack, 'Die Konstitutive Widersprüchlichkeit Der DDR: Oder: War Die DDR-Gesellschaft Homogen?', *Geschichte Und Gesellschaft*, 24 (1998), 110–31; Detlef Pollack, 'Modernization and Modernization Blockages in GDR Society', in *Dictatorship as Experience: Towards a Socio-Cultural History of the GDR*, ed. by Konrad H. Jarausch (New York: Berghahn Books, 1999), pp. 27–45.

60 Jarausch, 'Care and Coercion', pp. 57–64.

61 Kleßmann, p. 371.

62 Linda Fuller, 'Socialism and the Transition in East and Central Europe: The Homogeneity Paradigm, Class, and Economic Inefficiency', *Annual Review of Sociology*, 26 (2000), 585–609.

63 Patrick Major, *Behind the Berlin Wall: East Germany and the Frontiers of Power* (Oxford: Oxford University Press, 2010), p. 4; Patrick Major, 'Walled in: Ordinary East Germans' Responses to 13 August 1961', *German Politics and Society*, 99 (2011), 8–22.

64 Major, *Behind the Berlin Wall*, pp. 4–10.
65 Alf Lüdtke, *Eigen-Sinn: Industriealltag, Arbeitererfahrung und Politik vom Kaiser-reich bis zum Faschismus* (Hamburg: Ergebnisse, 1993); Thomas Lindenberger, *Herr-schaft und Eigen-Sinn in der Diktatur: Studien zur Gesellschaftsgeschichte der DDR* (Cologne: Böhlau, 1999).
66 Thomas Lindenberger, 'The Fragmented Society: "Societal Activism" and Authority in GDR State Socialism', *Zeitgeschichte*, 1 (2010), 3–20; Thomas Lindenberger, ' "Aso-ciality" and Modernity: The GDR as a Welfare Dictatorship', in *Socialist Modern: East German Everyday Culture and Politics*, ed. by Paul Betts and Katherine Pence (Ann Arbor, MI: University of Michigan Press, 2008).
67 Major, *Behind the Berlin Wall*, pp. 5–8.
68 Pollack, 'Die Konstitutive Widersprüchlichkeit Der DDR', p. 118.
69 Major, *Behind the Berlin Wall*, p. 6.
70 Major, *Behind the Berlin Wall*, p. 8. For the terminology of social performance that describes public behaviour as acting, see Goffman, *The Presentation of Self*; Goffman, *Behavior in Public Places*.
71 Mary Fulbrook, *Anatomy of a Dictatorship: Inside the GDR, 1949–1989* (Oxford: Oxford University Press, 1995); Mary Fulbrook, *The Divided Nation: A History of Germany, 1918–1990* (New York: Oxford University Press, 1992); Mary Fulbrook, *The People's State: East German Society from Hitler to Honecker* (London: Yale Uni-versity Press, 2005); *Power and Society in the GDR 1961–1979: The 'Normalisation' of Rule'?*, ed. by Mary Fulbrook (New York: Berghahn Books, 2009).
72 Mary Fulbrook, 'Living Through the GDR: History, Life Stories, and Generations in East Germany', in *The GDR Remembered: Representations of the East German State Since 1989*, ed. by Nick Hodgin and Caroline Pearce (Rochester, NY: Camden House, 2011), pp. 201–20.
73 Fulbrook, 'Living Through the GDR', p. 210. For more information, see Mary Ful-brook, 'The Concept of "Normalisation" and the GDR in Comparative Perspective', in *Power and Society in the GDR 1961–1979: The 'Normalisation of Rule'?*, ed. by Mary Fulbrook (New York: Berghahn Books, 2009), pp. 1–30; Dolores L. Augustine, 'The Power Question in GDR History', *German Studies Review*, 3 (2011), 633–52.
74 For Lindenberger's harsh criticism and Fulbrook's response, see Thomas Linden-berger, 'Normality, Utopia, Memory, and Beyond: Reassembling East German Soci-ety', *German Historical Institute London Bulletin*, 33 (2011), 67–91; Mary Fulbrook, 'Response to Thomas Lindenberger', *German Historical Institute London Bulletin*, 33 (2011), 92–8. Moreover, see the critical engagements with Fulbrook's concept by Eli Rubin, 'Review of Power and Society in the GDR, 1961–1979: The "Normali-sation of Rule"?, By Mary Fulbrook', *Central European History*, 1 (2011), 191–3; Augustine.
75 A recent study of women's experience with the baby pill during the GDR also utilises a generational approach. Annette Leo and Christian König, *Die 'Wunschkindpille': Weibliche Erfahrung und staatliche Geburtenpolitik in der DDR* (Göttingen. Wall-stein, 2015).
76 Betts, p. 18; Konrad H. Jarausch, 'Beyond Uniformity: The Challenge of Historicizing the GDR', in *Dictatorship as Experience: Towards a Socio-Cultural History of the GDR*, ed. by Konrad H. Jarausch (New York: Berghahn Books, 1999), pp. 3–14.
77 For an important overview of medicine in the context within societal developments dur-ing the nineteenth and twentieth centuries, see Roger Cooter, *Surgery and Society in Peace and War: Orthopaedics and the Organization of Modern Medicine, 1880–1948* (Basingstoke: Macmillan Press, 1993); *Medicine and Modern Warfare*, ed. by Roger Cooter, Mark Harrison, and Steve Sturdy (Amsterdam: Rodopi, 1999); *War, Medicine, and Modernity*, ed. by Roger Cooter, Mark Harrison, and Steve Sturdy (Stroud: Sutton, 1998); *Medicine in the Twentieth Century*, ed. by Roger Cooter and John V. Pickstone (Amsterdam: Harwood Academic, 2000).
78 Ernst.

79 Gabriele Moser, *'Im Interesse der Volksgesundheit. . .': Sozialhygiene und öffentliches Gesundheitswesen in der Weimarer Republik und der frühen SBZ/DDR. Ein Beitrag zur Sozialgeschichte des deutschen Gesundheitswesens im 20. Jahrhundert* (Frankfurt a.M.: VAS, 2002); Gabriele Moser, ' "Kommunalisierung" des Gesundheitswesens: Der Neuaufbau der Gesundheitsverwaltung in der SBZ/DDR zwischen Weimarer Reformvorstellungen und "Sowjetisierung" ', in *Geschichte der Gesundheitspolitik in Deutschland: Von der Weimarer Republik bis in die Frühgeschichte der 'doppelten Staatsgründung'*, ed. by Wolfgang Woelke and Jörg Vögele (Berlin: Duncker & Humblot, 2002), pp. 405–18; Gabriele Moser, *Ärzte, Gesundheitswesen und Wohlfahrtsstaat: Zur Sozialgeschichte des ärztlichen Berufsstandes in Kaiserreich und Weimarer Republik* (Freiburg: Centaurus, 2011).

80 Jeannette Madarász-Lebenhagen, 'Perceptions of Health After World War II: Heart Disease and Risk Factors in East and West Germany, 1945–75', in *Becoming East German: Socialist Structures and Sensibilities After Hitler*, ed. by Mary Fulbrook and Andrew I. Port (New York: Berghahn Books, 2013), pp. 121–40; Donna Harsch, 'Socialism Fights the Proletarian Disease: East German Efforts to Overcome Tuberculosis in a Cold War Context', in *Becoming East German: Socialist Structures and Sensibilities After Hitler*, ed. by Mary Fulbrook and Andrew I. Port (New York: Berghahn Books, 2013), pp. 141–57.

81 Donna Harsch, 'Medicalized Social Hygiene? Tuberculosis Policy in the German Democratic Republic', *Bulletin of the History of Medicine*, 86 (2012), 394–423.

82 Melanie Arndt, *Gesundheitspolitik im geteilten Berlin, 1948 bis 1961* (Cologne: Böhlau, 2009).

83 Arndt, pp. 14, 253, here p. 14.

84 Jessica Reinisch, *The Perils of Peace: The Public Health Crisis in Occupied Germany* (Oxford: Oxford University Press, 2013).

85 Anne Krüger, 'Review of Playing Politics with History: The Bundestag Inquiries into East Germany, by Andrew H. Beattie', *H-Soz-u-Kult*, 2009 <http://hsozkult. geschichte.hu-berlin.de/rezensionen/2009-2-148> [accessed 30 January 2019]. For a recent attempt, see *Aufarbeitung der Aufarbeitung: Die DDR im geschichtskulturellen Diskurs*, ed. by Saskia Handro and Thomas Schaarschmidt (Schwalbach/Ts.: Wochenschau, 2011).

86 'Vernehmungsprotokoll, 24. Dezember 1959': BStU, MfS, BV Dresden, AU 43/60, Bl. 118–19.

87 'Vernehmungsprotokoll, 24. Dezember 1959': BStU, MfS, BV Dresden, AU 43/60, Bl. 122–3.

88 'Vertraulich, betr. Herrn Oberarzt Dr. Korinek, 17. April 1950': StA DD, Dezernat Gesundheitswesen, 4.1.12, Nr. 21, Bl. 206.

Bibliography

Primary sources

Unpublished

BUNDESARCHIV (BARCH)

Ministry of Healthcare

BArch, DQ 1/12052 – Personalakte Walter Korinek, 1948–1967

ARCHIV DES BUNDESBEAUFTRAGTEN FÜR DIE UNTERLAGEN DES STAATSSICHERHEITSDIENSTES DER EHEMALIGEN DEUTSCHEN DEMOKRATISCHEN REPUBLIK (BSTU)

BStU, MfS, BV Dresden, AU 43/60

DRESDEN, STADTARCHIV (STA DD)

StA DD, Dezernat Gesundheitswesen, 4.1.12, Nr. 21

Published

Mecklinger, Ludwig, 'Der politische Auftrag des Gesundheitswesens: Aus der Rede des Ministers für Gesundheitswesen, OMR Prof. Dr. sc. med. Ludwig Mecklinger, auf der Kreisärztekonferenz', *humanitas*, 24 (1981), 1–3

Secondary sources

Arendt, Hannah, *On Violence* (New York: Harcourt Brace, 1970)
——, *The Origins of Totalitarianism* (London: Allen and Unwin, 1967)
Arndt, Melanie, *Gesundheitspolitik im geteilten Berlin, 1948 bis 1961* (Cologne: Böhlau, 2009)
Assmann, Aleida, *Der lange Schatten der Vergangenheit: Erinnerungskultur und Geschichtspolitik* (Munich: Beck, 2006)
——, *Geschichte im Gedächtnis: Von der individuellen Erfahrung zur öffentlichen Inszenierung* (Munich: Beck, 2007)
Augustine, Dolores L., 'The Power Question in GDR History', *German Studies Review*, 3 (2011), 633–52
Beattie, Andrew H., *Playing Politics with History: The Bundestag Inquiries into East Germany* (New York: Berghahn Books, 2008)
——, 'The Politics of Remembering the GDR: Official and State-Mandated Memory Since 1990', in *Remembering the German Democratic Republic: Divided Memory in a United Germany*, ed. by David Clarke and Ute Wölfel (Harmondsworth: Palgrave Macmillan, 2011), pp. 23–34
Bessel, Richard, *Germany 1945: From War to Peace* (London: Simon & Schuster, 2009)
——, 'Hatred After War: Emotion and the Postwar History of East Germany', *History & Memory*, 17 (2005), 195–216
Betts, Paul, *Within Walls: Private Life in the German Democratic Republic* (Oxford: Oxford University Press, 2010)
Black, Monica, *Death in Berlin: From Weimar to Divided Germany* (Cambridge: Cambridge University Press, 2010)
Cappelletto, Francesca, 'Introduction', in *Memory and World War II: An Ethnographic Approach*, ed. by Francesca Cappelletto (Oxford: Berg, 2005)
Confino, Alon, *Germany as a Culture of Remembrance: Promises and Limits of Writing History* (Chapel Hill, NC: University of North Carolina Press, 2006)
Cooter, Roger, *Surgery and Society in Peace and War: Orthopaedics and the Organization of Modern Medicine, 1880–1948* (Basingstoke: Macmillan Press, 1993)
Cooter, Roger, and John V. Pickstone, eds., *Medicine in the Twentieth Century* (Amsterdam: Harwood Academic, 2000)
Cooter, Roger, Mark Harrison, and Steve Sturdy, eds., *Medicine and Modern Warfare* (Amsterdam: Rodopi, 1999)
——, eds., *War, Medicine, and Modernity* (Stroud: Sutton, 1998)
Echternkamp, Jörg, and Stefan Martens, eds., *Experience and Memory: The Second World War in Europe* (New York: Berghahn Books, 2010)
Ernst, Anna-Sabine, *'Die beste Prophylaxe ist der Sozialismus': Ärzte und Hochschullehrer in der SBZ/DDR 1945–1961* (Münster: Waxmann, 1996)
Fulbrook, Mary, *Anatomy of a Dictatorship: Inside the GDR, 1949–1989* (Oxford: Oxford University Press, 1995)

————, 'Living Through the GDR: History, Life Stories, and Generations in East Germany', in *The GDR Remembered: Representations of the East German State Since 1989*, ed. by Nick Hodgin and Caroline Pearce (Rochester, NY: Camden House, 2011), pp. 201–20

————, ed., *Power and Society in the GDR 1961–1979: The 'Normalisation of Rule'?* (New York: Berghahn Books, 2009)

————, 'Response to Thomas Lindenberger', *German Historical Institute London Bulletin*, 33 (2011), 92–8

————, 'The Concept of "Normalisation" and the GDR in Comparative Perspective', in *Power and Society in the GDR 1961–1979: The 'Normalisation of Rule'?* ed. by Mary Fulbrook (New York: Berghahn Books, 2009), pp. 1–30

————, *The Divided Nation: A History of Germany, 1918–1990* (New York: Oxford University Press, 1992)

————, *The People's State: East German Society from Hitler to Honecker* (London: Yale University Press, 2005)

Fuller, Linda, 'Socialism and the Transition in East and Central Europe: The Homogeneity Paradigm, Class, and Economic Inefficiency', *Annual Review of Sociology*, 26 (2000), 585–609

Glaser, Daniel, *Dresden '91: Ein Beitrag zur Dialektik* (Filminitiative Dresden, 1991)

Goebel, Stefan, *The Great War and Medieval Memory: War, Remembrance, and Medievalism in Britain and Germany, 1914–1940* (Cambridge: Cambridge University Press, 2007)

Goffman, Erving, *Behavior in Public Places: Notes on the Social Organization of Gatherings* (New York: The Free Press, 1985)

————, *Frame Analysis: An Essay on the Organization of Experience* (Harmondsworth: Penguin Books, 1975)

————, *The Presentation of Self in Everyday Life* (New York: Anchor, 1959)

Grieder, Peter, *The East German Leadership, 1946–1973: Conflict and Crisis* (Manchester: Manchester University Press, 1999)

Halbwachs, Maurice, *On Collective Memory*, trans. by Lewis A. Coser (Chicago: University of Chicago Press, 1992)

Handro, Saskia, and Thomas Schaarschmidt, eds., *Aufarbeitung der Aufarbeitung: Die DDR im geschichtskulturellen Diskurs* (Schwalbach/Ts.: Wochenschau, 2011)

Harsch, Donna, 'Medicalized Social Hygiene? Tuberculosis Policy in the German Democratic Republic', *Bulletin of the History of Medicine*, 86 (2012), 394–423

————, 'Socialism Fights the Proletarian Disease: East German Efforts to Overcome Tuberculosis in a Cold War Context', in *Becoming East German: Socialist Structures and Sensibilities After Hitler*, ed. by Mary Fulbrook and Andrew I. Port (New York: Berghahn Books, 2013), pp. 141–57

Holtmann, Everhard, Uta Gerhardt, and Hans Braun, eds., *Die lange Stunde Null: Gelenkter sozialer Wandel in Westdeutschland nach 1945* (Baden-Baden: Nomos, 2007)

Jarausch, Konrad H., *After Hitler: Recivilizing Germans, 1945–1995*, trans. by Brandon Hunziker (New York: Oxford University Press, 2008)

————, 'Beyond Uniformity: The Challenge of Historicizing the GDR', in *Dictatorship as Experience: Towards a Socio-Cultural History of the GDR*, ed. by Konrad H. Jarausch (New York: Berghahn Books, 1999), pp. 3–14

————, 'Care and Coercion: The GDR as Welfare Dictatorship', in *Dictatorship as Experience: Towards a Socio-Cultural History of the GDR*, ed. by Konrad H. Jarausch (New York: Berghahn Books, 1999), pp. 47–69

————, 'Living with Broken Memories: Some Narratological Comments', in *The Divided Past: Rewriting Post-War German History*, ed. by Christoph Klessmann (Oxford: Berg, 2001), pp. 171–98

Jessen, Ralph, 'Die Gesellschaft im Staatssozialismus: Probleme einer Sozialgeschichte der DDR', *Geschichte und Gesellschaft*, 21 (1995), 96–110

Kansteiner, Wulf, 'Finding a Meaning in Memory: A Methodological Critique of Collective Memory Studies', *History and Theory*, 1 (2002), 179–97

Kleßmann, Christoph, 'Rethinking the Second German Dictatorship', in *Dictatorship as Experience: Towards a Socio-Cultural History of the GDR*, ed. by Konrad H. Jarausch (New York: Berghahn Books, 1999), pp. 363–78

Kocka, Jürgen, 'Eine durchherrschte Gesellschaft', in *Sozialgeschichte der DDR*, ed. by Hartmut Kaelble, Jürgen Kocka, and Hartmut Zwahr (Stuttgart: Klett-Cotta, 1994), pp. 547–53

———, 'The GDR: A Special Kind of Modern Dictatorship', in *Dictatorship as Experience: Towards a Socio-Cultural History of the GDR*, ed. by Konrad H. Jarausch (New York: Berghahn Books, 1999), pp. 17–26

Krüger, Anne, 'Review of Playing Politics with History: The Bundestag Inquiries into East Germany, by Andrew H. Beattie', *H-Soz-u-Kult*, 2009 <http://hsozkult.geschichte. hu-berlin.de/rezensionen/2009-2-148> [accessed 30 January 2019]

Leo, Annette, and Christian König, *Die 'Wunschkindpille': Weibliche Erfahrung und staatliche Geburtenpolitik in der DDR* (Göttingen: Wallstein, 2015)

Levine, Peter A., *Trauma and Memory: Brain and Body in a Search for the Living Past: A Practical Guide for Understanding and Working with Traumatic Memory* (Berkeley: North Atlantic Books, 2015)

Levy, Carl, and Mark Roseman, eds., *Three Postwar Eras in Comparison: Western Europe 1918–1945–1989* (Basingstoke: Palgrave, 2002)

Lindenberger, Thomas, ' "Asociality" and Modernity: The GDR as a Welfare Dictatorship', in *Socialist Modern: East German Everyday Culture and Politics*, ed. by Paul Betts and Katherine Pence (Ann Arbor, MI: University of Michigan Press, 2008)

———, *Herrschaft und Eigen-Sinn in der Diktatur: Studien zur Gesellschaftsgeschichte der DDR* (Cologne: Böhlau, 1999)

———, 'Normality, Utopia, Memory, and Beyond: Reassembling East German Society', *German Historical Institute London Bulletin*, 33 (2011), 67–91

———, 'The Fragmented Society: "Societal Activism" and Authority in GDR State Socialism', *Zeitgeschichte*, 1 (2010), 3–20

Lüdtke, Alf, *Eigen-Sinn: Industriealltag, Arbeitererfahrung und Politik vom Kaiserreich bis zum Faschismus* (Hamburg: Ergebnisse, 1993)

Madarász-Lebenhagen, Jeannette, 'Perceptions of Health After World War II: Heart Disease and Risk Factors in East and West Germany, 1945–75', in *Becoming East German: Socialist Structures and Sensibilities After Hitler*, ed. by Mary Fulbrook and Andrew I. Port (New York: Berghahn Books, 2013), pp. 121–40

Major, Patrick, *Behind the Berlin Wall: East Germany and the Frontiers of Power* (Oxford: Oxford University Press, 2010)

———, 'Walled in: Ordinary East Germans' Responses to 13 August 1961', *German Politics and Society*, 99 (2011), 8–22

Meuschel, Siegried, *Legitimation und Parteiherrschaft: Zum Paradox von Stabilität und Revolution in der DDR* (Frankfurt a.M.: Suhrkamp, 1992)

Mitscherlich, Alexander, and Margarete Mitscherlich, *The Inability to Mourn: Principles of Collective Behavior* (New York: Grove Press, 1975)

Moser, Gabriele, *Ärzte, Gesundheitswesen und Wohlfahrtsstaat: Zur Sozialgeschichte des ärztlichen Berufsstandes in Kaiserreich und Weimarer Republik* (Freiburg: Centaurus, 2011)

———, *'Im Interesse der Volksgesundheit. . .': Sozialhygiene und öffentliches Gesundheitswesen in der Weimarer Republik und der frühen SBZ/DDR: Ein Beitrag zur*

Sozialgeschichte des deutschen Gesundheitswesens im 20. Jahrhundert (Frankfurt a.M.: VAS, 2002)

——, ' "Kommunalisierung" des Gesundheitswesens: Der Neuaufbau der Gesundheitsverwaltung in der SBZ/DDR zwischen Weimarer Reformvorstellungen und "Sowjetisierung" ', in *Geschichte der Gesundheitspolitik in Deutschland: Von der Weimarer Republik bis in die Frühgeschichte der 'doppelten Staatsgründung'*, ed. by Wolfgang Woelke and Jörg Vögele (Berlin: Duncker & Humblot, 2002), pp. 405–18

Nora, Pierre, 'Introduction', in *Rethinking France: Les Lieux De Mémoire: Volume 4: Histories and Memories*, ed. by Pierre Nora (Chicago: University of Chicago Press, 2010), pp. VII–XIV

——, ed., *Rethinking France: Les Lieux De Mémoire: Volume 4: Histories and Memories* (Chicago: University of Chicago Press, 2010)

Pollack, Detlef, 'Die Konstitutive Widersprüchlichkeit Der DDR: Oder: War Die DDR-Gesellschaft Homogen?', *Geschichte Und Gesellschaft*, 24 (1998), 110–31

——, 'Modernization and Modernization Blockages in GDR Society', in *Dictatorship as Experience: Towards a Socio-Cultural History of the GDR*, ed. by Konrad H. Jarausch (New York: Berghahn Books, 1999), pp. 27–45

Port, Andrew I., 'The Banalities of East German Historiography', in *Becoming East German: Socialist Structures and Sensibilities After Hitler*, ed. by Mary Fulbrook and Andrew I. Port (New York: Berghahn Books, 2013), pp. 1–30

Reinisch, Jessica, *The Perils of Peace: The Public Health Crisis in Occupied Germany* (Oxford: Oxford University Press, 2013)

Renan, Ernst, 'Was ist eine Nation? Vortrag, gehalten an der Sorbonne am 11. März 1882', in *Was ist eine Nation? Und andere politische Schriften*, ed. & trans. by Henning Ritter and Walter Euchner (Wien: Folio, 1995), pp. 41–58

Rothman, David J., *The Discovery of the Asylum: Social Order and Disorder in the New Republic* (Boston: Little, Brown & Company, 1971)

Rousso, Henry, 'A New Perspective on the War', in *Experience and Memory: The Second World War in Europe*, ed. by Jörg Echternkamp and Stefan Martens (New York: Berghahn Books, 2010), pp. 1–9

Rubin, Eli, 'Review of Power and Society in the GDR, 1961–1979: The "Normalisation of Rule"? By Mary Fulbrook', *Central European History*, 1 (2011), 191–3

Schieder, Wolfgang, and Dietrich Papenfuß, eds., *Deutsche Umbrüche im 20. Jahrhundert* (Cologne: Böhlau, 2000)

Schmidt, Ulf, *Secret Science: A Century of Poison Warfare and Human Experiments* (Oxford: Oxford University Press, 2015)

Schroeder, Klaus, *Der SED-Staat: Geschichte und Strukturen der DDR* (Munich: Bayrische Landeszentrale für politische Bildungsarbeit, 1998)

——, *Die veränderte Republik: Deutschland nach der Wiedervereinigung* (Munich: Bayrische Landeszentrale für politische Bildungsarbeit, 2006)

Schroeder, Klaus, and Monika Deutz-Schroeder, *Soziales Paradies oder Stasi-Staat? Das DDR-Bild von Schülern – ein Ost-West-Vergleich* (Stamsried: Vögel, 2008)

Segalo, Puleng, 'Trauma and Gender', *Social and Personality Psychology Compass*, 9 (2015), 447–54

Timm, Annette F., 'The Legacy of Bevölkerungspolitik: Veneral Disease Control and Marriage Counselling in Post-WW II Berlin', *Canadian Journal of History/Annales Cannadienes d'histoire*, 2 (1998), 173–214

Weinke, Annette, *Die Verfolgung von NS-Tätern im geteilten Deutschland: Vergangen-heitsbewältigung 1949–1969, oder: Eine deutsch-deutsche Beziehungsgeschichte im Kalten Krieg* (Paderborn: Schöningh, 2002)

Wierling, Dorothee, 'The War in Postwar Society: The Role of the Second World War in Public and Private Spheres in the Soviet Occupation Zone and Early GDR', in *Experi-ence and Memory: The Second World War in Europe*, ed. by Jörg Echternkamp and Stefan Martens (New York: Berghahn Books, 2010), pp. 214–28

Winter, Jay, 'Conclusion: Metropolitan History and National History in the Age of Total War', in *Cities into Battlefields: Metropolitan Scenarios, Experiences, and Commemo-rations of Total War*, ed. by Stefan Goebel and Derek Keene (Farnham: Ashgate, 2011), pp. 219–23

——, *Remembering War: The Great War Between Memory and History in the Twentieth Century* (New Haven: Yale University Press, 2006)

——, 'Thinking About Silence', in *Shadows of War: A Social History of Silence in the Twentieth Century*, ed. by Efrat Ben-Ze'ev, Ruth Ginio, and Jay Winter (Cambridge: Cambridge University Press, 2010), pp. 3–31

Winter, Jay, and Emmanuel Sivan, 'Setting the Framework', in *War and Remembrance in the Twentieth Century*, ed. by Jay Winter and Emmanuel Sivan (Cambridge: Cambridge University Press, 1999), pp. 6–39

Wood, Nancy, *Vectors of Memory: Legacies of Trauma in Postwar Europe* (Oxford: Berg, 1999)

Yanni, Carla, *The Architecture of Madness: Insane Asylums in the United States* (Minneapolis, MN: University of Minnesota Press, 2007)

1 Treating the past

Narratives of the medical profession after 1945

Introduction

In July 1958, the MfS in Sebnitz, near Dresden, was informed about a doctors' gathering in a restaurant. An IM reported to the state security service that the adverse opinions of one tuberculosis clinician stood out, specifying:

> Regarding the last doctors' congress in Leipzig, Dr [Förster][1] stated that the Healthcare Minister, [Luitpold] Steidle allowed himself quite a lot there [in his speech attacking doctors]. After all, [Steidle] was also a Nazi since 1928 and eventually became [*Wehrmacht*] Colonel. [Förster] wondered how a human being like Steidle 'can betray his conviction' [. . .] [and] sell himself to be the Healthcare Minister today and that, above all, in the GDR.[2]

According to Förster, the new Health Minister – who had no medical training[3] – "stabbed the others [his comrades] in the back".[4] Like Steidle and many of the medical profession, Förster participated in the Second World War and had been an active member of the *Nationalsozialistische Deutsche Arbeiterpartei* [National Socialist German Workers' Party – NSDAP]. In his speech at the congress, however – which the GDR initiated as a counter-event to the doctors' conference that took place in West Germany in 1958 – Steidle argued in concordance with the *Sozialistische Einheitspartei Deutschlands* [Socialist Unity Party of Germany – SED]. He attacked both the involvement of doctors in the Third Reich, and also their 'class consciousness' and excessive financial and social demands, and consequently caused the protest of the pneumatologist.[5] Förster's anger reveals that the medical profession had always formed a strong social bond among its members – a mnemonic community – and was thus able to fend off state infiltrations and accusations, as well as lobby for concessions and professional rights.

In his 1983 book *The Nazi Party*, Michael H. Kater concludes that in the post-war period "[a] new and idealistic generation of physicians would be needed to rebuild a profession that by 1945 had sunk into total disrepute".[6] As shown in the preceding, the SBZ and also the Western Occupied Zones of Germany encountered a medical profession that had been heavily involved in Nazi organisations and medical crimes and thus was – among other professions – targeted by the policies of the Allies to transform German society after 1945. However, the health-threatening environment in postwar Germany was one motive of authorities and the medical profession for justifying concessions and the re-deployment of many former Nazi doctors.[7] Moreover, as Annette Weinke concludes, it was "Nazi incriminated people [referring to doctors, M.W.] of both German states [who] showed a disproportionately high willingness for adaptation and commitment".[8] The result was that the opportunity for doctors and other medical personnel to fall through the de-Nazification net was quite high at any given time.

For the SBZ, this endeavour came to a complete halt in Spring 1948, when the SMAD officially declared the end of de-Nazification with Command 35/48. However, despite their efforts, the preceding case highlights continuity of both state authorities and local doctors after 1945. Especially regarding 'euthanasia' crimes, both the GDR and the *Bundesrepublik Deutschland* [Federal Republic of Germany – FRG] faced a new round of de-Nazification procedures due to the belated discovery of incriminated doctors almost 20 years after the Second World War. Large investigations in West Germany during the 1960s affected East Germany, as trial inquiries mentioned names of doctors who still practised in the GDR.[9] Many of these had remarkable careers under the new socialist system that clashed with the state's 'anti-Fascist' paradigm and showed that a thorough de-Nazification of doctors could not be achieved on either side of the Iron Curtain.[10]

This chapter explores the postwar lives of physicians through a series of case studies: each example exposes diverse negotiation strategies and life-narratives that were employed by doctors to cope with the new socialist system. Therefore, I argue that the smooth transition of medical personnel from war to postwar was based on an individualised compromise between the doctor and local or state authorities. On the one hand, officials judged the degree of political and criminal involvement in the Third Reich from the available sources, compared to the current utility of a physician for curbing the epidemics after 1945. The result of this evaluation was decisive for the fate of doctors in postwar East Germany: prosecution, severe or mild sanctions towards, or the ability to continue, their medical practice. On the other hand, doctors used this occasion to depict themselves as indispensable for the state and society and created a life-narrative, omitting all memories that had the potential to compromise their future in postwar East Germany.

The medical memories of both medical personnel and state authorities could directly affect the career prospects of an individual. Therefore, medical memories describe the obtained medical career and skills of a doctor in the past, which were used, altered, or enhanced by the individual, mnemonic community or state after 1945. These reassembled life, institutional, and state narratives affected not only the professional life of the doctor, but also the relationship with, and the treatment of, the patient. This intertwined relationship between the state and its medical staff often enabled a person to mitigate membership in the NSDAP and even the involvement in war-crimes and atrocities.

In many cases, state authorities either buried people's Nazi past if the doctor was needed and demonstrated the will to adapt to the rules, or used this information to blackmail them. Especially for reputable doctors, however, Nazi links were often erased to sanitise their life paths in the GDR. Therefore, opportunist behaviour enabled the physician to secure a certain living standard and potentially provide for a family in the postwar era. This hypothesis is not uncommon, as people always have the desire to have security and pursue their personal goals in life. As a result, however, these postwar negotiations between individual doctors and the state proved to be pragmatic, mainly driven by the health predicaments in the postwar era.

Nonetheless, as Henry Leide suggests, these decisions were also embedded in the struggle for the legitimisation of the GDR as a proclaimed 'anti-Fascist state': a country where apparently no Nazis remained in influential positions after its de-Nazification procedures in the postwar era. On the one hand, East German state officials denounced and externalised the problem: in their political agitation, they established a state narrative in which the "Nazi was inherently a West German person".[11] Norbert Frei identifies this claim as an important part of East Germany's propaganda that targeted the Nazi past of West German politicians and officials for legitimisation purposes – it was a 'battle for memory' over how to deal with Germany's recent past and simultaneously accommodate the majority of people in the new state.[12]

On the other hand, the GDR authorities maintained their image of an 'anti-Fascist state' by using their intelligence apparatus to avoid any publicity about exposed Nazi cases or war-crimes, especially during the 1960s. This inherent legitimacy problem, embedded in the Cold War struggle between West and East Germany, ironically led to the fact that many former Nazis pursued their career, unmolested by criminal charges. Both competing states hesitated to initiate proceedings against them in the 1960s to evade the accusation of leniency towards former Nazis and war criminals applied during the postwar years by the other side, and the consequent international reputational damage.[13]

The chapter's core revolves around individuals, all of whom worked in the East German healthcare system with different specialisations, employed in hospitals, health clinics, and even prisons for at least some time after 1945. However, the data used in this study has its limitations. The vast majority of personal information was found in the archival files of the former secret police of the GDR. Therefore, the scope of cases is restricted to individuals who came under the scrutiny of the state. Ramifications of this issue include that the degree of political involvement before 1945 is higher than in the studies of Anna-Sabine Ernst and Kater.[14] Nevertheless, the data shows trends that the numbers from aforementioned authors confirm. Additional methodological problems lie in the accuracy of the biographical facts. The inherent fallacies of this data were circumvented with help from secondary and online sources about people where possible. In cases in which this study has to rely on archives, inaccuracies could occur and bias the analysis.

For comparison purposes, these people are split into four different age cohorts with striking differences in their biographies and transition from the Third Reich into the GDR. The creation of these generational cohorts is admittedly a retrospective endeavour and artificial construction.[15] Many historians refrain from using the term 'generation', as it is as vague as other homogenising historical concepts, such as class affiliation or nationhood.[16] No methodology or approach is sufficient to encompass all facets of a generation, which, by nature, are highly diverse.[17] However, as the following analysis shows, distinct experiences would vanish if the selected cases were analysed as a whole. Therefore, they are split into four age cohorts in line with Ernst's study, which analyses the NS-membership among professors of medicine in East Germany, shown in Table 1.1: the World War One Generation (born between 1886–1895), the Weimar Generation (1896–1905), the Generation of Depression and Upheaval (1906–1915), and the Nazi Generation (1916–1925).

The analytical context behind the ten-year cohorts is the identification of the contemporary events that, assumingly, most decisively shaped people's belief system and perception according to their age, and thus can be described as their primary socialisation – thus all of them had different experiences during their childhood or adolescence, which distinguishes them from one another.

With this foundation, the study follows the idea of identifying a "sense of generational distinctiveness" – for example, someone born in 1880 would have had a very different outlook towards the changing political systems than someone born in the midst of the First World War.[18] Therefore, the creation of these East German age cohorts, especially in line with Ernst's analysis, gives this study the chance to identify specific characteristics of each cohort.[19] This endeavour consequently enlightens the understanding of the interdependency between the socialisation, experience, and memory of the individual with its mnemonic community – a community of shared values and memories – and its social environment and state.

Fulbrook, for example, identified similar patterns in the life paths of individuals born in the late 1920s and early 1930s. These people were often at the forefront of the new 'socialist system' in East Germany, which Fulbrook described as the main feature of the '1929er' generation.[20] Among this historically constructed age cohort, a widespread postwar euphoria towards the new socialist project could be found, despite all the difficulties of life after the war. However, this enthusiasm eventually gave way to disenchantment due to everyday realities in the socialist state and Cold War context.[21]

Table 1.1 Distribution of medical professionals into generational cohorts from this study and the work of Ernst

Born between	Own study (N=128)		Ernst (N=207)	
	Abs.	*%*	*Abs.*	*%*
Cohort A – 1886–1895	16	12.5	41	19.8
Cohort B – 1896–1905	34	26.6	56	27.0
Cohort C – 1906–1915	64	50.0	79	38.2
Cohort D – 1916–1925	14	10.9	31	15

Source: See Appendix; Ernst, *'Die beste Prophylaxe ist der Sozialismus'*, p. 151, Table 13. Numbers of her generations between 1886 and 1925 added up lead to a total of 207 instead of the overall 262 with which Ernst worked in her study.

This statement equally applies to my own family: my grandfather, born in 1925, joined the *Hitlerjugend* [Hitler Youth – HJ], and after he had received his draft notice in 1942, he volunteered for the German Navy to avoid deployment at the eastern front. Shortly after the war, he became one of the *Neulehrer* [New Teachers],[22] and joined the *Freie Deutsche Jugend* [Free German Youth – FDJ], the *Freier Deutscher Gewerkschaftsbund* [Free German Trade Union – FDGB], the *Gesellschaft für Deutsch – Sowjetische Freundschaft* [German–Soviet Friendship Association – DSF], and finally the SED. He pursued a career in education, in which he started as a teacher and eventually became the head of a local school. As described in the preceding, he was a convinced proponent of the new state and even participated in the political realm with a seat in the *Rat des Kreises* [county council] – a typical biography of Fulbrook's 1929ers.

Like so many of his contemporaries, he believed in the slogans of 'anti-fascism', 'anti-capitalism', and 'anti-imperialism'. He saw the GDR as a new start, an alternative model of society, and a way to express his conviction that, ideally, there should be 'no more war' in Europe and the world. However, he gradually became disappointed, voiced criticism, and subsequently lost all his professional and political positions before the events that led to the German reunification in 1989/90. These nuances in people's lives are easily overlooked by a narrow view that focusses on the policy level. Therefore, this chapter investigates the complexity of individual lives and life decisions, negotiated with themselves, the mnemonic community, and the state, through the framework of medical memories and experiences.

Many of the case studies, scrutinised in the following, feature remarkable careers. Their integration into the 'new' emerging healthcare system not only illustrates the necessity of employing former NSDAP members to cope with epidemic diseases, but also exposes prospects, which the chaos of the postwar years and the uncertainty of the future offered to doctors. On the one hand, this chapter shows that physicians consciously used the postwar conditions to 'sanitise' their past or, as in Korinek's case, exploited the need for medical personnel to enhance their career prospects. On the other hand, the state also protected some of its physicians against accusations, 'defamation', and the domestic or international exposure of their former NSDAP membership or involvement in war-crimes.

The following question arises here: what was the social and political background that determined the political involvement of the physicians, pre- and post-1945? This issue especially targets all possible overlaps between the so-called 'two German dictatorships'. The answer to this question can be found in the following sections, which investigate how medical memories informed the decision-making of individuals, communities, and state authorities regarding a person's opportunities and fate in the postwar era. Furthermore, they discuss why a significant number of doctors rejected any state influence by referring to their profession as 'apolitical'.[23] This statement is in sharp contrast to the high degree of their involvement in Nazi organisations, but reflects the plummeting of political activity after 1945 in East Germany among the discussed cases (see Figure 1.1 on p. 57). It was not only an exoneration strategy, but also the unconscious feeling of something that can be called 'collective guilt'.[24] This term has been criticised for its pitfalls in recent historiographical debates[25] and by Hannah Arendt, who rather pointed towards the 'implicit' versus 'complicit' guilt as the new 'banality of evil';[26] however, it offers one perspective of why, according to Weinke, contemporaries of the late 1940s desperately sought for *Ruhe* [peace and quiet].[27] This chapter offers insight into the negotiation of doctors and the state within the context of postwar 'silence' and the imminent Cold War.

In this context, a generalisation of postwar career paths of the East German medical profession is thus untenable. Instead, the book shows that people like Dr Förster and the Health Minister Steidle from the opening quotation, who actively participated in the Third Reich, equally continued to shape the healthcare system at the local and state level in postwar East Germany. In this way, these people ensured that the past had its place in the present, and, potentially, in the future of the patient and the proclaimed 'new' socialist state.

Cohort A (1886–1895): the World War One Generation

Born in 1891, Reinhard Carrière, who after 1945 became the chief doctor of the psychiatric hospital in Zschadraß (Colditz), represents one example of the first generation who actively experienced the First World War. The war and its aftermath in Weimar had the biggest impact on people born between 1886 and 1895, defining their primary socialisation. These circumstances caused, according to Fulbrook, their high 'cultural availability for mobilisation' for future political projects, which she defines as a given inner predisposition: people were readily available to be mobilised for an ideology, depending on the degree of their convictions and beliefs.[28] The numbers of this study in Table 1.2 are, in comparison with Ernst and Kater, distorted. This deviance is due to the fact – as explained earlier – that most of the cases in the database were obtained from the MfS files, which concentrated their investigations on former members of Nazi organisations. However, this does not invalidate the findings altogether; they can offer some valuable conclusions for this particular generation.

As shown in Table 1.2, the degree of 'cultural availability for mobilisation' was high for this cohort. The defeat in the First World War, the unrest in Weimar, and the right-wing narrative about the 'stab in the back' by left-wing politicians fuelled their support and approval of Hitler's claims.[29] Whether the latter was also true for Carrière, who joined the NSDAP in 1933 and became a member of the *Nationalsozialistische Volkswohlfahrt* [National Socialist People's Welfare – NSV] and *Nationalsozialistischer Ärztebund* [National Socialist Doctors' Association – NSÄB], remains unclear.[30]

However, Carrière became the senior physician under the leadership of the well-known proponent of 'euthanasia' and forced sterilisations Paul Nitsche in the Psychiatric Hospital Pirna-Sonnenstein in 1936.[31] According to his son, Carrière joined the party only because it was a requirement for this position. However, he would have had to leave the institution already one year after, because he expressed criticism and thus was re-deployed to an administrative position in Leipzig. Therefore, he knew about the medical crimes during the Third Reich; his potential involvement cannot be judged.[32]

Table 1.2 Cohort A (1886–1895): overview of political involvement before 1945 in comparison to studies of Ernst and Kater

Pre-1945	Own study (N=16)		Ernst (N=41)		Kater (average from medical licensure period 1878–1924)[y]
	Abs.	%	Abs.	%	%
NSDAP	12	75.0	21	51.1	43.1
NSÄB	5	31.3	4[x]	9.8	39.5
SA	5	31.3	9	22.0	21.0
SS	2	12.5	1	2.4	3.9
Without	2	12.5	9	22.0	/

Source: See Appendix; Ernst, *'Die beste Prophylaxe ist der Sozialismus'*, p. 151, Table 13; Kater, *Doctors under Hitler*, p. 245, Table 2.4. (x) This number represents people who were only involved in NSÄB or similar Nazi organisations, without an NSDAP, SS, or SA membership. Therefore, this number is low compared to the actual involvement in the NSÄB. (y) Kater uses in his study the medical licensure period to separate his cohorts. For example, for Cohort A, when calculated from the birthdate, the medical licensure period was around 1912 to 1922. Therefore, the two studies are comparable only to a certain extent. However, Kater's analysis is important to contextualise and confirm the trends identified here.

One of his contemporaries, Friedrich Wilhelm Brekenfeld (*1887), also boosted his personal progress by joining the NSDAP in 1937 and becoming the *Deutsches Rotes Kreuz* [German Red Cross – DRK] *Generalhauptführer* [general head leader] and Leader of the *Landesstelle* [provincial office] III – Berlin and Brandenburg – of the DRK.[33] The statement in one of his works from 1939 proves that Brekenfeld's decision to join the Nazi party was not solely a pragmatic one:

> [The DRK] requires from its [male and female] leaders and sub-leaders other than the technical understanding of medical care also real leadership qualities and to be completely absorbed in the National Socialist ideology. [. . .] In the most difficult hours, the swastika also gives them strength and confidence in their actions as well as endurance[,] sense and aim: "All for Germany!"[34]

Both Carrière and Brekenfeld were in their 40s when Hitler assumed power in Germany – they are outstanding examples of careerists under the banner of Nazism, and at least Brekenfeld apparently was a proponent of its ideology, which opened his path to the top ranks of the DRK.

However, for them and others of this generation (1886–1895), the experience of another defeat – this time, a 'total' one, with foreign powers occupying Germany entirely after a war in which they were involved – might have caused a political disenchantment, the averting of unnecessary attention by the public and authorities, and the wish to retreat and concentrate on family life that prevented them from further political participation in the GDR.[35] Even if the sample size of 16 people in this cohort is not representative, the analysis shows that due to this situation, only around 44 per cent were organised in political parties, and 37.5 per cent even avoided any civil commitment after 1945 (see Table 1.3). By contrast, only 12.5 per cent were not politically active during the Third Reich, a number that is also confirmed by Ernst's study with 22 per cent (see Table 1.2).[36]

Brekenfeld, for example, was not involved in any political organisation in post-war East Germany. However, he became a professor at Humboldt University in Berlin and was the Director of the Head Department of Hygiene within the *Ministerium für Gesundheitswesen* [Healthcare Ministry – MfG] in the GDR. There he was, inter alia, responsible for blood donation regulations, including the issues surrounding syphilis transmissions through blood transfusion. Therefore, Breken-feld had negotiated a crucial position within the GDR healthcare system with a continuation of medical memories and experiences: his views on medical issues shaped the postwar East German healthcare system.[37] Even after his retirement from this position, he remained a scientific officer and advisor at the MfG and received prestigious awards for his work. This career path was possible despite the fact that he was not politically involved in the GDR but a former proponent of the Nazi regime in a high position.[38]

Brekenfeld and the first generation's general unwillingness to engage politically with the new system was mostly due to their primary socialisation and ideological predisposition, as well as their age being over 50 in 1945, which may have impeded any further commitment.[39] Egbert Schwarz (*1890) is an example of this tendency. Schwarz had a steady career in East Germany, despite the fact that he was heavily involved in Nazi organisations during the Third Reich: with memberships in the NSDAP, the NSÄB, and, most problematically, the *Schutzstaffel* [SS]. As archival sources suggest, his further commitment rested wholly on the 'scientific' side of his job as a professor at the Medical Academy in Erfurt and his membership and high position in the *Leopoldina* – a supposedly 'apolitical' scientific association of natural scientists founded in the seventeenth century.[40]

Consequently, Schwarz fell into the long tradition, exposed by Tobias Weidner, of the medical profession's claim to be 'apolitical' – somewhat elevated over the 'petty business of politics'.[41] This communication strategy of silence and denial – itself

Table 1.3 Cohort A (1886–1895): overview of political involvement after 1945

Post-1945	Own study (N=16)		Overlap pre-/post-1945 (N=16)		Percentage of total number of political organisation[(x)]
	Abs.	%	Abs.	%	%
SED	3	18.8	1	6.3	**33.3**
FDGB	6	37.5	4	25.0	**66.7**
DSF	1	6.3	0	0.0	**0.0**
Bloc-parties	4	25.0	3	18.8	**75.0**
Without	6	37.5	6	37.5	**100.0**

Source: See Appendix. (x) Percentages represent the proportion of people in this postwar party or organisation who were involved in pre-1945 Nazi organisations to various degrees.

highly political – was not limited to the medical personnel, but was also true for the East German engineers, as shown by Dolores L. Augustine.[42] She identifies that their retreat into an 'apolitical' disposition was "based partly on the defence mechanisms developed by technical professionals working for the Nazis to justify themselves after the war", as well as "rooted in [their] professional ideology".[43] These two statements represent a fundamental contradiction, as, in the 1960s, the short-lived technocrats worked on behalf of the state and fulfilled its economic and political goals.[44] In general, as Fulbrook concludes, it was the notion of "a profession of ignorance held up as a profession of innocence",[45] which contemporaries created in the postwar era. It exemplifies an important strategy of self-exoneration and reassembled life-narratives, which were shattered by the memories and experiences of defeat, chaos, and uncertainty, pre- and post-1945.

However, some individuals from this cohort decided to get involved in politics again – if out of conviction, pragmatism, or both is not always clear. Carrière, for example, joined the *Christlich-Demokratische Union (Ost)* [Christian Democratic Union (East) – CDU] after 1945. As shown in Table 1.3, membership in other parties, like the CDU, *National-Demokratische Partei Deutschlands* [National Democratic Party of Germany – NDPD], or *Liberal-Demokratische Partei Deutschlands* [Liberal Democratic Party of Germany – LDPD], is higher in this sample (25 per cent) than in the SED (19 per cent). Moreover, a substantially greater percentage of other parties' members were involved in Nazi organisations (75 per cent of other party members) than those who became part of the socialist vanguard (33.3 per cent of SED members).

This finding supports the hypothesis that the so-called *Blockparteien* [bloc-parties], composed of the CDU, NDPD, and LDPD, were deliberately created by the SED. Their aim was to integrate and accommodate former NSDAP members and contemporary right-wing or conservative groups within the new socialist society.[46] However, the political self-determination and policy influence of bloc-parties was limited, and the parties' sovereignty was increasingly dismantled by the SED's overruling demands of controlling the output of social organisations.[47] Nevertheless, this study shows that the creation of these parties was a success for the GDR when considering the medical profession's overall reluctance and even refusal of political activity in general and the first cohort in particular.

Karl Linser (*1895), on the other hand, was an example of a person who, apart from his memberships in the *Sturmabteilung* [Storm Unit – SA] and the NSV, could identify his views with the new socialist party.[48] In the postwar era, in particular, Linser was the architect behind the policies of curbing widespread sexually transmitted diseases (see Chapter 2). Therefore, he is another example of the continuity of medical concepts in the form of memory and experience: Linser used his knowledge of medicine and had an accelerated career in the GDR, which favoured these 'social hygienic' views that he derived from the Weimar Republic.[49] From a hospital in Dresden, he was promoted to become a professor in Leipzig in 1946, before he left for Berlin one year later. There Linser became the next Head of the *Deutsche Zentralverwaltung für das Gesundheitswesen in der sowjetischen Besatzungszone* [German Central Administration of Healthcare in the Soviet Occupied Zone – DZVGW] – a typically stellar postwar career of selected, reputable, and SED-conforming doctors.

Paul Konitzer (*1894) preceded Linser as the Head of the DZVGW and was another representative of the World War One Generation and SED member. For Moser, Konitzer represented the impersonated continuity of Weimar traditions, which he implemented with the help of the Soviet authorities.[50] However, after a short career at the top of the East German healthcare system, the Secret Police Department of the *Министерство внутренних дел* [Soviet Interior Ministry – MVD] arrested him due to the suspected involvement in harming Russian prisoners of war [POWs]. Konitzer died shortly after his incarceration – if by suicide or execution firing squad is not entirely clear.[51] Regardless of whether or not the accusation against Konitzer was true, it is a remarkable example of fast-moving postwar life. After initial success and development, an individual life could fall apart overnight due to, in this case, medical memories of soldiers, mistreated in a POW camp, and of Konitzer himself, which caught up with him. Either these memories and the expectation of punishment burdened him to such extent that he sought a way out through suicide, or these memories informed officials to decide that he was eligible to be eliminated.

This section has exposed the continuities between the National Socialist and the East German state in the form of local doctors and health officials from the first generation (1886–1895) – and with this, the survival of medical concepts and memories that would shape the postwar healthcare system accordingly. Nevertheless, a high number of medical personnel avoided any political commitment after 1945 (see Table 1.3). All members of Cohort A, who avoided political engagement during East Germany's socialist transformation, had a National Socialist past: a feature, though, which is not limited to this generation.

Cohort B (1896–1905): the Weimar Generation

In 1965, the MfS investigated the past of Leipzig's District Doctor Johannes Schneider (*1896) when his acquaintance with Herbert Becker (*1900)[52] – an alleged member of the Planning Department at the Nazi 'euthanasia' headquarters known as *Aktion T4* – made him suspicious to the authorities. During their research, the MfS discovered that

> At an assault of the SA on a summer house settlement [. . .] [he was] asked, don't you see Dr Schneider, how they maltreat humans here, and he answered, that is no concern of mine, I am not on duty.[53]

Schneider's former NSDAP membership, his public behaviour, and the memories of the local community, registered by the MfS during their investigations, made him appear unreliable for state authorities. He did not put up "[a] flag or propaganda [. . .] on his property", and neighbours described him as "presumptuous and aloof"[54] – thus these reports represent a parallel to the denunciations of neighbours to the Gestapo during the Third Reich.[55] However, as archival sources suggest, the MfS was not eager in following up this connection to clarify Schneider's activities, for example, as a former military doctor in Warsaw.[56]

These officially repressed medical memories of an individual by the East German intelligence apparatus were due to an inter-German incident: in West Germany in 1962, the lawsuit against Werner Heyde (*1902) and others, whom state prosecutors believed to be involved in 'euthanasia' during the Third Reich, received extensive media coverage. The reason for this broad interest was not least due to the suicide of the chief suspect, Heyde, and the incarceration of a media reporter on the grounds of "political defamation": the reporter was behind bars because he revealed that FRG state authorities knew about Heyde's false identity as early as the late 1950s.[57]

Due to this legal case, the efforts of the West German investigators stretched across the border to East Germany. In their official letter rogatory, they mentioned names of doctors who might have been involved in the 'Euthanasia Programme', but were still practising in the GDR. Becker was one of them and thus supposed to appear as a witness in West Germany. Evidence and the testimony of a former colleague were readily available, confirming that he worked as a member of the Planning Department in the *Aktion T4* programme.[58] However, East German state authorities circumvented cooperation with the West by initiating investigative efforts of their own. They used the results of these exertions to convince West German prosecutors that Becker was not needed on the witness stand – a typical strategy of the MfS and the SED in the 1960s to prevent uncomfortable revelations.[59] Therefore, Schneider and Becker's smooth transitions from the Third Reich into the GDR were ordinary life stories of the second cohort (1896–1905).

A high degree of participation during the Third Reich was, according to Fulbrook, characteristic of the 'First War Youth' or 'Weimar Generation'.[60] The experiences of defeat and the loss of older relatives shaped their primary socialisation and partially resulted in their prominent involvement in the right-wing violence of the Weimar years. However, Detlef Peukert illustrates the diversity of the Weimar youth, suggesting that only a small portion of adolescents were politically organised. Consequently, the influx of the Weimar Generation into the nationalistic youth needs to be contextualised: they had significantly fewer members than the socialist youth movement – and both were rather peripheral parts of the Weimar youth. Nevertheless, as Peukert concludes, "the influence [of these two youth groups] was certainly greater than their relatively low levels of memberships implied".[61] Fulbrook follows this argument, stating that the nationalistic youth movement was "a significant and highly visible minority of the first-war youth generation", which was driven by the desire to avenge the defeat.[62] Due to this context, they were easily influenced by Hitler's propaganda and predisposed to become the foundation of Nazi organisations.[63]

However, this section qualifies these judgements of Fulbrook and Peukert as only one part of the story of the Weimar Generation. As shown in the example of Becker and Schneider, their transition between the political systems was exceptional (see Tables 1.4 and 1.5). Many from the 34 people in this second generation of the sample were able to pursue remarkable careers in both the Third Reich, in their late 20s and early 30s, as well as the GDR, when they were in their 40s.

Table 1.4 Cohort B (1896–1905): overview of political involvement before 1945 in comparison to studies of Ernst and Kater

Pre-1945	Own study (N=34)		Ernst (N=56)		Kater (average from medical licensure period 1919–1932)[(y)]
	Abs.	%	Abs.	%	%
NSDAP	27	79.4	31	55.4	50.8
NSÄB	9	26.5	9[(x)]	16.7	46.2
SA	12	35.3	13	23.2	28.4
SS	3	8.8	1	1.8	7.4
Without	7	20.6	8	14.3	/

Source: See Appendix; Ernst, *'Die beste Prophylaxe ist der Sozialismus'*, p. 151, Table 13; Kater, *Doctors under Hitler*, p. 245, Table 2.4. (x) This number represents people who were only involved in NSÄB or similar Nazi organisations, without an NSDAP, SS, or SA membership. Therefore, this number is low compared to the actual involvement in the NSÄB. (y) Kater uses in his study the medical licensure period to separate his cohorts. For example, for Cohort B, when calculated from birthdate, the medical licensure period was around 1922 to 1932. Therefore, the two studies are comparable only to a certain extent. However, Kater's analysis is important to contextualise and confirm the trends identified here.

Table 1.5 Cohort B (1896–1905): overview of political involvement after 1945

Post-1945	Own study (N=34)		Overlap pre-/ post-1945 (N=34)		Percentage of total number of political organisation[(x)]
	Abs.	%	Abs.	%	%
SED	8	23.5	5	14.7	**62.5**
FDGB	15	44.1	12	35.3	**80.0**
DSF	8	23.5	6	17.6	**75.0**
Bloc-parties	6	17.6	6	17.6	**100.0**
Without	13	38.2	10	29.4	**76.9**

Source: See Appendix. (x) Percentages represent the proportion of people in this postwar party or organisation who were involved in pre-1945 Nazi organisations to various degrees.

Their age is significant here, as it can explain this transition: they were young careerists who often experienced unemployment during the Weimar Republic due to the economic crisis. The Third Reich, however, provided them with an upward mobility, which this cohort sought, due to the exploitation and segregation of minority groups.[64] In the postwar era, it was this group, composed of middle-aged, experienced, and skilled professionals, on which the Soviet and GDR authorities had to rely to curb epidemic diseases. Therefore, it was their skills in the form of medical memories and experiences which protected most of them from legal scrutiny, from de-Nazification procedures, and thus from bigger life or career breaks after 1945.

Johannes Kuniß (*1904) illustrates the ramifications of this finding and thereby represents another notable example of this highly unique, but diverse second generation. After his incarceration in the immediate postwar period, Kuniß regained high positions in the mental hospital in Waldheim from 1950 onwards. He had become an FDGB and DSF member before he joined the SED in 1960. However, Kuniß not only was greatly involved in the Third Reich politically – with memberships in the NSDAP, SA, NSÄB, and NSV – but he also worked in numerous mental institutions in high positions, which suggests his knowledge about, or even participation in, the 'Euthanasia Programme'.[65]

Furthermore, Kuniß was a psychiatric expert and medical consultant in public office in Leipzig.[66] In 1964, this former employment led to an incident which gives some insight into the internal procedures and the negotiation strategies in the GDR regarding reputable doctors and their questionable past. In his position as a psychiatric expert in Leipzig, Kuniß was supposedly responsible for committals to mental asylums, like Zschadraß, which often had political rather than medical reasons. With 47 petitions and inquiries[67] to different GDR and foreign state, media, and societal bodies, Anne Müller and her brother Bernd Müller[68] tried to initiate a prosecution of Kuniß. They accused him of being an SS doctor who carried out political crimes.[69] Anne Müller, claiming to be a convinced communist, suggested that Kuniß committed her to Zschadraß for political reasons after she had been publicly denounced. According to Müller, she was mistreated and doomed to be killed in this institution, a fate which was averted only by the intervention of her former husband, a dentist.[70]

The GDR authorities, however, reacted differently than expected from an 'anti-Fascist' state. Anne and Bernd Müller became a nuisance to the SED due to their wide-ranging activity and campaign to raise awareness of their cause inside and outside of East Germany. The state prosecution office decided to issue a warrant and put them under arrest.[71] Thereafter, they forcefully evicted Anne Müller from her apartment.[72]

As archival sources reveal, Anne and Bernd Müller had already come to the state's attention in the 1950s, which led to their expulsion from the socialist party.[73] These preconditions appeared to be one of the main reasons why the MfS directed its investigational efforts towards them instead of Kuniß. The result was that a witness report about Anne Müller's condition after her release from Zschadraß – stating that she had "bruised places spread over her body and a wound on her head, which was caused by tearing off a tuft of hair" – was apparently disregarded.[74] The state security service was more concerned about the impact of Anne Müller's arrest on the mood and rumours in the neighbourhood.[75]

In the end in 1965, Anne Müller faced institutionalisation due to a certificate that described her as having a "psychopathic personality", and her brother met "criminal proceedings for slandering the state or for the defamation and insult" of Kuniß.[76] At this moment, however, Bernd Müller turned against his sister and claimed that her "delusional ideas" blinded him.[77] Subsequently, the state dropped the accusations against Bernd, whereas Anne Müller did not face prosecution, but remained in a mental asylum.[78]

What Anne and Bernd Müller could not know is that Kuniß was a contracted psychiatric assessor of prisoners for the state security service. Regardless of whether or not the accusations against Kuniß were true, it was this connection to the MfS, combined with the GDR's hesitations to investigate their reputable doctors in the 1960s, which evidently protected Kuniß from any further consequences. Moreover, he must have been aware of his bargaining power in these negotiations because Kuniß refused any further work for the MfS if state authorities were unable to quash the accusations – they, in turn, did everything to calm him down and assure him of their protection.[79]

This case illustrates how medical memories and experiences of a doctor and the state worked hand in hand: the state was interested in concealing the past of a reputable doctor to its benefit, while the physician used his medical experiences and political integration to secure his position within the state. By contrast, the state classified the medical memories and experiences of the individual, here in the form of Anne Müller, as a nuisance and disregarded them accordingly; they even used them against her.[80] Kuniß's example – even if this circumstance can be described as extraordinary – represents one possible coping and negotiation strategy, which involved the cooperation with, and the protection from, the state, which did not stand alone, as similar cases in this chapter illustrate.

Nonetheless, the medical profession as an often enclosed mnemonic community not only enjoyed the protection of the GDR, but also faced prosecution. The medical memories of, and the negotiation between, the individual and the state led to a different political outcome if the authorities saw their chance to prosecute medical crimes and former Nazis. As Leide concludes for Otto Hebold's (*1896) case – an *Aktion T4* advisor – if the state decided that a doctor was dispensable, and if the potential negative internal and international impact of a trial was expected to be minimal, proceedings were possible.[81] The SED arrived at the same conclusion regarding Kurt Heißmeyer (*1905), who was involved in medical experiments during the Second World War. He represents another exceptional case of this cohort because he was able to practice undisturbed as a private doctor of pneumonic diseases for almost 20 years. However, in 1963, Heißmeyer faced prosecution and received a life sentence in 1966.[82]

Leide concludes that the SED and MfS employed the following calculation: the state would prosecute only cases in which a life sentence or capital punishment was the certain outcome. Moreover, it was important that the defendant could be portrayed as a "regrettable individual offender who skilfully understood how to disguise himself in the GDR society" during the procedures.[83] In Heißmeyer's case, another important fact seems to be decisive: he was neither in a high position nor politically involved and epitomised an ideologically undesirable private practitioner.[84]

Apart from this political calculation, this study adds medical memories and experiences to the precondition for any trials against doctors. The cases of Kuniß and Heißmeyer illustrate that their individual value to the state was determined by the political and social context of their 'medical experiences'. Dissimilar 'medical memories' of both – where one carried out medical experiments in a concentration camp, and the other was supposedly involved in 'euthanasia' and committed people to mental asylums for political reasons – resulted in contradictory decisions by the state. Therefore, this book refrains from generalising the postwar adaptation strategies of former Nazi members, as the framework of medical memories and experiences uncovers highly diverse life paths of individuals and reactions of the state or mnemonic community.

Apart from these singular cases, the political activity of the Weimar Generation (1896–1905) from this database within the socialist and the bloc-parties was, as for Cohort A, around 40 per cent in the postwar era. This relatively limited engagement in social and political affairs is in strong contrast to their far-reaching involvement in the NSDAP (around 80 per cent). This finding is in line with Fulbrook's analysis of the '1900er', who, according to her, would staff the Nazi organisations and thus carry the National Socialist movement disproportionately in contrast to other generations.[85] However, the 'First War Youth Generation', as Fulbrook calls this cohort, had a higher percentage of members in the SED (around 23 per cent) than in the bloc-parties (around 18 per cent), whereas individuals born between 1886 and 1895 preferred parties outside of the socialist camp (SED: around 19 per cent; bloc-parties: around 25 per cent).

Overall, and in contrast to the World War One Generation (1886–1895), the 34 people in the sample for Cohort B (1896–1905) had a very high transposition from the National Socialist into the GDR political and societal organisations, identified in all the preceding cases. Apart from another heavy drain of Nazi members into bloc-parties, as all of their members in the sample had a National Socialist past, the FDGB also shows with 80 per cent of people having former memberships in Nazi organisations, a very high political overlap (see Table 1.5). Already in a discussion at the state level in 1946, health officials debated if former NSDAP members should be excluded from the FDGB. However, they concluded that "they [doctors with a Nazi past] are too many. The trade union would not be able to work if 70 per cent of the doctors had to stay out".[86]

The main reason for these high numbers was that many doctors joined the trade union, as the SMAD quickly dissolved traditional chambers and medical associations in the postwar era. Subsequently, the medical profession was left without any representative body outside of the FDGB.[87] This transformation was another conscious decision by East German and Soviet authorities, which was informed by the aim of an egalitarian society, which included diminishing the high status of doctors in society. However, this political step was also rooted in medical memories, as officials suspected that the medical institutions and associations were involved in, or at least aware of, medical crimes carried out under the Nazi regime.

Cohort C (1906–1915): the Generation of Depression and Upheaval

At some point in her life, Elfriede Ochsenfahrt (*1914) decided to change her last name slightly from 'Ochsenfahrt' to 'Ochsenfarth'. It was a subtle change, which, as archival sources and recent media coverage suggest, had a profound origin – resting in her medical memories.[88] Ochsenfarth had a steady career path in the GDR: she became an SED member, and after the sudden death of Dresden's District Doctor in 1960, she was promoted to this high position. One year later, Dresden's District Board also elected her as a new member: the peak of her career.[89]

However, archival research into the MfS files of the aforementioned doctors Becker and Schneider, who supposedly were involved in the 'Euthanasia Programme' during the Third Reich, revealed a rare find: a handwritten report which questioned Ochsenfarth about her past. In this document, the MfS made her aware that they received the information that she worked in a mental asylum in the Third Reich and served as a witness in the Dresden Doctors' Trial in 1947. Obviously knowing that she could not refute this fact, Ochsenfarth admitted that she worked in Großschweidnitz – an asylum in which children and adults were euthanised and from which mentally handicapped people had been transported to Pirna-Sonnenstein, where they faced certain death. Ochsenfarth, however, immediately claimed that "[h]er former superior had always asserted that female doctors were not involved in euthanasia affairs" and thus knowledge of the crimes had reached her only via rumours, spread among the population.[90] This statement is contradictory and appears to be a typical reassembled life-narrative of a doctor, burdened by his or her past and medical memories.

During the Dresden Doctors' Trial, at which the prosecutor invited Ochsenfarth only to the witness stand, she faced heavy accusations from her former colleagues: a former wardress claimed that Ochsenfarth actively practised 'child euthanasia' in Großschweidnitz.[91] Despite this fact and that her name 'Ochsenfahrt' appears in many patient files of euthanised children as well as adults, Ochsenfarth apparently did not endure further investigation and was able to have a remarkable career.[92] The exposure in 1964 could not harm her anymore: at this point in her life, she had already completed rewriting her life-narrative and altered medical memories of the past to serve personal ends. Additionally, as mentioned earlier, the GDR consciously avoided any further National Socialist related trials, especially of reputable doctors like Ochsenfarth.[93]

Unfortunately, archival sources about the life of Ochsenfarth are almost non-existent, which is another possible indication that this case is of questionable character – and that the state made a conscious decision to sanitise a career path by apparently destroying evidence. By contrast, her friends said that she avoided any public gathering, despite her high positions. She supposedly led a reclusive life, where her memories tortured her, as a former acquaintance of Ochsenfarth stated in a recent newspaper article about her life: "For that, what she obviously did back then, she had to suffer heavily for the rest of her life".[94] This suffering, though, was highly personal as she never faced prosecution – and the relatives of her potential victims never received any form of compensation.

Nevertheless, whether or not the accusation against her was true, the case demonstrates that medical memories are composed of an external and internal component: externally, Ochsenfarth presumably established a convincing life story by altering her past and involvement, as well as her name. The modification of the 'h' in her name from 'Ochsenfahrt' to 'Ochsenfarth' represents a typical way of creating a false impression in the public realm, in line with Goffman's suggestion of public behaviour, performance, and disguise. The alteration was deliberately minimal, though, so that friends and family could easily identify her and she could claim that her name was misspelt. However, it was sizeable enough that she could also deny being the 'Ochsenfahrt' who could potentially appear in Nazi documents found in the postwar era – one can only speculate if this decision was made independently or instructed by state organs. Internally, it was the guilt, inherent in her past, which seems to be prevalent, determining her social and public behaviour. Ochsenfarth's case represents an important insight into the complex processes of coming to terms with someone's medical memories and experiences, which led to differentiated outcomes for internal and external coping strategies.

Ochsenfarth is an ordinary member of Cohort C, born between 1906 and 1915. Due to their primary socialisation, mainly during the crisis years of the Weimar Republic, and as the likely children of the World War One Generation (1886–1895), many individuals from this cohort show similar life paths. They were still largely involved in the Third Reich (see Table 1.6) and were more or less active participants in the Second World War. However, as visible in Table 1.7, their political activity after 1945 rose remarkably, whereas, in comparison to previous cohorts, NSDAP membership among the 64 people in this study's sample plummeted from almost 80 to fewer than 60 per cent (see Tables 1.2, 1.4, and 1.6). The percentages of political overlap between the Third Reich and the GDR are also much lower than that of the second generation. These findings confirm Fulbrook's conclusion which describes the 'First War Youth' or Cohort B (1896–1905) as an outstanding cohort regarding their 'cultural availability for mobilisation' due to socialisation, thus forming the backbone of Hitler's Reich.[95]

Like the previous two generations, this age cohort (1906–1915) shows a high political transition in people with an NS past (over 85 per cent) into the 'bloc-parties', and a large number of individuals who were not politically active after 1945 at all (around 39 per cent). It illustrates that the medical personnel, and especially doctors, either joined a party outside of the SED which might be more accommodating towards their beliefs, or tried to abstain from any further political commitments. The latter could be due to medical memories and experiences, which they obtained during the Third Reich. As elaborated before, their 'apolitical' attitude was a façade, which they developed in the postwar years while reassembling their life-narratives, shattered due to defeat and the ethical responsibility for their profession's criminal activities during the Second World War.[96] However, this finding needs some further research, extending Weidner's study about the 'apolitical medical profession in the long-nineteenth century' into the twentieth century.[97]

Nonetheless, there were other assimilation strategies, which the already discussed case of Walter Korinek (*1914) illustrates. Despite the fact that he never finished his medical studies, he was able to pursue a steady career as an orthopaedist in various clinics in and around Dresden after 1945. Authorities who asked for

Table 1.6 Cohort C (1906–1915): overview of political involvement before 1945 in comparison to studies of Ernst and Kater

Pre-1945	Own study (N=64)		Ernst (N=79)		Kater (average from medical licensure period 1933–1945)[y]
	Abs.	%	Abs.	%	%
NSDAP	37	57.8	42	53.2	43.7
NSÄB	7	10.9	4[x]	5.1	19.7[z]
SA	15	23.4	19	24.1	29.2
SS	7	10.9	2	2.5	10.1
Without	20	31.3	27	34.2	/

Source: See Appendix; Ernst, p. 151, Table 13; Kater, *Doctors under Hitler*, p. 245, Table 2.4. (x) This number represents people who were involved in only NSÄB or similar Nazi organisations, without an NSDAP, SS, or SA membership. Therefore, this number is low compared to the actual involvement in the NSÄB. (y) Kater uses in his study the medical licensure period to separate his cohorts. For example, for Cohort C, when calculated from the birthdate, the medical licensure period was around 1932 to 1942. Therefore, the two studies are comparable only to a certain extent. However, Kater's analysis is important to contextualise and confirm the trends identified here. (z) In the period 1939 to 1945, Kater provides for the NSÄB a proportion of membership as low as 7.4 per cent. According to Ralf Forsbach, the reason for this development was that the influence and significance of the NSÄB declined during the Second World War due to the increasing importance of the Association of Statutory Health Insurance Physicians of Germany [*Kassenärztliche Vereinigung Deutschlands*]. Rolf Forsbach, '"Pfleger der Gene" und "biologischer Soldat": Der Nationalsozialistische Deutsche Ärztebund (NSDÄB)', in *'Und sie werden nicht mehr frei sein ihr ganzes Leben': Funktion und Stellenwert der NSDAP, ihrer Gliederungen und angeschlossenen Verbände im 'Dritten Reich'*, ed. by Stephanie Becker and Christoph Studt (Berlin: LIT, 2012), pp. 223–36 (p. 235).

Table 1.7 Cohort C (1906–1915): overview of political involvement after 1945

Post-1945	Own study (N=64)		Overlap pre-/ post-1945 (N=64)		Percentage of total number of political organisation[x]
	Abs.	%	Abs.	%	%
SED	22	34.4	12	18.8	**54.5**
FDGB	26	40.6	14	21.9	**53.8**
DSF	6	9.4	1	1.6	**16.7**
Bloc-parties	7	10.9	6	9.4	**85.7**
Without	25	39.1	19	29.7	**76.0**

Source: See Appendix. (x) Percentages represent the proportion of people in this postwar party or organisation who were involved in pre-1945 Nazi organisations to various degrees.

his documents, such as his approbation and certificate of specialisation, received the following answer:

[I] ask you to be patient regarding the missing copies of my approbation and the recognition as specialist [*Facharztanerkennung*] for a few days. Since

I simultaneously applied for the permission to establish a private clinic as orthopaedist [. . .] both original documents are still with my application with the Lord Mayor of Bautzen, Health Administration. As soon as they have been given back, I will send you the missing documents.[98]

This apology is only one example of many, showing how Korinek circumvented the possible exposure of his fraud and how authorities often failed to follow up the issue.[99]

However, he increasingly came under the state's scrutiny during the 1950s – though for different reasons. Firstly, the SED excluded him from its ranks due to debts to the party. Secondly, he also was known to have an alcohol problem, was involved in fights, insulted police officers, and quit jobs overnight when his demands were not met – for example, to be put in a higher salary group.[100] All this made him a nuisance to the authorities, and thus he earned enemies among the city council, who tried to dismiss him in the mid-1950s. However, the chief doctor at the orthopaedic clinic continued to protect Korinek due to his apparent skills and the lack of specialists.[101]

Nevertheless, the situation changed quickly in the late 1950s. Korinek's connection to Ceccetti alias Czeck, who were both involved in illegal trade and narcotics imports from West Berlin, brought him to the attention of the MfS.[102] Moreover, after almost 15 years of his deception, Korinek felt the need to reveal his fraud to the district doctor, in the hope that he would receive the chance to repeat his exams and finally obtain his approbation.[103] All these facts – document forgery, deception, and illegal trade – as well as illegal abortions, performed on several women, led to his arrest during Christmas 1959, described at the beginning of this book.[104] However, after his trial and five months in prison, Korinek was released and able to continue his medical practice as the head of an orthopaedic clinic with only one restriction: he received the salary of a nurse until he provided his approbation.[105] During the following years, though, he was under continuous attack by fellow doctors, city authorities, and state officials. Korinek went through several disciplinary procedures, as he still used *Dr. med.* in his official letters – a fraud punishable by law.[106]

By contrast, Korinek persistently demanded to receive recognition and the opportunity to repeat his exams, which officials supposedly promised to him. In this context, he always referred to his experience with the MfS in a positive light:

I am still thankful for the fate that [the arrest by the MfS during Christmas 1959] happened because in this institution, which is often feared in an unjustifiable way, I found people and personnel, who followed up everything in the greatest detail and also intensively engaged with my medical matter [meaning, his missing approbation, the illegal abortions, and his medical skills].[107]

The sentiment in his writings exposes the intention to utilise the MfS against other authorities in order to fulfil his personal interests. Francesca Weil identified this motive as one of the main reasons to cooperate with the MfS from her sample of 493 IM doctors. Physicians developed this contact with the hope of increasing the standard of their working conditions, as well as enhancing their careers. Augustine has recognised a similar strategy for East German engineers and showed that "paradoxically, it was the Stasi informants themselves who at times addressed the big, thorny issues".[108] Consequently, as Weil concluded her study, "a large part of the IM doctors succumbed to the belief that they had forwarded their criticism to an influential and extensively influence-exerting institution".[109] However, the MfS was in no position to achieve any actual change on the policy level – either state or local – which disenchanted many of their IM in the 1960s and beyond.[110]

In Korinek's case, a similar outcome is recognisable. The Head of the MfS District Branch Dresden, Rolf Markert, who himself changed his name and birthdate in the 1940s,[111] refused to get involved again, and city authorities apparently were able to reach a conclusion in 1964: they removed him from any medical position and made his case public.[112] The last documents in Korinek's file in the Federal Archive are letters to the GDR *Handelsorganisation* [Trading Organisation – HO] Restaurant and Hotel Branches in Dresden in 1967. This correspondence shows that state officials tried to find a placement for him as a receptionist or waiter because he started an apprenticeship in a hotel in the 1930s – however, the branch refused his appointment, as Korinek never obtained a qualification for these jobs.[113] This correspondence represented the end of a remarkable postwar career, which lasted with minor curtailments for over 20 years. After being the head of an orthopaedic clinic, now he was not even eligible to obtain a job as a waiter.

In conclusion, Korinek, as an exceptional case in many ways, was able to use his medical memories and experiences, which he obtained during the 1930s and the Second World War, to establish a life-narrative, and abuse the postwar conditions to enhance both his opportunities and salary. However, the latter seemed not enough to him: Korinek got increasingly involved in illegal trade, narcotics smuggling, and illegal abortions for fees.[114] This extraordinary culmination of various criminal and ethical transgressions resulted in state and especially city officials increasingly judging him as dispensable, despite his medical experience and skills. However, medical predicaments of the postwar era, the protection of influential people, the difficulties of obtaining information about doctors, and the lack of medical specialists prolonged this process for over two decades. Therefore, this case also confirms the finding that state authorities were often unable to investigate an individual's past and medical memories in detail until the late 1950s and 1960s. This fact ultimately allowed incriminated former Nazi party members, but also fraudulent doctors, to slip through the net of East Germany's de-Nazification and licensure systems.

Cohort D (1916–1925): the National Socialist Generation

The ancient Charité in Berlin was the most prestigious hospital in the GDR. Hence, it was in the SED's interest to improve the working conditions in this institution continuously, concentrating the available material and financial resources on this prestige project to the detriment of other East German hospitals.[115] The prominence but also the adjacency of this institution to the West Berlin border made it a *Schwerpunkt* [focal point] for the MfS. This situation created the need for IM to safeguard the Charité from 'internal and external enemies'. From this background – as well as the Cold War context and the continuous stream of doctors from the East to the West – the MfS suggested in May 1960 to recruit the Professor of Internal Medicine Johannes Garten (*1920), who was a senior physician at the Medical Clinic II of the Charité.[116]

In their investigation, the MfS officers quickly realised that Garten hid his involvement in the *Deutsches Jungvolk* [German Youth Folk – DJV], which later became part of the HJ, and the NSDAP in his personal records after 1945. However, this disguise had no consequences for him. State authorities were more concerned about his wife, who shortly after the public upheaval of 17 June 1953, which was a political disaster for East Germany, obtained *Westpakete* [parcels from the West], claiming that her four children were 'undernourished'. The GDR customs officials, who caught her, wanted to make this case public. However, the SED, the MfS, and the chief director at Garten's clinic prevented the revelation due to the fear that Garten could leave for the West. Garten and his wife only received criticism in an internal procedure, as both were doctors with high salaries.[117]

This case illustrates how authorities were caught between their ideological claims and the everyday reality. 17 June 1953 was a crucial test of the stability of the young GDR. The East German state, however, would have failed this challenge if the Soviet Union had not nipped the protest in the bud with their tanks – and if the West had not hesitated to intervene due to the danger of war.[118] After the events of 1953, the oppression of any 'oppositional' and 'deviant' behaviour increased. Doctors, however, received growing concessions from the state as a result of the lack of personnel among their profession.[119] This predicament caused the SED's overall ambiguous enforcement of policies, swaying between granting concessions to doctors and implementing strict socialist principles, during the 1950s: an inconsistency that led to an increase of distrust and denial among the medical profession, rather than to the 'political-ideological' stabilisation of their attitudes towards the socialist project.[120]

Despite this incident and Garten's general reluctance to join any political organisation, or to make his political consciousness visible after 1945, the medical memories, in the form of his medical skills and Nazi past, as well as his high position within the mnemonic community of the Charité made him a potentially valuable IM for the MfS. Weil shows in her study of IM doctors that physicians with a known criminal past were of especially high value for the East German secret police. Their appreciation was derived from the fact that the state security service was able to blackmail affected doctors to work for them. Nevertheless, the main reason for the preferred deployment of incriminated physicians as IM was because colleagues viewed them as disloyal to the GDR. They were more open to express their real opinions in the presence of an apparently 'subversive' doctor in which the MfS were particularly interested.[121]

In Garten's case, their calculation of his 'usefulness' was that his long medical experience and the established network within this institution could safeguard future events – such as political assemblies – at this hospital. Furthermore, he could potentially be used to prevent 'illegal *Republikfluchten* [flights from the Republic]', as in 1959 alone, 13 doctors left for the West from this clinic.[122] To achieve a reliable cooperation, the MfS decided on a slow and careful procedure, the so-called "gradual recruitment on the basis of conviction".[123] Subsequently, they initiated the first meeting via Garten's supervisor. During this encounter, they elicited his opinions regarding physicians' escape to West Germany and other topics, about which Garten spoke openly after an initial hesitation towards the MfS officer. In the end, the MfS's strategy was successful as Garten agreed to meet the intelligence officer again.[124]

In this and the following 'meeting report', Garten showed signs of the belief that he could influence policies and procedures in the Charité for the better by cooperating with the MfS.[125] However, Garten seemed to be reluctant to share any details about colleagues – he always referred to his lack of knowledge in this regard, that he was not interested, or did not believe in the rumours spread about potential flight plans of doctors.[126] This fact shows that doctors – if not blackmailed – had some agency and leeway when cooperating with the MfS regarding the information they would share with their contact officers about patients and colleagues. Some doctors like Manfred Oertel (*1940), director of the psychiatric hospital in Großschweidnitz since 1980, were more than happy to pass on even whole patient files to the state security service of the GDR, which represents more than just a breach of their medical confidentiality.[127] No IM, whether an eager or reluctant informant, could estimate what the MfS would do with the information received and how this would affect the people denounced. Therefore, these two cases show that collaboration with the MfS has to be evaluated individually, without a judgement *a priori*.[128]

Nevertheless, Garten apparently agreed to the MfS officer's statement that "any unlawful departure from the GDR, regardless of whether or not one likes it, represents objectively a commitment to the West Zone State and its war policy".[129] This statement appears like a typically ideological SED claim. It could be seen as a defence strategy by Garten to keep his 'apolitical' disposition and simultaneously sustain cooperation with the MfS.

The state security service found in him a person who provided them with information, based on his medical memories and experiences, derived from his position within a mnemonic community of doctors, and thus he was of high significance. Garten's past and the concealment of his involvement in the Third Reich were never a topic in the meetings, negotiations, or for his evaluation.[130] Moreover, his 'gatekeeper' position and the consequent leverage must have been palpable for Garten as well: in the end, he used the protection and disguise of his willing cooperation with the MfS to leave the GDR for the West at the beginning of August 1961.[131] This case represents another story of an unsuccessful attempt by the SED and the MfS to penetrate the 'stubborn bourgeois' parts of the medical profession.

In general, the fourth generation (1915–1925) in this sample shows some similarities to Fulbrook's '1929ers', as well as common characteristics regarding their responses towards memories, experiences, and the primary socialisation which they went through. This generation was integrated into the youth organisations of the Third Reich, and some even joined the NSDAP (see Table 1.8). If possible, future doctors carried out their medical studies and received their approbation during the war years, after which almost all men were actively involved in the battles of the Second World War. Kater's study shows that especially the younger generations, who completed their studies between 1942 and 1945, joined the NSDAP – a fact that also reveals the privileged status of young physicians, whereas entry into the party for other social groups or older medical professionals was limited through restrictive party admission policies.[132] However, this is only partly true for all 14 people in this cohort of the sample. In particular younger members show life paths analogous to the '1929ers'. They had to join either the HJ or *Bund Deutscher Mädel* [German Girls' League – BDM], their members experienced a total war on the battlefield or the home front, and all of them faced the collapse of an ideology, which shaped their whole belief system from early childhood.

As in the case of my grandfather (*1925), many of the late-born individuals of this cohort were at the forefront of the new political systems in the East and West, which respectively promised a better future and a supposed clear break with the Nazi past. Fulbrook identifies that individuals born around 1929 would "try to change the world" and reject any legacies and projects of the preceding generations.[133] This predisposition quickly made them the main target for Soviet and East German authorities and 'culturally available for mobilisation' into the new socialist state and its (mass-)organisations.[134] Despite all fallacies in the data

Table 1.8 Cohort D (1916–1925): overview of political involvement before 1945 in comparison to studies of Ernst and Kater

Pre-1945	Own study (N=14)		Ernst (N=31)		Kater (average from medical licensure period 1939–1945)[(y)]
	Abs.	%	Abs.	%	%
NSDAP	5	35.7	7	22.6	44.1
NSÄB	0	0	2[(x)]	6.5	7.4
SA	0	0	0	0	21.8
SS	1	7.1	0	0	11.0
Without	8	57.1	21	67.7	/

Source: See Appendix; Ernst, *'Die beste Prophylaxe ist der Sozialismus'*, p. 151, Table 13; Kater, *Doctors under Hitler*, p. 245, Table 2.4. (x) This number represents people who were involved only in NSÄB or similar Nazi organisations, without an NSDAP, SS, or SA membership. Therefore, this number is low compared to the actual involvement in the NSÄB. (y) Kater uses in his study the medical licensure period to separate his cohorts. For example, for Cohort D, when calculated from the birthdate, the medical licensure period was around 1942 to 1952. Therefore, the two studies are comparable only to a certain extent. However, Kater's analysis is important to contextualise and confirm the trends identified here.

and the small number of the sample, this fact is proven by the high percentage of memberships across political and societal organisations of this generation (1916–1925) in the postwar era, as shown in Table 1.9 (over 85 per cent). Therefore, the 'National Socialist Generation' is the first in which political involvement was higher post-1945 than pre-1945 (around 42 per cent) – a novel feature compared to the previous three generations. The percentage of the last age cohort of the study that was not engaged in any political organisation after 1945, with 14.3 per cent, was almost as low as it was for the First World War cohort (1886–1895) before 1945, with 12.5 per cent. Ernst's study confirms this finding by providing that 67.7 per cent of people born between 1916 and 1925 had no political affiliation before 1945.[135]

Despite the diversity between older and younger members of this generational cohort, it can be assessed from the statistics that, compared to previous generations, they were the first generation that was overrepresented in the new organisations of the GDR. Moreover, members of this last cohort were likely to be the children of the Weimar Generation, born between 1896 and 1905; the latter, in contrast, was highly involved in Hitler's regime. This fact provides evidence to the finding that Cohort D (1916–1925) felt the need to distance itself from its parental generation, a conclusion that Fulbrook draws for her 1929ers as well.[136]

Support to this hypothesis is given by the fact that two prominent figures of the East German healthcare system were among this group: Hans-Jürgen Matthies (*1925) and Ludwig Mecklinger (*1919). Both reached high positions and had remarkable careers. After serving in the *Nationale Volksarmee* [National People's Army – NVA] as a professor of military medicine, Mecklinger became the Associate Minister in 1964 and then the Minister of Healthcare in 1971 – the first minister with a medical background in this position.[137] Before 1945, he was hardly involved in the Third Reich, but like many other doctors of his age finished his medical studies during the war and afterwards practised as an *Unterarzt* [a lower rank medic] in the *Wehrmacht* – thus Mecklinger was a typical representative of the older members of this cohort.[138]

Table 1.9 Cohort D (1916–1925): overview of political involvement after 1945

Post-1945	Own study (N=14)		Overlap pre / post-1945 (N=14)		Percentage of total number of political organisation[(x)]
	Abs.	%	Abs.	%	%
SED	4	28.6	1	7.1	25.0
FDGB	5	35.7	0	0	0
DSF	2	14.3	0	0	0
Bloc-parties	3	21.4	3	21.4	100.0
Without	2	14.3	2	14.3	100.0

Source: See Appendix. (x) Percentages represent the proportion of people in this postwar party or organisation who were involved in pre-1945 Nazi organisations to various degrees.

Matthies, by contrast, was six years younger, which resulted in a huge differ-ence in his life path. He was not only in the HJ, as it was compulsory for his age group, but also joined the NSDAP in 1943 and served in the Second World War.[139] For this reason and due to his age, Matthies was not able to start his medical stud-ies before the end of the war – he received his approbation in 1953.[140] Despite his greater involvement in the Third Reich, Matthies also had a steady career in the GDR. After he had joined the SED in the postwar years, he became a leading neuroscientist and pharmacologist, with seats in the *Ärztekommission beim Polit-büro des Zentralkomitees der SED* [Doctors' Commission at the Politburo of the SED Central Committee] and in the SED *Bezirksleitung* [Regional Directorate] in Magdeburg.[141] Both Mecklinger and Matthies show that the experiences and memories of total war, defeat, and the complete disregard of an ideology could have a very different outcome in comparison to the other cohorts analysed in this study. In their cases, the postwar era offered them a new project, a new future to work towards, which was also determined by their medical memories.

Nevertheless, a stellar career was not limited to socialist party members. In general, many of the people in this cohort occupied high positions within the healthcare system, despite being members of one of the bloc-parties or not being politically involved in the state at all. Reinhard Schwarzlose (*1918) and Char-lotte Bergmann (*1920) represent striking examples for this statement. Both were members of the NSDAP and youth organisations in the Third Reich – and both received their approbation during the Second World War.[142] After 1945, Schwar-zlose was involved in the State Brandenburg's Head Healthcare Department and joined the NDPD.[143] Later he served as Lieutenant-Colonel and Chief of the Medical Service at the *Kommando Luftstreitkräfte/Luftverteidigung* [Air Force Staff and Command as well as Air Defence – Kdo LSK/LV] of the NVA. He also was a member of the NDPD's Central Committee, a member of the Frankfurt/Oder's District Board, and a *Nachfolgekandidat* [succession candidate] for the GDR *Volkskammer* [People's Chamber].[144] Schwarzlose was one of the first to receive the prestigious award *Verdienter Arzt des Volkes* [honour given to doctors for special merits for the people] in 1949, which shows the fast progress in his career after 1945.[145]

Bergmann had a similar life path. After her participation in the BDM and NSDAP, she joined the LDPD in the postwar years. Her medical specialisa-tion was social hygiene, and with this expertise, Bergmann became a council-woman, as well as the Head of the Healthcare Department at Leipzig's District Board. Later she was a member of the LDPD's Central Committee and, like Schwarzlose, had a seat in the People's Chamber.[146] Both were outstanding cases in their development after 1945. Nevertheless, they confirm the general trend exposed in this study, as well as by Fulbrook, that this generation was the driving force of the new East German state.[147] For all cases, negotiations with the state over their present and future careers were in favour of these young generations of doctors, like the '1929ers'. Therefore, the state often exoner-ated their Nazi involvement in order to use their energy and enthusiasm for the new society – a fact that is further analysed in Chapter 3 for the 'war youth'. In conclusion, their medical memories and experiences, obtained during the war and particularly in the chaos and epidemics of the postwar era, would shape the new socialist healthcare system accordingly, which is shown in Chapter 2 for venereal diseases.

Conclusion

In 1964, one year after Hannah Arendt's report on the Eichmann Trial was published,[148] the American playwright and socio-critical essayist Arthur Miller observed the first Auschwitz Trial in West Germany as a journalist for the *New York Times* – a court case against 22 former SS members in Frankfurt/Main.[149] In his subsequent essay, he pointed towards the abstractness of the murders brought in front of this tribunal:

> Once the jackbooted masters of a barbed-wire world, they are now middle-aged Germans in business suits. [. . .] [They] could pass for anybody's German uncle. [. . .] Some [. . .] turned into successful business men, professionals and ordinary workers. They [. . .] reared families and even became civic leaders in their communities.[150]

For him this fact appeared as unreal: how could these people carry on with 'normal' lives after Auschwitz?

In this chapter, this question within the framework of medical memories and experiences was the main drive for investigating the negotiation between state authorities and the individual doctor about the past, present, and future. Many of the medical personnel from the sample used showed a high potential for assimilation to changes in political systems and ideology. They often pursued this endeavour due to personal interests, to sustain professional growth, or simply to survive the uncertainty and chaos of the postwar period.

In his essay, Miller offered two insightful examples for this process. The first was Oswald Kaduk, who became known as a very sadistic SS man: he shot inmates arbitrarily when drunk.[151] In the late 1950s, however, Kaduk was a respected nurse, and his patients called him fondly *Papa Kaduk* – they wrote a letter to the court in which they defended him. As Miller observed, Kaduk himself seemed "to be quite convinced that he is indeed Papa Kaduk and not at all the monster being painfully described from the witness chair".[152] The same was valid for Victor Capesius, who, as the camp pharmacist, was in charge of putting the right amount of *Zyklon-B* into the gas chambers.[153] After the war, he was able to obtain high positions in his local community and went on hunting expeditions to Africa. After the German police had arrested Capesius, the local gentry was surprised: "[h]ow, it was actually asked, could a gentleman of such sensibility have done such awful things?"[154]

Consciously or unconsciously, Miller identified the ability of those formerly involved in the Nazi Reich, incriminated or not, to establish a new, convincing life-narrative – and to cover their past with a coat of silence and forgetting. As shown in many of the preceding case studies, the selection of medical memories and experiences led to rewritten life paths that served their respective ends. They silenced their past, established a cover story, and enhanced their career prospects – not least through the subtle balance of inventing and omitting certain facts.[155]

Connected with this finding, the overarching purpose of these altered memories was self-protection – they helped to preserve the desired impression, behaviour, and life-narrative in the public realm, as defined by Goffman's theories. However, the question is that, even if they were able to establish a masquerade, like in the case of the fraud doctor Korinek, why did the state and the judicial bodies react so late or, as in many instances in this study, not at all?

Miller claimed that in West Germany police and the state were very reluctant to support the arrests of former Nazis and the prosecution efforts of the Frankfurt trials.[156] This study suggests that this was not solely a West German phenomenon, but similarly applicable to East Germany. The reason for this reluctance is derived from the social and political context of the Cold War era, in which both sides feared an international loss of reputation. In the GDR during the 1950s, the continuous 'brain drain', especially of doctors to the West, caused a scarcity of medical personnel that led to far-reaching concessions and an 'alliance policy', to the detriment of socialist ideals.[157]

Consequently, all case studies utilised in this chapter confirm Leide's thesis that "[i]n fact, the SED's integration policy towards the 'bourgeois intelligentsia' also offered Nazi incriminated [doctors], with a corresponding adaptation, a considerable protection from prosecution".[158] This development was possible only because of the predicament of the epidemic diseases and the scarcity of doctors and thus the pragmatism employed in the postwar years. One of the most important reasons for the leniency in the de-Nazification of doctors was that the healthcare system became an integral part of ideological struggles between West and East Germany.[159] Due to the epidemics of the postwar years and the continuous drain of medical personnel to the West during the 1950s, the GDR became increasingly hesitant to proceed against its doctors – especially fearing to exacerbate the shortage of medical staff.[160]

Another important context of this political dilemma is 17 June 1953 and the de-Stalinisation movements in Eastern Europe after Stalin's death in the same year, which heightened the SED's anxiety towards their people from this date onwards. This distrust led not only to an extension of the security and repression apparatus, but also to a greater sensitivity to changes in public opinion and mood. As shown, the lack of specialists and doctors could result in negative rumours, which the SED tried to avoid by averting incarcerations of former Nazis and applying a general leniency towards its medical personnel. The investigation of the medical profession as a mnemonic community in transition from pre- to post-1945, within the framework of medical memories and experiences, exposes the inherent pragmatism of all governmental decisions and policies towards this group, already identified by Ernst for doctors in particular and by Corey Ross for the population in general.[161] The direct result of these decisions and policies was that many former Nazi members within the medical profession experienced a smooth transition between the systems.

Nevertheless, the state's fear of its population had another layer. Miller observed in his trial report that, while being confronted with the testimonies of the Auschwitz Trial, "the German housewives who comprise most of the jury burst into tears or sit with open horror in their faces".[162] Here, the contradictory memories of the 'ordinary' German, the perpetrator, and camp inmates were uncovered. These testimonies did not fit into the narratives of 'German housewives', as Miller called them:

> [T]hey were shopping, putting their children to bed, going on picnics on sunny days, worrying about a daughter's wedding dress or a son's well-being in the army while mothers like themselves and children no different from their own were forced to undress, to walk into a barren hall, and breathe the gas which some of the defendants now sitting here carefully administered.[163]

This statement reveals memory repression about the events of the Third Reich and Second World War, which left its scars on any person, irrespective of their age and position. As Miller heard from the prosecutors, the opposition against this trial within the German population was as high as 90 per cent.[164] The result was not only an institutionalised resistance towards exposure, but also a widespread unwillingness to support the investigation against Nazi criminals, particularly among the local community. The notion was that the past should be laid to rest, to carry on with their lives in the present, and to have their view directed towards the future. Weinke identified this common mentality of *Ruhe* [peace and quiet] as well, which both East and West Germans applied regarding their Nazi past – the postwar silence.[165] Consequently, it was in the state's interest to uphold the 'anti-Fascist' façade as in the GDR and simultaneously serve this feeling – to give it a rest – among their people in order to legitimise the state.

However, not only the population but also – to Miller's surprise – the accused did not believe in their crimes: "none of the accused has suggested he may have done something wrong; there is no sign of remorse, and they appear to maintain a certain unity among themselves even now".[166] Similar to the medical profession, the former SS members formed a mnemonic community: a milieu in which social bonds were strong and supported their individual life-narratives with the help of their joint efforts in silencing and sanitising the past. Their defence strategy relied upon the Third Reich's hierarchical structure – analogous to Eichmann's claim that they all were only 'small cogs in a larger machine'.[167]

It was these arguments that Miller was hardly able to comprehend: "[w]hat scares some Germans, however, and makes the German to this day an enigma to many foreigners, is his capacity for moral and psychological collapse in the face of a higher command" [168] – an argument similar to Hannah Arendt's thesis about 'the banality of evil'.[169] This study shows that this mental predisposition of self-defence was especially true for the 'turncoats' within the sample: they could easily assimilate to new authorities and accordingly had stable or stellar careers due to their opportunistic behaviour and adaptation strategy.[170]

Fulbrook identifies for her generational analyses three major strategies of 'self-representation' in the postwar era.[171] Firstly, people claimed that they were just "taken in" by a charismatic leader and had "not known" about the cruelties of the regime.[172] However, as soon as they were informed, they would have been converted.[173] As Fulbrook stressed, this group had no sense of guilt in their life-narratives and excused their ignorance with innocence – a typical strategy of many doctors in this chapter. The second group claimed that they were consistent in the form that they had always been against the Third Reich and were only forced to appear as conforming to the state on the outside – another form of distancing the contemporary self from the memories. Fulbrook's last group was composed of all who consciously or unconsciously 'clung to' the National Socialist ideology in the postwar era.[174]

However, this chapter has refined Fulbrook's analysis by drawing attention to the adaptation strategies of medical personnel in the transition from the Third Reich into the East German state. It has shown that the negotiation process was highly individualised and depended on the time as well as the social and political context at the local, state, and international level. Therefore, this procedure and life decisions made by the doctor and the state often went in their complexity beyond the three general categories of 'self-representation' defined by Fulbrook. The result of the exposed continuity was that concepts and mentalities from the past continued to exist in the form of people, like doctors, who influenced the local level of society in the East and West. It is the primary purpose of this book to investigate ramifications of this transition from Nationalism to Socialism for the GDR.[175]

Therefore, Figure 1.1 illustrates the overall political involvement of the sample before 1945 on the left and after 1945 on the right. The second graph also details the transition between the political systems, showing what percentage of the members of political parties or organisations in the GDR had a Nazi or socialist past. However, analysing the data of the 128 people as a whole, as reflected in Figure 1.1, would have disguised many findings and glazed over the diverse characteristics if not split into the four generations. As Fulbrook illustrates, on the one side, this method is essential to understand different responses towards events, violence, and developments of the twentieth century among different age cohorts.[176] They also offer an insight into the creation of diverse medical memories and the effect of undergoing various medical experiences at different ages that would shape a person's future career and medical practice – and thus this chapter has developed Fulbrook's approach further.

On the other side, the state and the mnemonic community judged a person's past according to its contemporary 'usefulness'. The outcome of this assessment depended on the dynamics of Cold War struggles and potential national and international ramifications that any such revelation might have. In many ways, this framework and the findings in this chapter underline the judgement that the GDR was 'driven' by external and internal pressures – such as the 'anti-Fascist' paradigm, the flight of medical personnel, and the issue of legitimacy. The outcome was that the SED was unable to establish legitimacy proactively, was doomed to

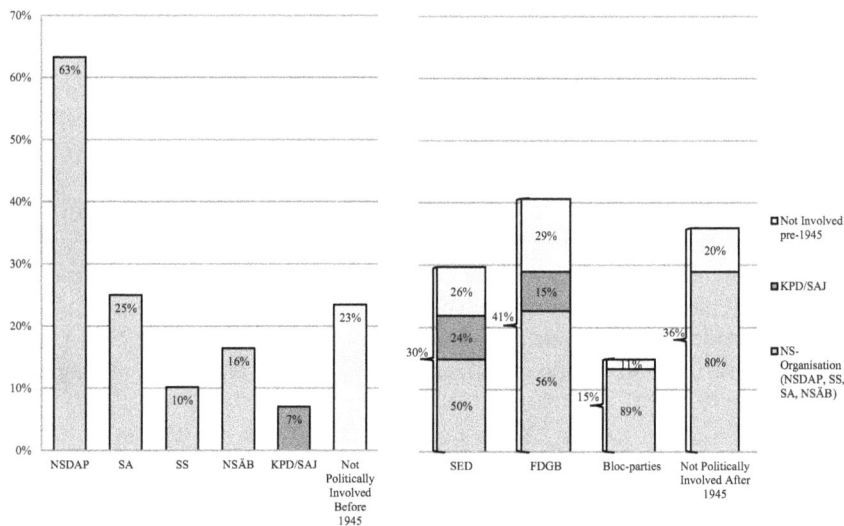

Figure 1.1 Overview of the overall political involvement of the 128 people in this study's sample before and after 1945

Source: See Appendix.

reactive measures, and partly relinquished its socialist ideals due to real predicaments at the local level of society.

Therefore, the SED's 'alliance policy' was a disguise and justified a rather pragmatic approach as well as negotiation strategies driven by current medical and political issues. It was also the result of legitimacy concerns that the SED faced, especially during the 1960s. As Weinke identifies, doctors' Nazi legacy became, in this context, a useable past, applied according to East Germany's needs.[177] However, the GDR's calculations ended in a self-made "dead end", as Leide concludes, and consequently, the medical profession was prevented from a transformation due to the political, social, and medical context of the postwar years.[178]

Subsequently, the keyword for this study must be 'continuity' in the broadest sense possible within the framework of medical memories and experiences. The sections of the chapter and Figure 1.1 reveal not only the high involvement of the sample in the Third Reich, but also their political opportunism towards the GDR. In comparison, the SED had slightly more former Nazi members (N=20) than the bloc-parties (N=18). This finding could confirm the conclusion of Leide that the SED was composed of more Nazis than the NDPD.[179] However, this study qualifies this claim and shows that the proportional overlap was much higher within the bloc-parties: almost 90 per cent of the people who were CDU, NDPD, or LDPD members were previously involved in the Third Reich. Despite the fallacies inherent in the database utilised here, this percentage proves that individuals with a right-wing disposition were more likely to join a nationalist rather than a socialist party. However, as visible in the second graph of Figure 1.1, there also were a high proportion of former Nazi members who refused to get politically involved in the GDR at all. This analysis illustrates that the SED was not able to accommodate and gain the support of everyone within the medical profession for the new cause – even so, supposedly 'apolitical' doctors were often able to negotiate unrestricted careers and reach high positions in the postwar years and beyond.

In 1969, the Associate Health Minister of the GDR Mecklinger – one of the cases explored in this study – discussed with MfS officials the procedure against doctors who had supposedly been involved in politically motivated sterilisations during the Third Reich. However, even in the late 1960s, state authorities showed great reluctance to investigate the medical profession, as this would draw public attention and could have adverse effects on the planned legalisation of abortions in the GDR.[180]

In conclusion, as late as 25 years after the Second World War, many of the ethical crimes carried out by medical personnel during the Third Reich remained unpunished, and affected doctors were able to carry on supposedly 'normal' lives. The ramifications that these findings had for the doctor-nurse-patient relationship were, as Kater identifies, fear, distrust, and suspicion on the patient's side, and are one of the main topics throughout the book.[181] For medical memories and experiences, personnel continuity meant a broad continuity of medical concepts, clichés, patterns of stigmatisation, prejudices, language, symbols, and mentalities, which become especially noticeable when looking at the medical and social treatment of sexually transmitted diseases in Chapter 2 and the medical war experiences of children in Chapter 3.

Notes

1 The name was made anonymous due to public and archival restrictions. Therefore, the fictitious name Dr Förster will be used to enhance comprehension in the following.
2 'Informationsbericht, 1. Juli 1958': BStU, MfS, BV Dresden, KD Sebnitz, 4409, Teil 1, Bl. 19.
3 'Steidle, Luitpold (CDU), 20. Juni 1960': BStU, MfS, HA XX, 5752, Bl. 158–61.
4 'Informationsbericht, 1. Juli 1958': BStU, MfS, BV Dresden, KD Sebnitz, 4409, Teil 1, Bl. 19.
5 'Bericht über die Lage im Gesundheitswesen, 29. August 1958': BStU, MfS, ZAIG, 122, Bl. 40–1; Melanie Arndt, *Gesundheitspolitik im geteilten Berlin, 1948 bis 1961* (Cologne: Böhlau, 2009), p. 183.
6 Michael H. Kater, *The Nazi Party: A Social Profile of Members and Leaders, 1919–1945* (Oxford: Basil Blackwell, 1983), p. 137.
7 Richard Bessel, *Germany 1945: From War to Peace* (London: Simon & Schuster, 2009), pp. 321–2, 330–1, 334, 343–53, 386–8; Jessica Reinisch, *The Perils of Peace: The Public Health Crisis in Occupied Germany* (Oxford: Oxford University Press, 2013), p. 1. For the demand of doctors in postwar East Germany, see Anna-Sabine Ernst, *'Die beste Prophylaxe ist der Sozialismus': Ärzte und Hochschullehrer in der SBZ/DDR 1945–1961* (Münster: Waxmann, 1996), pp. 145, 180, 185–7.
8 Annette Weinke, *Die Verfolgung von NS-Tätern im geteilten Deutschland: Vergangenheitsbewältigung 1949–1969, oder: Eine deutsch-deutsche Beziehungsgeschichte im Kalten Krieg* (Paderborn: Schöningh, 2002), p. 330.

9 Weinke, pp. 326–32; Henry Leide, *NS-Verbrecher und Staatssicherheit: Die geheime Vergangenheitspolitik der DDR* (Göttingen: Vandenhoeck & Ruprecht, 2005), pp. 332–53.
10 'Betr.: Euthanasie-Prozeß in Westdeutschland, 3. April 1963': BStU, MfS, HA XX, 4980, Bl. 158.
11 Leide, p. 12; Gabriele Moser, *'Im Interesse der Volksgesundheit. . .': Sozialhygiene und öffentliches Gesundheitswesen in der Weimarer Republik und der frühen SBZ/DDR: Ein Beitrag zur Sozialgeschichte des deutschen Gesundheitswesens im 20. Jahrhundert* (Frankfurt a.M.: VAS, 2002), p. 171.
12 Norbert Frei, *Adernauer's Germany and the Nazi Past: The Politics of Amnesty and Integration*, trans. by Joel Golb (New York: Columbia University Press, 2002), pp. 311–12.
13 Leide, pp. 12, 176, 413–18.
14 Ernst, pp. 151, Table 13; Michael H. Kater, *Doctors Under Hitler* (Chapel Hill, NC: University of North Carolina Press, 1989), pp. 245, Table 2.4.
15 Karl Mannheim, 'Das Problem der Generationen', *Kölner Vierteljahrshefte für Soziologie*, 7 (1928), 157–85, 309–30; Herbert Butterfield, *The Discontinuities Between the Generations in History: Their Effect on the Transmission of Political Experience* (Cambridge: Cambridge University Press, 1972).
16 For the original meanings of class and nation, see the works of Karl Marx, *Karl Marx: Economy, Class, and Social Revolution*, ed. & trans. by Zbigniew A. Jordan (London: Joseph, 1971); Max Weber, *From Max Weber: Essays in Sociology* (London: Routledge, 2009).
17 Mark Roseman, 'Introduction: Generation Conflict and German History 1770–1968', in *Generations in Conflict: Youth Revolt and Generation Formation in Germany 1770–1968*, ed. by Mark Roseman (Cambridge: Cambridge University Press, 1995), pp. 1–46; Stephen Lovell, 'Introduction', in *Generation in the Twentieth-Century Europe*, ed. by Stephen Lovell (Houndmills: Palgrave Macmillan, 2007), pp. 1–18; Dorothee Wierling, 'Generations and Generational Conflicts in East and West Germany', in *The Divided Past: Rewriting Post-War German History*, ed. by Christoph Klessmann (Oxford: Berg, 2001), pp. 69–89.
18 Lovell, p. 3.
19 Ernst, p. 151, Table 13.
20 Mary Fulbrook, *Dissonant Lives: Generations and Violence Through the German Dictatorships* (Oxford: Oxford University Press, 2011), chapter 7, especially 7.3.; Richard Bessel, 'Hatred After War: Emotion and the Postwar History of East Germany', *History & Memory*, 17 (2005), 195–216.
21 Fulbrook, p. 473.
22 Fulbrook illustrates the significance of the 'New Teachers' for the GDR and its own narrative, as well as for the 1929er generation, which mostly benefited from this over proportional 'upwards mobility', regardless of social background, in her book, Fulbrook, pp. 304–5, 335.
23 Tobias Weidner, *Die unpolitische Profession: Deutsche Mediziner im langen 19. Jahrhundert* (Frankfurt a.M.: Campus, 2012). For another recent, general overview of the cultural implication of the 'unpolitical German' in the postwar era and beyond, see Sean A. Forner, 'Reconsidering the "Unpolitical German": Democratic Renewal and the Politics of Culture in Occupied Germany', *German History*, 32.1 (2014), 53–78.
24 Katharina von Kellenbach, *The Mark of Cain: Guilt and Denial in the Post-War Lives of Nazi Perpetrators* (New York: Oxford University Press, 2013).
25 Lars Rensmann, 'Collective Guilt, National Identity, and Political Processes in Contemporary Germany', in *Collective Guilt*, ed. by Nyla R. Branscombe and Bertjan Doosje (Cambridge: Cambridge University Press, 2004), pp. 169–90.
26 'German "Collective Guilt" a Fallacy, Arendt States at Ford Hall Forum', *The Harvard Crimson*, 1964 <www.thecrimson.com/article/1964/3/16/german-collective-guilt-a-fallacy-arendt/> [accessed 30 January 2019].

27 Weinke, p. 333; Alexander Mitscherlich and Margarete Mitscherlich, *The Inability to Mourn: Principles of Collective Behavior* (New York: Grove Press, 1975).
28 Fulbrook, pp. 483–4.
29 Fulbrook, p. 260.
30 'Dr. Reinhard Carrière, 02. März 1963': BStU, MfS, HA XX, 5749, Bl. 164.
31 Thomas Schilter, *Unmenschliches Ermessen: Die Nationalsozialistische 'Euthanasie'-Tötungsanstalt Pirna-Sonnenstein 1940/41* (Leipzig: Kiepenheuer, 1999).
32 Anke Hinrichs, 'Die Carrières', *Eppendorfer: Zeitung für Psychiatrie*, 26.2 (2011), 3.
33 'Dr. Friedrich-Wilhelm Brekenfeld, 2. März 1963': BStU, MfS, HA XX, 5749, Bl. 134–6.
34 'Dr. Friedrich-Wilhelm Brekenfeld': BStU, MfS, HA XX, 5749, Bl. 135.
35 Fulbrook, p. 260.
36 Ernst, p. 151, Table 13.
37 'Anordnung über das Blutspendewesen, 8. September 1951': BArch, DQ 1/2209, Bl. 276.
38 'Dr. Friedrich-Wilhelm Brekenfeld, 2. März 1963': BStU, MfS, HA XX, 5749, Bl. 134–6.
39 'Bericht über die Lage im Gesundheitswesen der DDR, 29. August 1958': BStU, MfS, ZAIG, 122, Bl. 24
40 'Prof. Dr. Schwarz, Egbert, 21. April 1959': BStU, MfS, HA XX, 5752, Bl. 130–2.
41 Weidner, pp. 392–3.
42 Dolores L. Augustine, *Red Prometheus: Engineering and Dictatorship in East Germany, 1945–1990* (Cambridge, MA: MIT Press, 2007), pp. XVIII–XIX.
43 Augustine, pp. XVIII–XIX.
44 Jeffrey Kopstein, *The Politics of Economic Decline, 1945–1989* (Chapel Hill, NC: University of North Carolina Press, 1997), pp. 45–8; Thomas A. Baylis, *The Technical Intelligentsia and the East German Elite: Legitimacy and Social Change in Mature Communism* (Berkeley: University of California Press, 1974), pp. 262–4; John C. Torpey, *Intellectuals, Socialism, and Dissent: The East German Opposition and Its Legacy* (Minneapolis, MN: University of Minnesota Press, 1999), p. 57.
45 Fulbrook, p. 477.
46 Roland Höhne, 'Von der Wende zum Ende: Die NDPD während des Demokratisierungsprozesses', in *Parteien und Wähler im Umbruch: Parteiensystem und Wählerverhalten in der ehemaligen DDR und den neuen Bundesländern*, ed. by Oskar Niedermayer and Richard Stöss (Wiesbaden: VS, 1994), pp. 113–42; Christoph Schreiber, *'Deutsche, auf die wir stolz sind.' Untersuchungen zur NDPD* (Hamburg: Dr. Kovac Verlag, 2018).
47 Höhne, pp. 113–15.
48 Peter Schneck, *Linser, Karl*, 2009 <www.bundesstiftung-aufarbeitung.de/wer-war-wer-in-der-ddr-%2363%3B-1424.html?ID=2117> [accessed 30 January 2019].
49 'Rat der Stadt Dresden, Dezernat Gesundheitswesen an Herrn Präs. Prof. Dr. Linser, DWK, HA GW, 7. Dezember 1948': BArch, DQ 1/128, Bl. 214.
50 Moser, pp. 177–8.
51 Peter Schneck, *Konitzer, Paul*, 2009 <www.bundesstiftung-aufarbeitung.de/wer-war-wer-in-der-ddr-%2363%3B-1424.html?ID=1834> [accessed 30 January 2019]; Clive Freeman and Gwynne Roberts, *Der kälteste Krieg: Professor Frucht und das Kampfstoff-Geheimnis* (Berlin: Ullstein, 1982), pp. 42–3.
52 BStU, MfS, HA IX/11, RHE-West 178/1 and 178/2; Leide, pp. 338–40.
53 'Ermittlungsauftrag Nr. 1697, 15. Juni 1956': BStU, MfS, HA XX, 3310, Bl. 84.
54 'Ermittlungsauftrag Nr. 1697, 15. Juni 1956': BStU, MfS, HA XX, 3310, Bl. 84.
55 Frank McDonough, *The Gestapo: The Myth and Reality of Hitler's Secret Police* (London: Coronet, 2015), chapter 5; Paul Betts, *Within Walls: Private Life in the German Democratic Republic* (Oxford: Oxford University Press, 2010), pp. 42–50.
56 'Ermittlungsauftrag Nr. 1697, 15. Juni 1956': BStU, MfS, HA XX, 3310, Bl. 83–5; 'Sachstandsbericht – Betr.: Operativ-Vorlauf "Vergangenheit", 9. Juni 1964': BStU, MfS, BV Leipzig, AOP 746/66, Bl. 185.

57 'Heyde-Mitwisser: Die Schatten weichen', *Der Spiegel*, 6 (1962), 30–1; 'Heyde/ Sawade – Verstummte Zeugen', *Der Spiegel*, 23 (1960), 35–8; 'Euthanasie – Die Kreuzelschreiber', *Der Spiegel*, 19 (1961), 35–44; Nina Grunenberg, 'Der merkwürdige Fall Heyde: Sollte der „Euthanasie"-Prozeß nicht stattfinden?', *Die Zeit*, 21 February 1964 <https://www.zeit.de/1964/08/der-merkwuerdige-fall-heyde> [accessed 30 January 2019].

58 Leide, pp. 339–40. 'Auskunftsbericht, 22. Dezember 1965': BStU, MfS, HA XX, 3310, Bl. 89–93; BStU, MfS, HA IX/11, RHE-West 178/1 and 178/2

59 'Abschlußbericht zum Vorlauf-Operativ "Vergangenheit", 28. Februar 1966': BStU, MfS, BV Leipzig, AOP 746/66, Bl. 307–9. For a similar conclusion, see Leide, p. 340.

60 Fulbrook, p. 488.

61 Detlev J. K. Peukert, *The Weimar Republic: The Crisis of Classical Modernity* (London: Lane, 1991), pp. 89–95, here 91.

62 Fulbrook, p. 488.

63 Fulbrook, pp. 488–9.

64 Fulbrook, p. 488.

65 'Betr.: Euthanasie-Prozeß in Westdeutschland, 3. April 1963': BStU, MfS, HA XX, 4980, Bl. 158.

66 'Auskunftsbericht. Kunis, Johannes, 13. August 1964': BStU, MfS, AP 6338/77, Bl. 15–17.

67 'Vernehmungsprotokoll, 8. April 1965': BStU, MfS, BV Lpz, AU 1924/65, Bd. 2, Bl. 166–73, here 169–70.

68 Names were made anonymous due to public and archival restrictions. Therefore, the fictitious names Anne Müller and Bernd Müller are used to enhance comprehension in the following.

69 'Fristverlängerung, 8. Juni 1965': BStU, MfS, BV Lpz, AU 1924/65, Bd. 1, Bl. 297–8.

70 '[Anne Müller] Heute – nach fast zwanzig Jahren – zeige ich nochmal das furchtbarste Kapitel meines Lebens auf, 25. April 1964': BStU, MfS, BV Lpz, AU 1924/65, Bd. 1, Bl. 11–18.

71 'Haftbeschluß/Haftbefehl [Anne Müller], 22. Februar 1965': BStU, MfS, BV Lpz, AU 1924/65, Bd. 2, Bl. 10–11.

72 'Aktennotiz, 18. März 1965': BStU, MfS, BV Lpz, AU 1924/65, Bd. 2, Bl. 136.

73 'Ermittlungsbericht [Anne Müller], 1. September 1964': BStU, MfS, BV Lpz, AU 1924/65, Bd. 1, Bl. 45–6; 'Ermittlungsbericht [Bernd Müller], 3. September 1964': BStU, MfS, BV Lpz, AU 1924/65, Bd. 1, Bl. 47–8.

74 'Bericht, 19. März 1965': BStU, MfS, BV Lpz, AU 1924/65, Bd. 2, Bl. 147.

75 'Beschuldigte [Anne Müller], 19. März 1965': BStU, MfS, BV Lpz, AU 1924/65, Bd. 2, Bl. 148 and reports 149–53.

76 'Betr.: Anzeigeerstattung des [Bernd Müller], in Sachen seiner Schwester [Anne Müller] gegen den Dr. H. Kuniß, Waldheim, 24. August 1964': BStU, MfS, AP 6338/77, Bl. 19–23, here 22 and 23.

77 'Abschlußbericht, 5. Juli 1965': BStU, MfS, BV Lpz, AU 1924/65, Bd. 2, Bl. 214–18, here 217–18.

78 'Verfügung, 31. Juli 1965': BStU, MfS, BV Lpz, AU 1924/65, Bd. 2, Bl. 220.

79 'Betr.: Anzeigeerstattung des [Bernd Müller], in Sachen seiner Schwester [Anne Müller] gegen den Dr. H. Kuniß, Waldheim, 24. August 1964': BStU, MfS, AP 6338/77, Bl. 19–23, here 21–2.

80 For another example, see Leide, pp. 293–6.

81 Leide, pp. 136–44.

82 'Anklageschrift, 30. Juni 1966': BStU, MfS, HA XX, 16974, Bl. 3–22.

83 Leide, p. 416; Weinke, pp. 331–2.

84 'Information zu einigen Fragen betreffend ehemalige Mitglieder der NSDAP und anderer faschistischer Organisationen, die heute zum Teil in der DDR tätig sind, 27. April 1964': BStU, MfS, HA XX, 5755, Bl. 30–50, here 40; Gerhard Naser, *Hausärzte in der DDR: Relikte des Kapitalismus oder Konkurrenz für die Polikliniken?* (Bergatreute: Eppe, 2000), pp. 304–12, here 311.

85 Fulbrook, pp. 488–9.
86 'Betr.: Erweiterte Vorstandssitzung vom 4.6.46, 4. Juni 1946': BArch, DQ 1/139, Bl. 131.
87 Ernst, p. 334; *Bewährtes Bündnis: Arbeiterklasse und medizinische Intelligenz auf dem Weg zum Sozialismus*, ed. by Horst Jentzsch (Berlin: VEB Verlag Volk und Gesundheit, 1987), pp. 50–1.
88 'Bericht: Befragung der Bez.-Ärztin Dresden, OMR Dr. Ochsenfarth, 23. Mai 1964': BStU, MfS, BV Leipzig, AOP 746/66, Bl. 147–8; Oliver Reinhard, 'Das Geheimnis der Bezirksärztin', *Sächsische Zeitung* (Dresden, 20 November 2014), p. 3.
89 'Stellungnahme zu dem mir am 2.8.1963 durch Herrn Chefarzt Dr. med. Schmeiser und Herrn Merkel eröffneten Beschluß, 12. August 1963': BArch, DQ 1/12052, unpaginated; Reinhard, p. 3.
90 'Bericht: Befragung der Bez.-Ärztin Dresden, OMR Dr. Ochsenfarth, 23. Mai 1964': BStU, MfS, BV Leipzig, AOP 746/66, Bl. 147.
91 Reinhard, p. 3.
92 See, for example, the patient file of Emma Frieda Mickel, who was euthanised before Christmas 1944. 'Emma Frieda Mickel, geb. Wiedmer': HSA DD, Landesanstalt/ Fachkrankenhaus Großschweidnitz, 10822, Nr. F 5376.
93 For another example, see Leide, p. 418.
94 Reinhard, p. 3.
95 Fulbrook, p. 489.
96 Reinisch, p. 2.
97 Weidner.
98 'Walter Korinek an Rat der Stadt Dresden, Hauptgesundheitsamt, 2. August 1948': BArch, DQ 1/12052, unpaginated.
99 'Einschätzung zu Operativ-Vorgang "Spinne", 15. Dezember 1959': BStU, MfS, BV Dresden, AU 43/60, Bl. 18.
100 'Betr. Schlägerei der Herren Dr. Korinek und Dr. [. . .], 19. April 1950': StA DD, Dezernat Gesundheitswesen, 4.1.12, Nr. 21, Bl. 49; 'Vertraulich, Betr. Herrn Oberarzt Dr. Korinek, Krhs. [. . .], 17. April 1950': StA DD, Dezernat Gesundheitswesen, 4.1.12, Nr. 21, Bl. 206.
101 'Niederschrift, 27. September 1950': StA DD, Dezernat Gesundheitswesen, 4.1.12, Nr. 21, Bl. 48; 'Betr. Antrag des Herrn Dr. med. Walter Korinek auf Rücknahme der fristlosen Kündigung bezw. Wiedereinstellung in städtische Dienste, 30. Oktober 1950': BArch, DQ 1/12052, unpaginated; 'Herrn Dr. med. Walter Korinek, geb. 19.4.14, 22. Dezember 1950': BArch, DQ 1/12052, unpaginated.
102 'Einschätzung zu Operativ-Vorgang "Spinne", 15. Dezember 1959': BStU, MfS, BV Dresden, AU 43/60, Bl. 9–20.
103 'Aktennotiz, August 1959': BArch, DQ 1/12052, unpaginated.
104 'Sachstandsbericht, 7. Januar 1960': BStU, MfS, AU 43/60, Bl. 95, 99–100, 104–10.
105 'Wiedereinstellung als Arzthelfer, 10. Mai 1960': BArch, DQ 1/12052, unpaginated; 'An Frau Bezirksärztin, Medizinalrat Dr. Ochsenfarth, Betr.: Walter Korinek, geb. 19.4.14, 17. Mai 1962': BArch, DQ 1/12052, unpaginated.
106 'Eröffnungsbeschluß zur Durchführung eines Disziplinarverfahrens gegen den Arzthelfer Walter Korinek, 24. Juli 1963': BArch, DQ 1/12052, unpaginated.
107 'Stellungnahme zu dem mir am 2.8.1963 durch Herrn Chefarzt Dr. med. [. . .] und Herrn [. . .] eröffneten Beschluß': BArch, DQ 1/12052, unpaginated.
108 Augustine, p. 347.
109 Francesca Weil, *Zielgruppe Ärzteschaft: Ärzte als inoffizielle Mitarbeiter des Ministeriums für Staatssicherheit* (Göttingen: Vandenhoeck & Ruprecht, 2008), pp. 287–92, here 292.
110 Weil, pp. 292–3.

111 Ilko-Sascha Kowalczuk, *Stasi konkret: Überwachung und Repression in der DDR* (Munich: Beck, 2013).

112 ' "Doktor ohne Promotion. Strafbare Anmaßung eines akademischen Grades", *Sächsisches Tagesblatt*, 29. April 1964': BArch, DQ 1/12052, unpaginated. 'Walter Korinek – Zulassung zum medizinischem Staatsexamen, 12. Mai 1964': BArch, DQ 1/12052, unpaginated.

113 'MfG – Recht – an HO-Gaststätten- und Hotelbetrieb Dresden, Betr.: Walter Korinek, geb. 19.4.1914, 7. Februar 1967': BArch, DQ 1/12052, unpaginated; 'Schreiben der HO-Gaststätten- und Hotelbetrieb Dresden an das MfG – Recht –, 14. Februar 1967': BArch, DQ 1/12052, unpaginated.

114 'Sachstandsbericht, 7. Januar 1960': BStU, MfS, AU 43/60, Bl. 100.

115 Wiebke Janssen, 'Medizinische Hochschulbauten als Prestigeobjekt der SED: Das Klinikum Halle-Kröllwitz', *Deutschland Archiv*, 4 (2012), 703–12.

116 'Vorschlag zur Anwerbung eines GI, 4. Mai 1960': BStU, MfS, HA IX/11, ZA 7294, Objekt 13, Bl. 30–3.

117 BStU, MfS, HA IX/11, ZA 7294, Objekt 13, Bl. 13–16; 'Vorschlag zur Anwerbung eines GI, 4. Mai 1960': BStU, MfS, HA IX/11, ZA 7294, Objekt 13, Bl. 31.

118 Ilko-Sascha Kowalczuk, *17. Juni 1953* (Munich: Beck, 2013).

119 Ernst, p. 341; Klaus-Dieter Müller, 'Die Ärzteschaft im staatlichen Gesundheitswesen der SBZ und DDR 1945–1989', in *Geschichte der deutschen Ärzteschaft*, ed. by Robert Jütte (Cologne: Deutscher Ärzte-Verlag, 1997), pp. 243–73.

120 For more details, see Markus Wahl, *"It Would Be Better, If Some Doctors Were Sent to Work in the Coal Mines": The SED and the Medical Intelligentsia Between 1961 and 1981* (New Zealand: University of Canterbury, 2013).

121 Weil, pp. 288–9.

122 'Vorschlag zur Anwerbung eines GI, 4. Mai 1960': BStU, MfS, HA IX/11, ZA 7294, Objekt 13, Bl. 31–3.

123 'Vorschlag zur Anwerbung eines GI, 4. Mai 1960': BStU, MfS, HA IX/11, ZA 7294, Objekt 13, Bl. 33.

124 'Bericht über erfolgte Kontaktaufnahme, 24. Juni 1960': BStU, MfS, HA IX/11, ZA 7294, Objekt 13, Bl. 34–5.

125 'Treffbericht, 10. November 1960': BStU, MfS, HA IX/11, ZA 7294, Objekt 13, Bl. 39–41. Augustine, p. 347; Weil, pp. 91–8, 287–92.

126 'Bericht über erfolgte Kontaktaufnahme, 24. Juni 1960': BStU, MfS, HA IX/11, ZA 7294, Objekt 13, Bl. 34–5; 'Treffbericht, 10. November 1960': BStU, MfS, HA IX/11, ZA 7294, Objekt 13, Bl. 39–41.

127 See his IM file, 'IM Akte "Bernd Richter" ': BStU, MfS, BV DD, AIM 402/92.

128 Kowalczuk, *Stasi konkret*.

129 'Treffbericht, 10. November 1960': BStU, MfS, HA IX/11, ZA 7294, Objekt 13, Bl. 40.

130 'Bericht über erfolgte Kontaktaufnahme, 24. Juni 1960': BStU, MfS, HA IX/11, ZA 7294, Objekt 13, Bl. 34–5; 'Treffbericht, 10. November 1960': BStU, MfS, HA IX/11, ZA 7294, Objekt 13, Bl. 39–41.

131 'Meldung einer Republikflucht, 4. August 1961': BStU, MfS, HA IX/11, ZA 7294, Objekt 13, Bl. 50.

132 Kater, *The Nazi Party*, pp. 54–7 and 245, Table 2.4.

133 Fulbrook, p. 489.

134 Fulbrook, pp. 291–308, 488–9.

135 Ernst, p. 151, Table 13.

136 Fulbrook, p. 489.

137 *Das Gesundheitswesen der DDR in der Periode der weiteren Gestaltung der entwickelten sozialistischen Gesellschaft und unter dem Kurs der Einheit von Wirtschafts- und*

Sozialpolitik (1971–1981), ed. by Horst Spaar (Berlin: Interessengemeinschaft Medizin und Gesellschaft, 2002), p. 25.

138 Peter Schneck, *Mecklinger, Ludwig*, 2009 <www.bundesstiftung-aufarbeitung.de/ wer-war-wer-in-der-ddr-#63;-1424.html?ID=2117> [accessed 30 January 2019].

139 'Prof. Matthies, Hans-Jürgen': BStU, MfS, HA XX, 5751, Bl. 228.

140 Werner Hartkopf, *Matthies, Hansjürgen*, 1992, p. 233 <www.bbaw.de/bbaw/ MitgliederderVorgaengerakademien/AltmitgliedDetails?altmitglied_id=1764> [accessed 30 January 2019]; Harry Waibel, *Diener vieler Herren: Ehemalige NS-Funktionäre in der SBZ/DDR* (Frankfurt a.M.: Lang, 2011), p. 212.

141 'Prof. Matthies, Hans-Jürgen': BStU, MfS, HA XX, 5751, Bl. 228; Hartkopf, p. 233.

142 'Dr. med. Charlotte Bergmann (LDP)': BStU, MfS, HA XX, 5749, Bl. 75; 'Dr. Reinhard Schwarzlose, 20. Juni 1960': BStU, MfS, HA XX, 5752, Bl. 144. For comparison, see BArch-BDC, Personenbezogene Unterlagen der Reichskulturkammer (RKK), R 9361-V/83367, Reinhard Schwarzlose.

143 Frederike Sattler, *Wirtschaftsordnung im Übergang: Politik, Organisation und Funktion der KPD/SED im Land Brandenburg bei der Etablierung der zentralen Planwirtschaft in der SBZ/DDR 1945–1952, Teil 2* (Münster: LIT, 2002), p. 906.

144 'Dr. Reinhard Schwarzlose, 20. Juni 1960': BStU, MfS, HA XX, 5752, Bl. 144.

145 Dirk Hubrich, *49/21, Schwarzlose, Dr. Reinhard*, 2013 <www.deutsche-gesellschaft-fuer-ordenskunde.de/DGOWP/wp-content/uploads/2013/06/VL-VAdV-1949-1978. pdf> [accessed 30 January 2019].

146 'Dr. med. Charlotte Bergmann (LDP)': BStU, MfS, HA XX, 5749, Bl. 75.

147 Fulbrook, pp. 291–308.

148 Hannah Arendt, *Eichmann in Jerusalem: A Report on the Banality of Evil* (New York: Penguin Books, 1994).

149 This trial was the first of many subsequent Auschwitz Trials. Even at the beginning of 2016, German courts sued an Auschwitz guard, who had been identified recently. Gisela Friedrichsen, 'Prozess gegen früheren KZ-Wachmann: "Vernichtung durch Lebensverhältnisse"', *Der Spiegel*, 2016 <www.spiegel.de/panorama/justiz/ auschwitz-prozess-in-detmold-vernichtung-durch-lebensverhaeltnisse-a-1076943. html> [accessed 30 January 2019].

150 Arthur Miller, 'The Nazi Trials and the German Heart', in *Echoes Down the Corridor: Arthur Miller: Collected Essays 1944–2000*, ed. by Steven R. Centola (London: Methuen, 2000), pp. 62–68.

151 For further information about Oswald Kaduk, see Ernst Klee, 'Kaduk, Oswald', in *Auschwitz: Täter, Gehilfen, Opfer und was aus ihnen wurde: Ein Personenlexikon* (Berlin: Fischer, 2013).

152 Miller, pp. 62–3, here 63.

153 For further information about Victor Capesius, see Dieter Schlesak, *Capesius, der Auschwitzapotheker* (Bonn: Dietz, 2006).

154 Miller, p. 63.

155 For a definition of this phenomenon, see Nigel C. Hunt, *Memory, War, and Trauma* (Cambridge: Cambridge University Press, 2010), pp. 115–18.

156 Miller, p. 64. Frei draws the same conclusion in his analysis about the West German practice regarding the Nazi past of politicians and officials. Frei, pp. 303–12.

157 For the concessions granted to the medical profession by the SED, see 'Zu Fragen des Gesundheitswesens und der medizinischen Intelligenz, 16. September 1958', in *Dokumente der Sozialistischen Einheitspartei Deutschlands: Beschlüsse und Erklärungen des Zentralsekretariats und des Parteivorstandes, Band VII* (Berlin: Dietz, 1961), pp. 348–52; 'Kommuniqué des Politbüros des Zentralkomitees über Maßnahmen zur weiteren Entwicklung des Gesundheitswesens und zur Förderung der Arbeit der medizinischen Intelligenz, 16. Dezember 1960', in *Dokumente der Sozialistischen Einheitspartei Deutschlands: Beschlüsse und Erklärungen des Zentralsekretariats und des Parteivorstandes, Band VIII* (Berlin: Dietz, 1962), pp. 303–6.

158 Leide, p. 353; Weinke, p. 46. Moser also emphasises the importance of East Germany's alliance efforts especially towards the 'old elites' of the medical profession. Moser, p. 153.
159 Ludwig Mecklinger, 'Der politische Auftrag des Gesundheitswesens: Aus der Rede des Ministers für Gesundheitswesen, OMR Prof. Dr. sc. med. Ludwig Mecklinger, auf der Kreisärztekonferenz', *humanitas*, 24 (1981), 1–3.
160 According to Ernst, 927 doctors left the GDR for the West in 1958, which represented around 7 per cent of all available doctors in East Germany – a dangerous development for the SED. Ernst, pp. 34, 55.
161 Ernst, p. 180; Corey Ross, *Constructing Socialism at the Grass-Roots: The Transformation of East Germany, 1945–65* (Houndmills: Palgrave, 2000), p. 184.
162 Miller, p. 62.
163 Miller, p. 62.
164 Miller, p. 62.
165 Weinke, p. 333.
166 Miller, p. 66.
167 Arendt, p. 57.
168 Miller, p. 65.
169 Arendt, pp. 4–6.
170 For further information on the issue of turncoats, see Weinke, p. 330. Another example is offered by Klaus Mann's novel *Mephisto*. There he describes an opportunistic actor in transition between the Weimar Republic and the Third Reich, whose real counterpart also had a remarkable career in the GDR. Therefore, the actor was able to accommodate himself with three different political systems. Klaus Mann, *Mephisto: Roman einer Karriere* (Berlin: Rowohlt, 2000).
171 Fulbrook, p. 280.
172 Fulbrook, pp. 280–1.
173 Fulbrook, pp. 280–1.
174 Fulbrook, p. 281.
175 Already Moser identifies that continuity of medical personnel meant a continuity of language towards refugees, lower classes, and other marginalised groups. Moser, p. 165.
176 Fulbrook, pp. 482–9, here 488.
177 Assmann also discusses Friedrich Nietzsche's notion of a "useable past" by the state, the mnemonic community, and the individual. Aleida Assmann, 'History and Memory', *International Encyclopedia of the Social & Behavioral Sciences* (Elsevier, 2001), pp. 6822–29.
178 Leide, p. 418.
179 Leide, p. 46.
180 'Bericht über eine Aussprache mit dem stellv. Minister für Gesundheitswesen, Prof. Dr. Mecklinger am 20.2.1969, 25. Februar 1969': BStU, MfS, HA XX, 527, Bl. 581–5, here 585.
181 Kater, *Doctors under Hitler*, p. 237.

Bibliography

Primary sources

Unpublished

BUNDESARCHIV (BARCH) – SAMMLUNG BERLIN DOCUMENT CENTRE (BDC)

BArch-BDC, Personenbezogene Unterlagen der Reichskulturkammer (RKK), R 9361-V/83367, Reinhard Schwarzlose

BUNDESARCHIV (BARCH)

Ministry of Healthcare

BArch, DQ 1/128 – Schriftwechsel mit Landes- und Provinzialverwaltungen; Sachsen, 1945–1949

BArch, DQ 1/139 – Bekämpfung von Geschlechtskrankheiten, Mitteilungen und Richtlinien der Deutschen Zentralverwaltung für Gesundheitswesen, Bd. 3, 1946–1947

BArch, DQ 1/2209 – Bekämpfung der Geschlechtskrankheiten, 1948–1951

BArch, DQ 1/12052 – Personalakte Walter Korinek, 1948–1967

ARCHIV DES BUNDESBEAUFTRAGTEN FÜR DIE UNTERLAGEN DES

STAATSSICHERHEITSDIENSTES DER EHEMALIGEN DEUTSCHEN DEMOKRATISCHEN

REPUBLIK (BSTU)

BStU, MfS, AP 6338/77

BStU, MfS, AS 2453/67

BStU, MfS, AU 131/60

BStU, MfS, BV DD, AIM 402/92

BStU, MfS, BV Dresden, AIM 1272/82

BStU, MfS, BV Dresden, AU 43/60

BStU, MfS, BV Dresden, KD Sebnitz, 4409

BStU, MfS, BV Leipzig, AOP 143/55

BStU, MfS, BV Leipzig, AOP 746/66

BStU, MfS, BV Leipzig, AU 1924/65

BStU, MfS, BV Leipzig, KD Leipzig-Land, 3738

BStU, MfS, GH, 19/59

BStU, MfS, HA II/10, 1037

BStU, HA VII, 2125

BStU, MfS, HA IX/11, AK 1453/75

BStU, MfS, HA IX/11, AK 1454/75

BStU, MfS, HA IX/11, AV 4/74

BStU, MfS, HA IX/11, AV 8/84

BStU, MfS, HA IX/11, RHE 1/66 VRP

BStU, MfS, HA IX/11, RHE 57/79 DDR

BStU, MfS, HA IX/11, RHE-West, 178/1

BStU, MfS, HA IX/11, RHE-West, 178/2

BStU, MfS, HA IX/11, RHE-West 203

BStU, MfS, HA IX/11, ZA 7294, Objekt 13

BStU, MfS, HA IX/11, ZA 11853/Objekt 13

BStU, MfS, HA IX/11, ZA 12.212/55, Objekt 12

BStU, MfS, HA IX/11, ZA I, Akte 145

BStU, MfS, HA IX/11, ZA I 7413, Akte 1

BStU, MfS, HA IX/11, ZA I 7414, Akte 31

BStU, MfS, HA IX/11, ZA VI 654, Akte 24

BStU, MfS, HA IX/11, ZB II 4553, Akte 1

BStU, MfS, HA IX/11, ZB II 4553, Akte 2

BStU, MfS, HA IX/11, ZB II 5842, Akte 1

BStU, MfS, HA IX/11, ZUV 49

BStU, MfS, HA XX, 527
BStU, MfS, HA XX, 3310
BStU, MfS, HA XX, 3364
BStU, MfS, HA XX, 3828
BStU, MfS, HA XX, 4244
BStU, MfS, HA XX, 4980
BStU, MfS, HA XX, 5628
BStU, MfS, HA XX, 5749
BStU, MfS, HA XX, 5750
BStU, MfS, HA XX, 5751
BStU, MfS, HA XX, 5752
BStU, MfS, HA XX, 5755
BStU, MfS, HA XX, 16974
BStU, MfS, ZAIG, 122

DRESDEN, HAUPTSTAATSARCHIV (HSA DD)

HSA DD, Landesanstalt/Fachkrankenhaus Großschweidnitz, 10822, Nr. F 5376

DRESDEN, STADTARCHIV (STA DD)

StA DD, Dezernat Gesundheitswesen, 4.1.12, Nr. 21
StA DD, Dezernat Gesundheitswesen, 4.1.12, Nr. 22

LEIPZIG, STADTARCHIV (STA LPZ)

StA Lpz, Stadtverwaltung und Rat, Nr. 1611

Published

'Euthanasie – Die Kreuzelschreiber', *Der Spiegel*, 19 (1961), 35–44
Grunenberg, Nina, 'Der merkwürdige Fall Heyde: Sollte der „Euthanasie"-Prozeß nicht stattfinden?', *Die Zeit*, 21 February 1964 <https://www.zeit.de/1964/08/der-merkwuerdige-fall-heyde> [accessed 30 January 2019]
'Heyde-Mitwisser: Die Schatten weichen', *Der Spiegel*, 6 (1962), 30–1
'Heyde/Sawade – Verstummte Zeugen', *Der Spiegel*, 23 (1960), 35–8
Jentzsch, Horst, ed., *Bewährtes Bündnis: Arbeiterklasse und medizinische Intelligenz auf dem Weg zum Sozialismus* (Berlin: VEB Verlag Volk und Gesundheit, 1987)
'Kommuniqué des Politbüros des Zentralkomitees über Maßnahmen zur weiteren Entwicklung des Gesundheitswesens und zur Förderung der Arbeit der medizinischen Intelligenz, 16. Dezember 1960', in *Dokumente der Sozialistischen Einheitspartei Deutschlands: Beschlüsse und Erklärungen des Zentralsekretariats und des Parteivorstandes, Band VIII* (Berlin: Dietz, 1962), pp. 303–6
Mecklinger, Ludwig, 'Der politische Auftrag des Gesundheitswesens: Aus der Rede des Ministers für Gesundheitswesen, OMR Prof. Dr. sc. med. Ludwig Mecklinger, auf der Kreisärztekonferenz', *humanitas*, 24 (1981), 1–3

'Zu Fragen des Gesundheitswesens und der medizinischen Intelligenz, 16. September 1958', in *Dokumente der Sozialistischen Einheitspartei Deutschlands: Beschlüsse und Erklärungen des Zentralsekretariats und des Parteivorstandes, Band VII* (Berlin: Dietz, 1961), pp. 348–52

Secondary sources

Arendt, Hannah, *Eichmann in Jerusalem: A Report on the Banality of Evil* (New York: Penguin Books, 1994)

Arndt, Melanie, *Gesundheitspolitik im geteilten Berlin, 1948 bis 1961* (Cologne: Böhlau, 2009)

Assmann, Aleida, 'History and Memory', *International Encyclopedia of the Social & Behavioral Sciences* (Elsevier, 2001), pp. 6822–29

Augustine, Dolores L., *Red Prometheus: Engineering and Dictatorship in East Germany, 1945–1990* (Cambridge, MA: MIT Press, 2007)

Baylis, Thomas A., *The Technical Intelligentsia and the East German Elite: Legitimacy and Social Change in Mature Communism* (Berkeley: University of California Press, 1974)

Bessel, Richard, *Germany 1945: From War to Peace* (London: Simon & Schuster, 2009)

———, 'Hatred After War: Emotion and the Postwar History of East Germany', *History & Memory*, 17 (2005), 195–216

Betts, Paul, *Within Walls: Private Life in the German Democratic Republic* (Oxford: Oxford University Press, 2010)

Butterfield, Herbert, *The Discontinuities Between the Generations in History: Their Effect on the Transmission of Political Experience* (Cambridge: Cambridge University Press, 1972)

Ernst, Anna-Sabine, *'Die beste Prophylaxe ist der Sozialismus': Ärzte und Hochschullehrer in der SBZ/DDR 1945–1961* (Münster: Waxmann, 1996)

Forner, Sean A., 'Reconsidering the "Unpolitical German": Democratic Renewal and the Politics of Culture in Occupied Germany', *German History*, 32 (2014), 53–78

Freeman, Clive, and Gwynne Roberts, *Der kälteste Krieg: Professor Frucht und das Kampfstoff-Geheimnis* (Berlin: Ullstein, 1982)

Frei, Norbert, *Adernauer's Germany and the Nazi Past: The Politics of Amnesty and Integration*, trans. by Joel Golb (New York: Columbia University Press, 2002)

Friedrichsen, Gisela, 'Prozess gegen früheren KZ-Wachmann: "Vernichtung durch Lebensverhältnisse"', *Der Spiegel*, 2016 <www.spiegel.de/panorama/justiz/auschwitz-prozess-in-detmold-vernichtung-durch-lebensverhaeltnisse-a-1076943.html> [accessed 30 January 2019]

Fulbrook, Mary, *Dissonant Lives: Generations and Violence Through the German Dictatorships* (Oxford: Oxford University Press, 2011)

'German "Collective Guilt" a Fallacy, Arendt States at Ford Hall Forum', *The Harvard Crimson*, 1964 <www.thecrimson.com/article/1964/3/16/german-collective-guilt-a-fallacy-arendt/> [accessed 30 January 2019]

Hartkopf, Werner, *Matthies, Hansjürgen*, 1992 <www.bbaw.de/bbaw/Mitgliederder Vorgaengerakademien/AltmitgliedDetails?altmitglied_id=1764> [accessed 30 January 2019]

Hinrichs, Anke, 'Die Carrières', *Eppendorfer: Zeitung für Psychiatrie*, 26 (2011), 3

Höhne, Roland, 'Von der Wende zum Ende: Die NDPD während des Demokratisierungs-prozesses', in *Parteien und Wähler im Umbruch: Parteiensystem und Wählerverhalten in der ehemaligen DDR und den neuen Bundesländern*, ed. by Oskar Niedermayer and Richard Stöss (Wiesbaden: VS, 1994), pp. 113–42

Hubrich, Dirk, *49/21, Schwarzlose, Dr. Reinhard*, 2013 <www.deutsche-gesellschaft-fuer-ordenskunde.de/DGOWP/wp-content/uploads/2013/06/VL-VAdV-1949-1978.pdf> [accessed 30 January 2019]

Hunt, Nigel C., *Memory, War, and Trauma* (Cambridge: Cambridge University Press, 2010)

Janssen, Wiebke, 'Medizinische Hochschulbauten als Prestigeobjekt der SED: Das Klinikum Halle-Kröllwitz', *Deutschland Archiv*, 4 (2012), 703–12

Kater, Michael H., *Doctors Under Hitler* (Chapel Hill, NC: University of North Carolina Press, 1989)

————, *The Nazi Party: A Social Profile of Members and Leaders, 1919–1945* (Oxford: Basil Blackwell, 1983)

Klee, Ernst, 'Kaduk, Oswald', in *Auschwitz: Täter, Gehilfen, Opfer und was aus ihnen wurde: Ein Personenlexikon* (Berlin: Fischer, 2013)

Kopstein, Jeffrey, *The Politics of Economic Decline, 1945–1989* (Chapel Hill, NC: University of North Carolina Press, 1997)

Kowalczuk, Ilko-Sascha, *17. Juni 1953* (Munich: Beck, 2013)

————, *Stasi konkret: Überwachung und Repression in der DDR* (Munich: Beck, 2013)

Leide, Henry, *NS-Verbrecher und Staatssicherheit: Die geheime Vergangenheitspolitik der DDR* (Göttingen: Vandenhoeck & Ruprecht, 2005)

Lovell, Stephen, 'Introduction', in *Generation in the Twentieth-Century Europe*, ed. by Stephen Lovell (Houndmills: Palgrave Macmillan, 2007), pp. 1–18

Mann, Klaus, *Mephisto: Roman einer Karriere* (Berlin: Rowohlt, 2000)

Mannheim, Karl, 'Das Problem der Generationen', *Kölner Vierteljahrshefte für Soziologie*, 7 (1928), 157–85, 309–30

Marx, Karl, *Karl Marx: Economy, Class, and Social Revolution*, ed. & trans. by Zbigniew A. Jordan (London: Joseph, 1971)

McDonough, Frank, *The Gestapo: The Myth and Reality of Hitler's Secret Police* (London: Coronet, 2015)

Miller, Arthur, 'The Nazi Trials and the German Heart', in *Echoes Down the Corridor: Arthur Miller: Collected Essays 1944–2000*, ed. by Steven R. Centola (London: Methuen, 2000), pp. 62–8

Mitscherlich, Alexander, and Margarete Mitscherlich, *The Inability to Mourn: Principles of Collective Behavior* (New York: Grove Press, 1975)

Moser, Gabriele, *'Im Interesse der Volksgesundheit. . .': Sozialhygiene und öffentliches Gesundheitswesen in der Weimarer Republik und der frühen SBZ/DDR: Ein Beitrag zur Sozialgeschichte des deutschen Gesundheitswesens im 20. Jahrhundert* (Frankfurt a.M.: VAS, 2002)

Muller, Klaus-Dieter, 'Die Ärzteschaft im staatlichen Gesundheitswesen der SBZ und DDR 1945–1989', in *Geschichte der deutschen Ärzteschaft*, ed. by Robert Jütte (Cologne: Deutscher Ärzte-Verlag, 1997), pp. 243–73

Naser, Gerhard, *Hausärzte in der DDR: Relikte des Kapitalismus oder Konkurrenz für die Polikliniken?* (Bergatreute: Eppe, 2000)

Peukert, Detlev J. K., *The Weimar Republic: The Crisis of Classical Modernity* (London: Lane, 1991)

Reinhard, Oliver, 'Das Geheimnis der Bezirksärztin', *Sächsische Zeitung* (Dresden, 20 November 2014), p. 3

Reinisch, Jessica, *The Perils of Peace: The Public Health Crisis in Occupied Germany* (Oxford: Oxford University Press, 2013)

Rensmann, Lars, 'Collective Guilt, National Identity, and Political Processes in Contemporary Germany', in *Collective Guilt*, ed. by Nyla R. Branscombe and Bertjan Doosje (Cambridge: Cambridge University Press, 2004), pp. 169–90

Roseman, Mark, 'Introduction: Generation Conflict and German History 1770–1968', in *Generations in Conflict: Youth Revolt and Generation Formation in Germany 1770–1968*, ed. by Mark Roseman (Cambridge: Cambridge University Press, 1995), pp. 1–46

Ross, Corey, *Constructing Socialism at the Grass-Roots: The Transformation of East Germany, 1945–65* (Houndmills: Palgrave, 2000)

Sattler, Frederike, *Wirtschaftsordnung im Übergang: Politik, Organisation und Funktion der KPD/SED im Land Brandenburg bei der Etablierung der zentralen Planwirtschaft in der SBZ/DDR 1945–1952, Teil 2* (Münster: LIT, 2002)

Schilter, Thomas, *Unmenschliches Ermessen: Die Nationalsozialistische 'Euthanasie'-Tötungsanstalt Pirna-Sonnenstein 1940/41* (Leipzig: Kiepenheuer, 1999)

Schlesak, Dieter, *Capesius, der Auschwitzapotheker* (Bonn: Dietz, 2006)

Schneck, Peter, *Konitzer, Paul*, 2009 <www.bundesstiftung-aufarbeitung.de/wer-war-wer-in-der-ddr-%2363%3B-1424.html?ID=1834> [accessed 30 January 2019]

——, *Linser, Karl*, 2009 <www.bundesstiftung-aufarbeitung.de/wer-war-wer-in-der-ddr-%2363%3B-1424.html?ID=2117> [accessed 30 January 2019]

——, *Mecklinger, Ludwig*, 2009 <www.bundesstiftung-aufarbeitung.de/wer-war-wer-in-der-ddr-#63;-1424.html?ID=2117> [accessed 30 January 2019]

Schreiber, Christoph, *'Deutsche, auf die wir stolz sind,' Untersuchungen zur NDPD* (Hamburg: Dr. Kovac Verlag, 2018)

Spaar, Horst, ed., *Das Gesundheitswesen der DDR in der Periode der weiteren Gestaltung der entwickelten sozialistischen Gesellschaft und unter dem Kurs der Einheit von Wirtschafts- und Sozialpolitik (1971–1981)* (Berlin: Interessengemeinschaft Medizin und Gesellschaft, 2002)

Torpey, John C., *Intellectuals, Socialism, and Dissent: The East German Opposition and Its Legacy* (Minneapolis, MN: University of Minnesota Press, 1999)

von Kellenbach, Katharina, *The Mark of Cain: Guilt and Denial in the Post-War Lives of Nazi Perpetrators* (New York: Oxford University Press, 2013)

Wahl, Markus, *"It Would Be Better, If Some Doctors Were Sent to Work in the Coal Mines": The SED and the Medical Intelligentsia Between 1961 and 1981* (New Zealand: University of Canterbury, 2013)

Waibel, Harry, *Diener vieler Herren: Ehemalige NS-Funktionäre in der SBZ/DDR* (Frankfurt a.M.: Lang, 2011)

Weber, Max, *From Max Weber: Essays in Sociology* (London: Routledge, 2009)

Weidner, Tobias, *Die unpolitische Profession: Deutsche Mediziner im langen 19. Jahrhundert* (Frankfurt a.M.: Campus, 2012)

Weil, Francesca, *Zielgruppe Ärzteschaft: Ärzte als inoffizielle Mitarbeiter des Ministeriums für Staatssicherheit* (Göttingen: Vandenhoeck & Ruprecht, 2008)

Weinke, Annette, *Die Verfolgung von NS-Tätern im geteilten Deutschland: Vergangenheitsbewältigung 1949–1969, oder: Eine deutsch-deutsche Beziehungsgeschichte im Kalten Krieg* (Paderborn: Schöningh, 2002)

Wierling, Dorothee, 'Generations and Generational Conflicts in East and West Germany', in *The Divided Past: Rewriting Post-War German History*, ed. by Christoph Klessmann (Oxford: Berg, 2001), pp. 69–89

2   Treatments from the past

Continuities in treating venereal diseases

Introduction

In January 1950, Susan Schneider[1] received a letter from an *Ambulatorium* for STDs in Dresden which stated that she should come to this health clinic immediately. Upon entering the doctor's room, she was told that the result of her smear test came back positive. Confused and anxious, Schneider explained to the doctor the whole story. As her partner got infected with gonorrhoea in Berlin and had received treatment, she wanted to get checked as well. Apparently out of embarrassment, she went to a doctor who was personally known to her partner, asking him for a favour: Walter Korinek, the doctor who has accompanied this book since the introduction.

Korinek agreed and privately tested Schneider for sexually transmitted diseases without any charge. In addition to the three swab tests from his patient, however, he added another one from himself: he must have presumed that he had been infected, not least as it was his swab that came back positive. Due to Korinek's knowledge that this was his test result, he told Schneider truthfully that she was disease-free. However, Dresden's health administration, which registered the positive case under her name, contacted Schneider and told her to come to a clinic immediately, eventually revealing the whole incident.[2] City authorities interrogated Korinek, who admitted his actions. He tried to conceal his own infection in order to avoid his registration as a person suffering from an STD. Against this background, he asked the authorities to delete the entry of Schneider in the STD file "that she does not incur any disadvantages from these [circumstances]", as she never was infected.[3]

In the end, Korinek received only an admonishment, despite the assessment that "in this particular case of a patient [Schneider], [Korinek] could have given a reason to initiate doubt towards the reliability of civic institutions".[4] Therefore, also this incident had no real effect on Korinek's career, even if he circumvented the strict laws and reporting system to curb the spread of venereal diseases in the postwar era. His medical memories and experiences in the form of his acquired skills helped him not only to obtain a job as a doctor, but also to retain high positions due to the lack of specialists. For the patient Schneider, on the contrary, the health administration decided to leave her in the belief that she suffered from gonorrhoea, and, subsequently, she experienced the medical and social treatment of people with STDs, which is illustrated in the following.[5]

In this chapter, I analyse the mentalities, social boundaries, and medical memories and experiences surrounding STDs in postwar East Germany, some of which the entry example already implied. It delineates how the East German population and administrative bodies reacted towards, and dealt with, the war-related STD epidemic. It argues that the smooth transition of greater parts of the medical personnel from the war to postwar era, revealed in Chapter 1, caused the persistence of medical concepts, stigmas, clichés, and languages. Consequently, the management of the postwar STD epidemic reveals significant continuities as well as tacit legacies of medical concepts and mentalities from previous political systems.

This chapter asserts that the medical memories of authorities and doctors shaped peoples' medical experiences in their present, and even the perceptions of their future – their career and personal life. For many people, a sexual infection was followed by alienation and profound medical and state interventions. This medical and social treatment often violated the integrity of individuals.

Therefore, the efforts of East Germany against the STD epidemic indicate that Harsch and Moser's term 'medicalised social hygiene' is applicable for this analysis. By utilising their concept, this chapter offers an important historiographical insight into sexual health during the postwar era in East Germany. However, it also reveals the limitations of their concept for the local level, such as Dresden and Leipzig. Therefore, the following analysis furthers our understanding of the mechanisms of society, memory, mentality, and the emerging 'new socialist state' and their proclaimed 'superior' healthcare system.

The chapter consists of four intertwining sections, which address sexuality and sexual health, the institution of health clinics for STDs, night raids, as well as the state's efforts to combine educational campaigns with the persistent stigmatisation of the STD sufferer to stop the spread of these diseases. The first part of this chapter examines the general situation of sexual health in East Germany in the transition from war to postwar, building on the works of Dagmar Herzog and Jennifer Evans.[6] In addition, the studies of Lesley Hall and Paul Weindling supply the broader context of the first half of the twentieth century.[7] The first section stresses the plurality and simultaneous existence of contradicting sexual mores, which contributed to the postwar perception of the Third Reich as an immoral period. This view was supported by the epidemic spread of STDs, which was part of the general public health crisis in East Germany and across Europe.[8] Therefore, the analysis of postwar sexuality and sexual health proves the continuity of mentalities, in the form of medical memories and experiences of the people, from Weimar to the GDR, which shaped the establishment of a 'new' healthcare system.[9]

After investigating the 'medicalised' response of the state to STDs during the postwar period, the second section focuses on the revival of the Weimar Republic's specialised outpatient health clinics as an example of institutionalised medical memories and experiences. By utilising archival files from Dresden and Leipzig, it discusses the leverage gained by local authorities to implement policies, and thus revealing the limitations of state interventions.

These clinics showed continuity not only in their conceptual framework, but also in their organisational procedures, buildings, and personnel. The experience of people within this institution thus corresponded to this persistent mentality towards patients suffering from STDs. Due to the health crisis, infected people were often deprived of their rights, which would contradict the ethical standards of today.

Therefore, the analysis of these STD health clinics demonstrates that medical memories and experiences had been institutionalised. This hypothesis is supported by the examination of complaints submitted by patients about treatment and the state-granted *Ekelzulage* [disgust-bonus] – an additional monthly payment received by medical personnel for treating 'disgusting' STDs and other skin diseases from 1953 onwards.

For all sections – but especially for the third – Harsch's study offers a valuable source of comparison with Tbc, the disease that caused the most deaths during the postwar era.[10] In the case of both STDs and Tbc, East Germany executed immense state interventions, not solely limited to the premises of health institutions, but also into people's everyday lives. Consequently, the third section examines the night raids carried out by health workers and the police forces. These raids targeted bars, nightclubs, and hotels to find the so-called 'promiscuous individuals' who were suspected of suffering from STDs.

The terminology employed needs to undergo a deeper analysis as labels such as prostitutes, 'clandestine prostitutes', and individuals 'with frequent promiscuous behaviour' were blurred, open to interpretation, and enforced differently. Their implementation often depended on the locality – the people in charge, as investigated in Chapter 1 – and was subject to continuous change. Moreover, these categories suggest that the health authorities' main target was women, whereas the role of males in the process of spreading STDs was neglected.

Therefore, the section concludes that medical experiences in people's everyday lives were highly dependent on gender, social status, and reputation within the local community. Particularly at this community level, the policies introduced, as well as the mentalities and stigmatisations enforced, suggest that the East German authorities intentionally created a system of denunciation. Evidence for this claim was found in personal petitions, subsequent reactions of local and state officials, as well as changes in policies, language, and terminology over time.

The concluding section merges the discussed themes of stigmatisation and education to argue that moralising campaigns combined with public awareness programmes about sexual health were used to accelerate the elimination of the STD epidemic. For this purpose, the section elucidates these often contradictory strategies by examining exhibitions and educational campaigns organised by the German Hygiene Museum in Dresden. It asserts that after years of silence regarding sexual health, there was a shift towards an open discourse about venereal diseases intended not only in East Germany, but also in various other countries. In the immediate postwar era, the attendance of exhibitions and lectures about sexual health suggest a high interest and demand among the population. Conversely, a persistent and even state-supported stigmatisation survived despite all educational efforts, which influenced policy-making locally and nationally. This twofold strategy of stigmatisation and education resulted in both an accelerated decline of STD cases, as well as unique medical experiences of patients with STDs, according to their societal judgement.

The overall purpose of this chapter is to show the impact of medical memories and experiences on the development of mentalities and policies towards the patient, exemplified by the issue of sexual health in the postwar period. As indicated in the introduction, it argues that East German health concepts and ideas were mainly taken from the Weimar Republic and social hygienic movements, rather than dictated by the Soviet occupation authorities. Furthermore, the use of official language reveals the continuity of the Third Reich in the medical and social treatment of patients suffering from STDs, a fact which was valid not only for East Germany, but also for all German-speaking countries.[11] Therefore, the chapter exposes the significance of the nuances and diverse medical experiences of people with STDs, which depended on the locality, officials, and medical personnel in charge, as well as the individual's reputation and social surroundings: a contribution to the 'grassroots' historiography of recent GDR scholarship.[12]

Shaping memory through experience: the official narrative of sexual activity and health from war to postwar

At the beginning of 1940, the City Police Department of Dresden complained about 'used' contraceptives littering the outer suburbs, forests, and the vicinity of military institutions. The authorities were particularly concerned, as these means were seen as a risk of infection if children unconsciously played with them.[13]

> The case of a 10-year-old child, infected with gonorrhoea [. . .] gave cause for me to stress again that on the forest edges, especially near military barracks and the city in general, used means of protection were left lying around or even hung up on the fences, shrubs and trees.[14]

This statement alone challenges the hypothesis that sexual prudery, vast sexual restrictions, and an ascribed silence around STDs were characteristic for the Third Reich. Instead, this section argues in accordance with Evans and Herzog that sexual mentalities demonstrate continuity in attitudes that were resilient to any supposed significant turning points in history.[15]

Social definitions of 'abnormality' are in no other area as moralised as for the subjects of sexuality, sexual health, and relationships. 'Normal behaviour', as analysed by Goffman, is, however, dependent on the societal context and period.[16] The resulting classification and stigmatisation of people at the margins of society were part of identification and legitimation procedures for the state narrative, demarcating, in this case, the 'normal' from the 'abnormal'. Similarly, labelling people as 'promiscuous' was in the state's interest to curb the STD epidemic. Therefore, this section sets up the basis for analysing medical memories and experiences of the medical profession, patients, and population with these diseases, by investigating the state narrative, derived from its medical memories, surrounding the recognised public health predicament.

In retrospect, Wolfgang Höfs claimed in his paper from 1952 that "[t]he wreckage of the Second World War extends to that area of interpersonal relationships where these are realised most frequently [. . .] namely to that of sexual life".[17] During his time as the Head of a Marriage and Sexual Counselling Centre for Men at the University Hospital in Leipzig, Höfs observed that – apart from the mental burden of war-related injuries – many 'unharmed' men were psychologically affected in a similar way. The examination of both groups, he continued, showed "that the psychologically induced sexual dysfunction evidently increased after the war".[18] However, according to Höfs' conclusion, not only did these mental conditions have a limiting effect on their sexual life, but they also caused the total opposite: people "also drifted into *Haltlosigkeit* [promiscuity], occasionally or partly continually" – meaning that some individuals reacted with a raised libido to their war experiences and pursued a 'sexually deviant behaviour'.[19]

In his account, Höfs emphasised medical, sexual, as well as social issues deriving from war; others, however, attributed the observed 'uninhibited' sexual activity to an overall immorality during the Nazi era, which was the more common narrative for East German officials in the postwar period.[20] The Head of the STDs Department at the DZVGW Max Klesse, for example, claimed that after Hitler came to power in 1933, people's 'normal sexual behaviour' had begun to dissolve. He stated that due to rearmament "[h]undreds of thousands of young married couples [were] disrupted; millions of young men [were] forced together in the military barracks, labour camps and for the construction of the strategic *Autobahnen*, and [thus] estranged from their normal relations".[21] Whether deliberately or not, Klesse did not only point to an increased 'promiscuous behaviour' in general, but also alluded to 'homoerotic spheres' during the Nazi period. The two statements of Höfs and Klesse challenge the commonly held opinion – widespread and dominant until the turn of the twenty-first century – that the Third Reich was strictly conservative in sexual matters, and that procreation regulations were purposefully applied only to serve their aim of racial superiority and Aryan domination of the world.[22]

Nonetheless, accepting the notion of sexual pleasure was, according to Herzog, part of the Third Reich as well, even if only for 'state-approved human beings'. By referring to a Nazi doctor who estimated an average use of 72 million condoms per year and stressed the problematic rise of premarital sex among the youth, Herzog illustrates that the limited view of Nazi policies towards 'reproduction' of Aryan families is untenable.[23]

Nazi Germany simultaneously enforced procreation and repressed promiscuity, while supporting sexual pleasure. Opinions were polarised between progressive and conservative sexual mores within the party, the church, and the population.[24] Therefore, by referring to the theories of Michel Foucault, Herzog reveals that facilitating the positive effects of experiencing pleasure consolidated Nazi power – especially by promoting pre-, intra-, and extramarital sex.[25] Sexual pleasure and satisfaction heightened the morale and loyalty to the *Führer*, which often contradicted the aim to break down the Weimar Republic's sexual legacy.

The purposeful utilisation of sex to strengthen personal ties to the regime, on the one hand, and the experience of sexual pleasure, on the other, may appear as contradictory. However, the Nazis offered a broad state narrative of sexual activity by defining sexual freedom and restriction according to race, moral views, and personal desires, and thus opportunities for the individual and mnemonic communities to assimilate with the regime. This conduct has been described as one of the most important reasons for Hitler's popularity in the recent literature.[26]

The heterogeneous nature of the narrative created by the Third Reich regarding the sexualities of various people with diverse ethnic or class backgrounds and the subsequent medical experiences of individuals had an impact on postwar mentalities and attitudes. This starting point is used for investigating the statistics of, and reasons for, the epidemic spread of STDs, which forms the basis for analysing the narrative and responses of state or local authorities. The resulting policies shaped the medical memories and experiences of the patients suffering from STDs within and outside health clinics.

Klesse's historical overview and report on venereal diseases in postwar East Germany concluded by stating that "[w]ar and commerce were, in the past as well as today, the *Schrittmacher* [pacemaker] of STDs".[27] In his statement, Klesse identified two reasons for the increase of STDs: war and the resulting displacement of people, especially caused by bombardment, battle, incarceration, expulsion, and resettlement.[28] However, these social issues and the rapid rise of venereal diseases were never a unique SBZ problem, and thus a comparison with the West Zone is essential to contextualise the analysis.

In Lower Saxony in the British Occupied Zone of Germany, for example, a report of the State Ministry of Labour, Rebuilding, and Health from 1948 also attributed the increase of STD cases to the "social disruption" of their population:[29]

> The 15- to 30-year-olds of the fluctuating population are the best breeding ground [for STD infections], regardless of whether or not the rootlessness of the population was or is caused by expulsion, escape, bombing, hunger, unemployment, or unwanted work commitments.[30]

The report concluded that these parts of the population had to find a residence first in order to register and effectively treat the STDs – consequently, they urged stricter regulations against the roving parts of the population.[31]

All occupied zones in Germany suffered from similar problems. East and West officials targeted immorality and promiscuity, which were supposedly prevalent among their respective populations. The official East German explanation for the low STD infections in February reveals this prejudice by stating that "the persisting cold weather back then [resulted in] fewer opportunities for outdoor, extramarital sex".[32] By contrast, authorities feared the summer and especially the spring seasons for their rise of 'sexually deviant behaviour', emphasising that issue in numerous reports.[33]

Pre- and extramarital sex remained highly stigmatised and was seen as a danger to society – a conclusion from which the state derived its right to intrude on the private spheres of its citizens. Nonetheless, as Hall similarly analyses for the UK, it was the qualitative judgement, rather than the quantitative amount of sexual activity, which changed during the 1940s: in the same way as in the SBZ, moralised judgements were the reaction of the state narrative towards a palpable and dangerous increase of STDs in the postwar UK.[34]

The threat of STDs and the reason for the subsequent reaction of health officials can be found in the age distribution of new infection cases.[35] Figure 2.1 shows that the age cohort of over 25-year-olds was the largest group which suffered from STDs in 1948. However, this fact has to be qualified as this group made up the largest part of the population. Therefore, their morbidity was relatively low, compared to the nearly 40 per cent of all new STD cases that occurred in 18- to 25-year-olds in Saxony in 1948 (Figure 2.1) – a development which authorities recognised as the biggest issue for the public health of the future generation.

It appears more threatening when considering the changed demography of postwar East Germany. War ensured that especially the numbers of men, but also of women, of this age group were significantly reduced during this conflict. The result was that STDs were disproportionally widespread within this cohort, which led to a high risk for their members to get infected.[36] Consequently, the state narrative targeted adolescents, suggesting that they were the most morally 'uprooted' and 'socially deviant' people in the period following the Third Reich. However, the new East German state also needed to rely on this generation for its legitimisation and construction. Therefore, authorities implemented policies for medically and socially controlling this generation in order to 'lead' them to 'the right path of Socialism': a reoccurring theme in this chapter, as well as Chapter 3.

Calculated from the overall percentage of new STD infections, the annual report of 1948 illuminated that for the over 18-year-olds 52 per cent were single, 37 per cent were married, and 11 per cent were separated or divorced.[37] This statistic also quantified that from these STD cases, only 17.5 per cent acquired their disease through marital sex; most transmissions (72.6 per cent) occurred pre- or

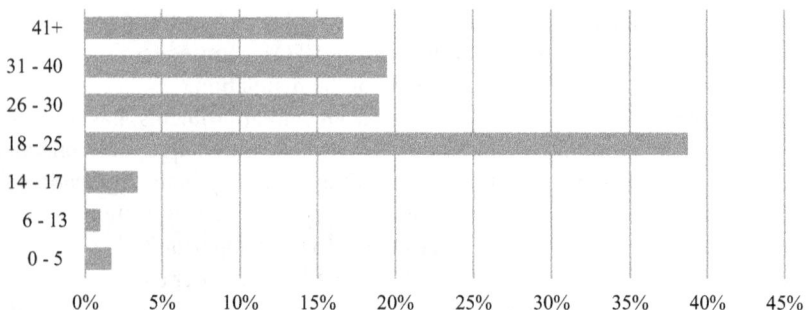

Figure 2.1 Age distribution of new STD cases in Saxony in 1948

Source: BArch, DQ 1/5440, Bl. 174–218.

extramarital with 'well known' or 'casual' contacts. By contrast, only 17 cases were registered in the Saxon statistics in 1948, in which a prostitute was supposedly the source of infection.[38] This low number contradicts the common view among the authorities that 'prostitutes' were the main problem for the STD epidemic, and thus challenges the policies implemented and stigmatisation enforced towards this group. However, the possibility that 'prostitutes' were hidden in the 'casual contacts' category is quite tenable, as people tried to avoid disclosing paying for sexual intercourse. As a result, the category of 'casual contacts' led the official narrative to the second main target: the 'frequently promiscuously behaving' person – findings that need further consideration in the following sections.

Continuing the analysis of Figure 2.1, the numbers of the group of the under 17-year-olds cannot be explained by an increase in 'immoral' sexual activity among adolescents alone. However, the state narrative mostly facilitated this argument that the youth's behaviour was the cause of the high STD infection rates among this group. Evaluating the statistics, the registered cases of birth and possible 'smear' infections are insufficient for justifying the total of 257 cases in the age group of the 0- to 5-year-olds and 149 in the 6- to 13-year-olds, especially as the reports provided proof for only 37 infections by birth.[39] Evans also refers to a case in postwar West Berlin where a 4-year-old boy developed an STD after he was raped by American soldiers. However, the occupiers never faced prosecution – the boy and his parents had to live with this incidence, without official support.[40] Consequently, behind these statistics, the concealed sexual abuse of minors by contemporaries is hidden and became part of 'war children's' medical war experiences, investigated in Chapter 3.

The analysis of the transition from war to postwar has illustrated that interpretations of sexuality and the connection with the STD epidemic in purely 'conservative' and 'repressive' terms appear untenable. As identified for the Third Reich, pre- and extramarital sex was common and partly encouraged by the regime due to its power-securing intentions. With the beginning of the Second World War, the Nazis established, for example, state-run brothels for the *Wehrmacht* to strengthen soldiers' battle morale. However, they also built similar facilities for forced foreign labour, and even for concentration camp prisoners. According to Timm, the Nazis' motivation was purely strategic: a sexually satisfied inmate or worker would be more productive for the Reich.[41] In the postwar years, health authorities continuously targeted prostitution – a so-called social hygienic burden of the 'old class system and bourgeois society'.[42]

In general, the quantity of sexual intercourse hardly changed with the end of the war. The change occurred in the qualitative judgement, here in the form of a state narrative of the nascent East German nation. Therefore, the so-called 'promiscuity' of adolescents, unmarried, and married people was a nuisance to, and thus constantly policed by, social and healthcare officials. In the case of Saxony, the local level analysis has revealed not only a widespread 'deviance' in sexual activity, but also some traits of sexual violence against minors. An acquired STD was often the only sign of sexual abuse, but was hardly registered as such by authorities in the postwar period. By contrast, a repeatedly addressed issue was the disproportionally high infiltration of STDs into the most fertile cohort of the population: the 18- to 25-year-olds. Due to this fact, East German authorities tried to push for a more conservative attitude and narrative towards sex, which initially propagated 'early marriage' and condemned any 'abnormality' as a Third Reich legacy and blamed it upon their lack of morality.[43] These arguments and the discussed statistics prove that medical memories significantly influenced the reaction of the state, which was reflected in the medical experiences of patients with the new postwar East German healthcare system and its institutions, for example, the *Ambulatorium*.

Institutionalised medical memories and experiences: the revival of *Ambulatorien*

The Head of the STD Department at the DZVGW, Klesse proclaimed in 1946 that "[t]he hitherto existing medical confidentiality has been restricted in this area because higher state interests and the welfare of others are at stake".[44] With this statement, Klesse basically justified that state interventions could not respect the borders of the private sphere in postwar East Germany – in particular if someone was suspected of having an STD. In the name of preserving public health, the state felt compelled and concurrently allowed to restrict individual liberties. Klesse's statement and the preceding section have shown the relation between the recognition of a predicament – the STD epidemic – and the implementation of forced and compulsory measures, such as hospitalisation and institutionalisation, which shaped the state narrative. This dualism, consisting of policies that intruded upon people's privacy, was considered a requirement for successfully curbing the continuous spread of the diseases.

At the conference of state venereologists in July 1946, the President of the DZVGW Paul Konitzer – discussed in Chapter 1 – agreed with Klesse's arguments. He called for more responsibility among doctors in the 'fight' against STDs in the sharpest tones:

> [The SMAD Command 030] means for you [here, addressing doctors responsible for curbing the STDs] the *most serious duty of your life*. There will be no further command, but there will be punishments, and in fact very resolute punishments. *I warn you! Take the command as seriously as possible* [emphasis as in the original, M.W.].[45]

Konitzer made clear to his colleagues that the process of implementing the Command 030 was comprehensively monitored by the SMAD: from the DZVGW director down to the provincial physician. The emphasis of their orders rested on fighting bureaucracy and introducing a far-reaching system of medical and social control.[46] Therefore, this section illustrates how the SMAD Commands, the East German state narrative, as well as central and local health authorities, such as Konitzer, Linser, or Klesse, and their medical memories shaped the resurrection of a health clinic that was set up to contain the STD epidemic in the postwar era. The emergence of this institution was a conscious continuity of the Weimar Republic. However, the investigation into this clinic also reveals legacies of the Third Reich, especially in regards to the use of language. The latter was partly due to the ability of medical personnel to continue their practice after 1945, as shown in Chapter 1, on the local level, which staffed this health institution and subsequently influenced the medical experiences of the patients as well.

Based on the SMAD order 25 from August 1945,[47] local authorities in Dresden decreed that the prophylaxis, diagnosis, as well as actual treatment of STDs "ha[d] to be carried out *initially regardless of costs* by every institution [emphasis as in the original, M.W.]", indicating that health officials were well aware of the predicament.[48] Moreover, they implemented laws that every patient with an STD had to be hospitalised and that doctors, patients, and the population as a whole had to be punished if they did not comply with the regulations. However, these initial orders were quickly identified to be insufficient, as German authorities, as well as medical professionals, proved to be reluctant partners to the SMAD. Six months after their initial orders, the Soviet officials complained that hospitalisation, investigating sources of infection, and especially the "fight against prostitution, as the fundamental cause for all STDs" were nonexistent. Therefore, the SMAD issued Command 030 in February, as well as Secret Order 0194 in July 1946, which would shape the medical landscape for the following years.

By enforcing a comprehensive 'combat' against STDs, the SMAD instructed that all local health authorities had to significantly expand the number of centres for educating, preventing, diagnosing, and treating STDs until March 1946.[49] Their use of words or phrases like "the comprehensive fight to defend the metropolitan area of Dresden" against STDs, in the official language, suggests a militaristic approach towards containing epidemics.[50] However, the postwar era showed not only a continuity of warfare language, especially regarding contagious diseases, but also a continuity of Weimar Republic and Third Reich medical concepts and descriptions of patients – a legacy in the form of medical memories and mentalities within the postwar East German society.[51]

Based on Command 030, the Soviet Commander of the SMAS, General Dubrovsky, released a state-specific decree at the end of February 1946. Apart from similar formulations as in the SMAD Command, Dubrovsky mainly attacked private practitioners in the Saxon state. According to him, they would "need for diagnosing an inadmissibly long time", and "bear no responsibility for the measures to fight diseases and carry out an adequate treatment".[52] Therefore, state health authorities were required to monitor private practitioners and control the accuracy of their work. Furthermore, to fulfil Dubrovsky's order to increase health clinics in rural areas, private practitioners were also obliged to work at least 4 hours in outpatient or inpatient STD institutions.[53]

Due to the large number of buildings destroyed or damaged in postwar Dresden, local officials instructed that "[p]rivate clinics of Dermatology and STD specialists and if necessary also those of GPs should be seized for this purpose" to fulfil Dubrovsky's request.[54] This procedure was tantamount to a nationalisation under the disguise of the STD epidemic. The reason why private practitioners faced these multifaceted restrictions and interventions into their practice was not only that the SMAD and the East German health officials favoured a state-run healthcare system, but also partly due to the medical memories of the East German state and the individual doctor: almost two-thirds of the private practitioners in Saxony during the Third Reich were members of the NSDAP or other Nazi organisations.[55] As a result, the East German state aimed to eliminate private clinics and create an entirely state-run healthcare system as early as 1946 – however, the GDR saw itself forced to apply a pragmatic de-Nazification and grant concessions, not least due to the constant drain of doctors to West Germany until the construction of the wall in 1961.[56]

Following the introduction of a state healthcare system, SMAS Order 64 from the beginning of March 1946 determined that every district had to establish health clinics for STDs, providing a comprehensive network throughout Saxony.[57] These medical institutions quickly became the focal point for all efforts to curb STDs in the postwar era. Their tasks included the treatment, counselling, prevention, aftercare, as well as comprehensive monitoring and reporting of cases.[58]

"*Ambulatorien* [health clinics] [is a] better name than *Beratungs- und Behandlungsstellen* [counselling and treatment centres]", remarked Konitzer in an extended board meeting at the DZVGW in June 1946.[59] Consequently, East German, and not SMAD, health authorities decided to revive *Ambulatorien*. Together with the other outpatient institute – the *Poliklinik* [polyclinic][60] – these types were nothing but new versions of an old concept: they were a conscious emphasis of the social and socialist hygiene legacies, partly realised in the Weimar Republic.[61] Therefore, the implementation of the health officials' medical memories into postwar East Germany shows their agency and contests the historiographical view of a pure dictation by Moscow.[62] For the SBZ and later the GDR, *Ambulatorien* were one important part of the free and universally accessible outpatient, state-run healthcare system. Health authorities established a separate clinic not only for STDs but also for Tbc, which was a novel feature of the Weimar Republic and yet was introduced to East Germany.[63]

To fulfil the manifold responsibilities of the *Ambulatorium*, health officials emphasised the work of *Fürsorgerinnen* [female carers and nurses], who were mainly entrusted with social hygiene tasks, such as caring for, and observing, patients, as well as carrying out administrative tasks. Apparent here is the desired shift of roles and competencies within the traditional hierarchies in clinics, which were often in conflict with the engraved institutional memories. However, compared to the FRG and previous periods, nurses gained a higher status within the provision of healthcare in the GDR, which was also reflected in their addition to the so-called 'doctor–nurse–patient relationship'.[64] State health officials, for example, showed their continuous appreciation of *Fürsorgerinnen* by introducing the so-called *Ekelzulage* [disgust-bonus] in August 1953. The GDR created this 'hardship allowance' for its medical personnel in the dermatology and STD institutes for the duration of 'nauseating work'.[65] However, apart from the state's appreciation of work carried out by its health personnel, this example exposes the mentalities towards people with skin diseases, and, especially, venereal diseases.

Therefore, the research of this type of medical institution offers some insight into the perception of individuals involved in the debates surrounding the medical and social treatment of STD patients. Already after the establishment of the health centres in 1946, some health officials voiced their discontent with the special clinics for STDs. They argued that *Ambulatorien* were "too public", infringing upon the intimacy and trusting atmosphere of the doctor's examination room.[66] Authorities recognised people's fears that visiting these clinics often resulted in the stigmatisation of the individual. The entry to the institutional space of the *Ambulatorium* signalled to the social environment that one might be 'promiscuous' and was thus accompanied with a danger of being 'shamefully' treated by others.[67]

Therefore, state and local officials intended to merge *Ambulatorien* into existing *Polikliniken* as one of their sub-departments to reduce the reluctance of patients to attend the STD clinic. However, the DZVGW argued that it was:

> not advisable to carry out the examinations, or possibly the police summoning, of promiscuous people in the polyclinic's premises. This certainly leads to objections of other patients who thereby are prevented from attending the outpatient clinic.[68]

This DZVGW statement immediately lends credence to the finding that contemporaries viewed people with STDs and the 'promiscuous' as public nuisances. Furthermore, it exemplifies the lack of anonymity – an essential prerequisite for the treatment of moralised diseases like STDs – and thus the disrespect of people's private sphere in these health institutions that shaped the medical experience of the individual patient within this clinic.

Nonetheless, after the GDR was founded, the state revisited the plan to integrate the health clinic for STDs into the polyclinic for financial reasons.[69] In particular, Saxony was in favour of this "because then the well-known and notorious name *Ambulatorium* would be omitted, which often gives cause for complaints".[70] The institution gained a bad reputation among the local population not least because of the mentioned organisational problems, and thus local authorities sought to rebrand the institution to disguise its medical memories and experiences.

The mentality and apparent treatment which patients experienced within these specialised institutes were an important reason for people's critical perceptions towards *Ambulatorien*. Already in September 1946, the city health department approached all health clinics for STDs in Dresden on this matter. By referring to numerous complaints by the local community, they stressed:

> that also the treatment of patients in the STD clinics and *Ambulatorien* has to be done in a way, which otherwise is common in hospitals as well. It has to be especially avoided that a *Polizei- und Kasernenton* [police and military tone] gains the upper hand while dealing with patients. We cannot forget, that we as doctors are facing patients. This, however, does not exclude that we in cases, in which we have to rely on force, indeed take drastic measures.[71]

This letter illustrates that patients in these institutions had adverse medical experiences. Not only within the population but also within these specialised clinics, patients with STDs faced stigmatisation, and doctors and nurses treated them as such.

Moreover, this was not a singular case in the local sphere of Dresden. The exposed mentality here that patients suffering from an STD were not regarded and treated as 'normal' patients with, for example, a cold was rather a common issue throughout the SBZ and later the GDR. In a meeting in March 1950 in the new Ministry of Labour and Healthcare, state health officials stressed "that the term *'Ambulatorium'* is not bearable anymore because the word alone evokes inhibitions among patients".[72] Therefore, they planned to 'camouflage' these special clinics and suggested to integrate them as departments of dermatology into hospitals. The recognised issues with the STD clinic's name resulted in its change in Dresden in July 1952 – from *Ambulatorien für Haut- und Geschlechtskrankheiten* to simply *Hautabteilung*, consciously avoiding STDs in the title.[73]

As this section has shown, the short life of the *Ambulatorien* for STDs between 1946 and 1952 was accompanied by organisational issues and questionable legacies from the past. Even if proposed and officially treated as such, these institutions were never the predominant form of STD clinics at any stage. The main burden was put on the shoulders of the numerous private practitioners who were restricted in their practice. Their premises were forcefully utilised by the state, and private doctors were compelled to undertake additional work in the state health sector from 1946 onwards.[74] Therefore, the example of curbing STDs exposed the struggle in the postwar years between and within local and central government bodies, between city officials, private and state doctors, and local health authorities, as well as the population and the new healthcare system – especially over the medical memories and experiences institutionalised in the *Ambulatorium*. In many respects, however, the reaction of the state and the population failed to end the taboo topic – acknowledging the possibility of acquiring sexually transmitted diseases – and thus to overcome the stigmatisation of STD sufferers.

This section has identified how the medical memories of health officials, doctors, nurses, and the population shaped the medical experience of patients suffering from STDs when attending specialised *Ambulatorien*. However, the uncovered mentalities were not limited to the institutional boundaries of a certain building, space, and place, but revealed themselves even more outside of these health clinics, discussed in the following section.

Experiencing medical memories: policing sources of infection

"The population probably still perceives the [STD] bureau as a prosecuting authority, which with its measures could apparently be a hindrance or even harmful to the sick person's private and work life for many years to come", stated the Dresden STD Department in its annual report of 1947.[75] This proves that people's behaviour and their perception of postwar medical institutions were a concern of the state as early as 1948.[76] This finding stands in contrast to Harsch's claim that patients' moods in East Germany were not analysed until 1963. However, if not in a psychological-analytical way, state departments had to ask themselves why people were reluctant to visit the previously discussed *Ambulatorien*. The case of Dresden reveals that health officials were aware of the necessary popular support to successfully curb STDs. They urged educational campaigns and exhibitions, thereby addressing people's fears of being "registered with the office [. . .] as well as [of being] forcefully hospitalised".[77] Nevertheless, health officials hastily stigmatised people as 'asocial' rather than studying the social and psychological background of their reluctant behaviour. The example shows, however, that the mood and perception of the 'ordinary' patient had to be considered if authorities sought to sell the new socialist healthcare system to the people – not least to convince them of the necessity of restricting personal liberty and applying forceful public health policies.

This section looks at the mentalities palpable in policing potential STD patients in postwar East Germany by discussing the arrival of Penicillin, the *Aktivausschuss* [Committee of Action], and the nightly raids in bars and clubs to find sources of infection. People's fears that these measures intruded upon their private sphere were a realistic perception. In January 1947, the Saxon STD Department reported 326 police-enforced admissions to hospitals or health clinics, as well as 38 punishments "due to the negligent spread of an STD".[78]

I argue that the department reinforced a widespread system of denunciation among the population that health officials viewed as a welcome support for their efforts to contain venereal diseases. It is shown that the authorities used the medical memories of STDs, in the form of persistent, out-dated medical concepts and mentalities, in order to prevent 'promiscuity'. In turn, the application of intrusive methods shaped the medical experience of patients, which, however, resulted in a rise in criticism of the state and subsequently increased their reluctance to consult doctors or seek medical treatment.

Additionally, the institutionalised and internalised medical memories, as illustrated for the space and personnel of the *Ambulatorium*, had an impact on the private and work life of an individual that influenced his or her prospects. The last point links the opening statement to the main analysis, and leads to the hypothesis of an extended monitoring, patronising, and reporting system, particular for the efforts to curb STDs, in comparison to previous political systems – not least, due to the continuity of medical personnel at the local level from the Third Reich into postwar East Germany, as introduced in Chapter 1.

However, these developments were embedded in the international context and in line with other, non-socialist countries. Therefore, the contextualisation of using force against, and the stigmatising of, people suffering from an STD reveals the persistence of views and mentalities believed to be obsolete. As Harsch concludes for Tbc, the forceful measures against, and the restricted personal freedoms of, Tbc patients did not become a subject of criticism or agitation in the struggle between the Cold War parties.[79] Consequently, this section illustrates people's everyday experience caused by the medical memories in the form of local efforts to curb STDs inside and outside of the *Ambulatorium* in postwar East Germany.

In the GDR, the advancement of medicine in the area of STDs was seen as a threat – a danger for the fundamental social hygienic concepts: educating, reporting, and monitoring.[80] Doris Foitzik shows for Hamburg that Penicillin had been sufficiently available for treating STDs since 1946, but it was not broadly available in East Germany until the beginning of the 1950s due to an insufficient pharmaceutical industry.[81] As most of the pharmacy industry was located in West Germany after the war, the GDR had to import 90 per cent of drugs from the West in 1949.[82]

However, the introduction of Penicillin as standard therapy for STDs was not always welcomed. At the conference of county doctors in October 1953, Dresden's *Bezirksvenerologe* [County Venereologist] Hörig – who was simultaneously the Medical Director of the *Fürsorgeheim Leuben* [Care Home Leuben] – emphasised that, owing to Penicillin, gonorrhoea had "lost much of its scare".[83] He criticised his colleagues' optimism and belief that STDs were a matter of the past due to the new drug. By contrast, Hörig argued that the easy curability resulted in increased levity and the renewed growth of fresh STD infections. Therefore, he concluded, the one-day outpatient treatment with Penicillin was insufficient.[84]

At the conference of district venereologists in 1951, Hörig's views were shared by others, such as a doctor who proudly remarked that no 'promiscuity' occurred in his area, and no forceful measures were necessary. His patients "beware of acquiring another STD" due to the differentiated application of treatment. Patients whom this doctor suspected to be 'promiscuous' did not receive Penicillin, but the old, more dangerous, painful, and prolonged treatment with (Neo-)Salvarsan, as well as Bismuth and Mercury preparations: a deterrent lesson with an out-dated medical treatment.[85] This ethically questionable and ultimately arbitrary application – using a medical treatment as punishment or deterrent for assumed 'promiscuous behaviour' – was, however, widespread in the GDR, even if challenged at the state level.[86]

As a result, patients with STDs had entirely different medical experiences with the healthcare system than people with the flu in the postwar era. Especially, where medical memories of previous systems prevailed, patients potentially faced far-reaching interventions into their rights, as well as harmful treatments, despite the fact that a simplified therapy was readily available and commonly used. The rumours of these procedures resulted in people's reluctance and criticism of not only the therapy's arbitrariness in particular, but also the obligation to hospitalise in general.

The questionable treatment, however, was also based on the blurry categories of the East German state for identifying the 'promiscuous'. The category of prostitutes, for example, was the main target for curbing STDs – an approach common throughout Europe in the nineteenth and twentieth centuries.[87] As Klesse recognised in his report from 1946, in the past "the regulations targeted only the [female] seller but not the customer of sexual pleasure, which partly resulted in corruption and acts of caprice".[88] However, the proclaimed shift to 'de-gender' the medical concept of STDs – even if engraved into policies – hardly occurred either locally or nationally.

The issue was that, on the one side, the people in charge of policing suspected STD cases in the local area were often the same as before 1945.[89] On the other hand, many state authorities also maintained the mentality and narrative that women were the main source of infection – thereby preventing a fundamental change in this regard.[90] Facing the remnants of previous systems in the form of medical and social treatment, real and suspected prostitutes often escaped to an unknown residence, hid from health authorities, or fled to the West.[91] The latter, however, did not change their situation, as the policies against prostitution were as restrictive in West Germany as in the East.[92]

Another category of people which East German officials saw as much as a threat for spreading STDs as prostitutes was the so-called person with *häufig wech-selnden Geschlechtsverkehr/-partner* [frequent promiscuous behaviour – hwG] – a term that was already in use in the Third Reich and was common in West Germany as well.[93] As authorities established a list not only of (suspected) prostitutes, but also of (suspected) hwG people, their medical experiences with the healthcare system were similar – especially regarding the restriction of personal rights and liberties. However, neither before 1945 nor during the postwar period existed a clear, nationwide definition of this category, a fact that led to highly diverse and arbitrary interpretations, but also false denunciations, and ultimately variegated the medical experiences of patients in different parts of East Germany.[94]

The SMAD Secret Command 0194 from 1946 required that a so-called *Akti-vausschuss* [Committee of Action] had to be established in every district to manage the hwG list. This committee was composed of members from the SED, bloc-parties, FDGB, FDJ, medical and teaching professions, as well as other state and political authorities, and thus was intended to be a cross-section of the socialist society – similar to the de-Nazification committees in every district.[95] In their monthly conventions, the *Aktivausschuss* determined which person had to be included or released from the list – a decision that decided whether or not someone would be under medical and social surveillance. New 'entries' were informed that they had to appear in the *Ambulatorium* for a weekly medical check-up from this date onwards. In cases in which the people did not follow this instruction, they were picked up by the police and forcibly brought to the health clinic. Secondly, if the STD test was positive, they immediately faced institutionalisation because they were deemed to be 'lingering', 'idle', and 'asocial elements'.[96]

The protocol of a meeting of the *Aktivausschuss* in a small town near Dresden in summer 1948 reveals that these committees possessed a far-reaching authority over suspected 'promiscuously behaving' people. In this session, all hwG individuals of this area were discussed, and it was decided who could be released from the list. However, committee members suggested new cases as well: two women "who supposedly perform a very striking change of their moral conduct" and whom "the criminal police are instructed to observe inconspicuously [. . .] for four weeks and report more details at the next meeting".[97] Furthermore, they discussed a single case of a 'promiscuous' woman, who was punished with blocking her ration card due to her refusal to work, and complained about her disappearance.[98]

Considering the meeting's procedure, this committee represented a fulfilment of social hygienic dreams. It did not only have authority over police actions and decided who had to be put under medical and social control, but also cooperated with the *Ambulatorien*, social, welfare, and judicial offices. In the case of a person disobeying their orders, these committees invaded every part of a person's life in the name of 'protecting society from the individual'. Consequently, the delegates decided over the fate of patients within the healthcare system – and with this, they defined their medical experiences.

Not least, with the established authority of the *Aktivausschuss*, a 'denunciation system' was created. Its arbitrariness and often personally motivated 'blackmailing' of people went so far that East German authorities realised in 1948 that these committees had escalated out of control: they admitted that, in many cases, "the term 'hwG-person' is probably assigned due to a too premature judgment".[99] To avoid these issues in the future, they sought to introduce guidelines, targeting "only the actual hwG-behaving people in the sense of clandestine prostitution" – meaning unregistered and 'part-time' prostitutes.[100] The situation report of Saxony from 1949, however, revealed the failure of the state intervention, not least, as the categories hwG person, 'clandestine prostitute', and 'real prostitute' overlapped and were insufficient in their definition. In this document, authorities spoke of 5,000 registered hwG-people in Saxony, 1,000 of which had been infected twice or more with an STD. This large number of people, who were caught in the medical and social monitoring systems of Saxony, made even the recipient, a state official, comment in disbelief: "?? Is this number correct?[sic]"[101]

In comparison, in January 1947 the Saxon health authorities reported to the SMAD a number of 124 prostitutes and 3,123 hwG people, composed of 153 men and 2,970 women.[102] A similar distribution can be found in succeeding reports, which proves that a decrease of denounced hwG individuals after the state intervention did not occur. Furthermore, while considering the surplus of the female population after the war, this distorted distribution exposes the biased implementation of the strict rules for curbing STDs, especially as most targeted men were the similar publicly targeted gays and so-called *Stricher* [rent-boys], rather than heterosexual males.[103]

These prolonged debates about terminology and subsequent punishments for people identified as 'promiscuous' expose the resistance of mentalities to shifts towards an equal understanding of sexual partners.[104] Their equal share of fault in the case of an infection, and a 'de-gendering' of STDs as a medical concept, did not occur – a continuity of medical memories of the past, and the subsequent medical experiences of patients in their present. Despite policies targeting both genders since 1946,[105] in reality, mainly the female participant of sexual acts faced – if infected with an STD and viewed as potentially 'promiscuous' – hospitalisation and eventual institutionalisation, even during the 1950s.[106]

Furthermore, blurred terminology supported a system of denunciation within society – as the category of being 'promiscuous' often depended on someone's social status, reputation among the community, party affiliation, and especially gossip – which was created with the intention to enhance preventative efforts, especially in the rural but also in the urban areas. As far as the archival files reveal, most of the stigmatised women belonged to the lower classes, those without regular income, who were often homeless, and without any close relatives. Therefore, the SMAD and the East German officials sought to police these women by night to curb not only STDs, but also 'social deviance'.

In the SBZ and in the West of occupied Germany, authorities relied on the execution of raids in the nightlife of their cities to support efforts to find sources of infections. Initially introduced by the occupation powers in both zones, West German authorities halted this measure in June 1947.[107] By contrast, East Germany continued raids far into the 1950s, but their efficiency and their outcomes caused concerns among SBZ health officials as early as 1945. In Dresden, for example, they made 66 raids in the year 1947, during which an overall number of 1,844 individuals were brought to an *Ambulatorium* for medical examination. However, only 1.3 per cent of these people were infected with an STD.[108] Therefore, the continuous use of raids represents an example of persistent mentalities towards women, a problematic legacy of procedures since the late-nineteenth century and Nazi Germany, as well as enforced social hygienic concepts in a patronising socialist state.

In general, the purpose of raids was to find 'promiscuous' people, carriers of STDs, and patients who eluded treatment, and thus they had to be carried out regularly in 'disreputable establishments' by health workers with help from police forces at night.[109] However, the disproportion between the efforts, the cost of resources, and the actual outcome was quickly realised and criticised by state health officials.[110] As Foitzik has shown for Hamburg, West German health authorities also condemned random raids by the British military police; however, it was not the degrading nature of raids, but their lack of efficiency, which was criticised.[111] This ignorance of popular opinion was not valid for East Germany, but they undertook raids for a longer period than the West.

In the Saxon mining town Aue, citizens complained to a national newspaper about the raids carried out during January 1948. According to the letter, officials not only "made large-scale raids in all establishments, even in the most reputable ones" but also "forced all attending guests to have a medical examination in an *Ambulatorium*".[112] The newspaper informed the DZVGW, which in turn criticised the Saxon and local health officials in Aue. In their letter to Saxony, they emphasised that "haphazardly implemented major raids only lead to the irritation of the population and thereby have rather disadvantageous effects on curbing STDs".[113] Already during the year 1947 and even more in 1948, state officials initiated a shift towards smaller, targeted raids, after they had realised the minimal outcome of STD cases, as well as the disturbance of greater parts of the population. East German authorities, in particular, were wary to avoid people's perception that they were put under 'general suspicion'.[114]

Despite its reputation, raids were still viewed as essential for curbing STDs. If the success rate was minimal, state officials – while recognising the overall decrease of STD cases – blamed local health authorities and the police for preparing the raids insufficiently, rather than acknowledged the issues inherent in this procedure.[115] The raids and nightly surveillance by police and health officials, however, represented a remnant of policies from previous political systems. Also in the Third Reich in Dresden in 1938, authorities established a special undercover force to observe and register hwG women in bars at night.[116] This legacy, however, did not prevent local officials from continuously using raids during the 1950s, albeit in a decreased number. The following examples from Bitterfeld and Leipzig reveal the connection between the forceful character, the legacy of the Third Reich, as well as the mentality of the people involved and targeted by these raids.

A report from Leipzig regarding the raids during the spring fair in 1955 stated that "[i]n *Schmidt's Bierstuben*, the audience was of such kind that almost all women should have been taken to a medical examination".[117] The bias inherent in this report was most evident in its claim that in Leipzig's bars "many women [. . .] obviously want to attract men through tempting dances".[118] Therefore, they targeted not only the suspected 'promiscuous' cases known to the *Ambulatorien* health workers, but also women in general, quickly identifying them as hwG individuals.

Despite the fact that most of the *Fürsorgerinnen* [health workers] and the city venereologist in Leipzig who wrote this report were female, the denunciation of, and the prejudices towards, women attending bars and dance halls reveals that they had no empathy for other women's desires – instead they often came to a much harsher judgement than men. Hall also identifies a similar pattern for the UK, stating that female police were stricter in sexual matters towards other women than male police.[119] For the GDR context, Betts' study also shows that mostly women denounced others and submitted petitions to the local and state authorities.[120] In the particular case of the mentioned female health workers in Leipzig, the general mentality towards women in the form of prevalent medical memories was in line with their views – 'the woman was the problem', and thus, the city's venereologist concluded, the raids needed to be intensified.[121]

Nonetheless, according to the report from Bitterfeld in 1951, the people targeted by these raids and denunciation system reacted in a challenging way for the young GDR state. The presence of the *Volkspolizei* [People's Police – VP], youth, and health workers in a beer garden resulted in verbal altercations and later physical violence. Attending adolescents refused to present their personal ID cards, which was seen by the police as 'impudent' behaviour; after they had used force, the situation escalated into a brawl, resulting in a couple of arrests. In a different pub on the same day, guests refused the inspection, and a renewed wave of accusations against the police and health officials led to a dispute. In the end, people who attended this pub punctured a tyre of the car belonging to a health worker, who, after experiencing this treatment, refused any further participation in future raids.[122]

These examples demonstrate that people began to reject being under the scrutiny of a paternalistic state in the 1950s: they targeted, blamed, and even attacked local officials, who were the representatives of the new socialist system. These conditions reflect the general conflict situation on the eve of the popular uprising in June 1953 in the GDR.[123] Another report from Leipzig about the autumn fair in 1955 also documented that "[o]ur measures were called undemocratic and unsuitable for our state today".[124] People realised the problematic connection of these raids with similar procedures during the Third Reich and beyond, tackling the widely pronounced 'democratic' character of the new socialist state. This represented a dangerous opinion for the GDR, as it undermined both the state narrative that described raids against 'asocial elements' as a necessity for the new order, and thus the legitimisation strategy of East Germany to gain popular support in the long-term.

This section has examined STD sufferers' experience of medical memories in the form of policing sources of infection, as well as its impact on the individual and on the perception of the medical profession and the state. Inherent to the measures was the social hygienic concept for curbing STDs through restricting the freedom of the affected people. The consequence was the establishment of a 'denunciation system', in which stigmatisation and false accusations led to actual implications for the targeted person. The Committee of Action decided that the individual should be put under surveillance by police forces, and if the suspected *Leumund* [reputation] of this person proved to be 'true', forceful measures were imposed upon her. Being registered with the health offices was accompanied with a stigma and could result in having an impact on someone's private and working life.

The belief that mainly women could be defined as 'promiscuous' or a hwG person was, however, found across all social and institutional ranks. Females accused other females, neighbours accused neighbours,[125] men accused women, state officials accused local officials, and so forth – a system of denunciation was created. According to Betts, this was a remnant of former political systems, especially the Third Reich, which used this form of local social control to enforce political conformity and stability at the local level.[126]

However, people started to refuse the openly patronising, monitoring, and intruding measures of the new socialist state during the 1950s – in a phase of political instability for the GDR and the imminent intensification of secret surveillance by the MfS. The atmosphere also challenged the state narrative, which legitimised the enforced public health measures. Therefore, officials stressed the importance of people's education by exhibitions and health campaigns, which simultaneously should reduce the need to hospitalise and police East Germany's citizens.

Conclusion: sexual education and stigmatisation in East Germany

This chapter has discussed intrusive state and public health measures that stigmatised and educated the individual. With this dualism, the East German authorities, firstly, sought 'specific preventive effects' that deterred the individual from 'socially deviant behaviour'. Secondly, they also heavily relied on the 'general preventive effect', accomplished with public educational campaigns which targeted 'promiscuity' as a prophylactic measure for the general population.

"Idleness, long sleeps, in order to pursue promiscuity at night. And the awakening was bitter: severe illness and now in a fast-tracked procedure in front of the court", stated the *Tagespost* about a show trial in a hospital in 1946.[127] Here, the two concepts – stigmatisation and education – were used as a tool to support the efforts of curbing STDs. Health officials, not limited to East Germany, viewed 'idleness' and 'promiscuity' as mutually dependent. The 'promiscuous' individual was seen as a public health hazard. 'Socially deviant behaviour' supposedly caused STDs and negligent sexual conduct, which was punishable by law.

However, due to the intrusive nature of the measures, discussed in the last section, the opinion and rumours among the population were monitored and used to assess the popularity of East German health policies. To gain the support of the masses, officials stressed the importance of educational campaigns to all strata of society. In retrospect, Hörig concluded in 1953 that "raising the general standard of living, eliminating the reluctance to work and unemployment, as well as the awareness campaign for broad segments of the population" were the reasons for the swift decrease of STDs.[128] The combination of education, propaganda, and re-socialising people through work was the main strategy, whereas West Germany concentrated its efforts, according to Foitzik, solely on re-socialisation until the end of the 1940s.[129]

Therefore, the SBZ, and later the GDR, formed a whole educational system, which was placed around health institutions like *Ambulatorien* and their forceful measures. The final part of this chapter concludes the features – education and stigmatisation – of the previous sections by analysing different forms of sexual health education. These public engagements were not only supposed to have a 'general preventive effect', but also to encourage 'healthy' marriages and the upbringing of the new generation. For this hypothesis, this section assesses exhibitions, posters, and the availability of prophylactics. The analysis illustrates how medical memories, in the form of mentalities and medical concepts, were reflected in educational campaigns and thus featured women as the main target similar to all policies previously discussed. Nevertheless, health officials used the tool of educating and stigmatising not only for creating fear, deterrence, and moral judgments regarding STD sufferers among the population, but also for increasing prevention, knowledge, and raising awareness. Therefore, revisiting Moser and Harsch's concept of 'medicalised social hygiene', this study suggests a mix of both fear and (medical) knowledge as an important feature of exhibitions. These have their roots in previous political systems and especially in the policies of the *Deutsche Gesellschaft zur Bekämpfung der Geschlechtskrankheiten* [German Association for Combating STDs] under the auspices of Albert Neisser and Alfred Blaschko since 1902.[130]

The preceding discussion showed how medical memories of the state, health officials, and doctors shaped the medical experiences of the STD patient, especially if identified as 'promiscuous'. However, the analysis would be incomplete without highlighting the diversity of medical experiences. An example from Dresden exposes a more differentiated societal approach to people with STDs. In this case, East German health officials intervened, stating that "[w]e cannot allow that a person suffering from an STD is dismissed from the public health service only due to her STD".[131] State officials stressed to local authorities that this disease was like any other illness and should be 'treated' correspondingly. However, they also inquired whether or not the STD transmission occurred due to "inferiority of character or moral unreliability [. . .] or if she caused damage to the reputation of the office".[132] In these cases, the dismissal was rightful, "[t]hough then the reason for the dismissal is not the disease but the ignoble behaviour of the employee".[133] Therefore, East German officials not only aimed to remove the silence surrounding STDs, but also maintained the stigma attached to 'promiscuity'.

The dualism of stigmatisation and education thus was part of people's everyday lives. In this narrow and biased scheme, patients with STDs, on the one hand, experienced comprehensive medical services, unseen in previous decades. On the other hand, as soon as the blurry line of 'promiscuity' was crossed by the individual in the opinion of the doctor, the health official, or even the neighbourhood, the medical experiences, as seen throughout this chapter, were composed of the deprivation of rights, institutionalisation, and harmful treatments – thereby impacting the personal and working lives of the affected individual. It was a social stamp that many of the inmates of the *Fürsorgeheim Leuben*, analysed in Chapter 4, potentially had to carry for the rest of their lives.

The last part of this chapter utilises exhibition material and street posters about sexual health, which incorporated all the previously discussed features of education and stigmatisation in order to prevent the spread of STDs. In many cases, the poster illustrations were medical memories put on display, and the most noticeable means of the East German campaign to reach all strata of society. The main producer of this material was the *Deutsches Hygiene Museum in Dresden* [German Hygiene Museum in Dresden – DHMD], founded in 1912. This institution represented a continuity of medical memories in its on-going existence throughout all political systems of twentieth-century Germany. The conceptual survival of this institution took the form of the building, space, staff, exhibition material used, and audience addressed. According to a report of the DHMD, the first large exhibition, which travelled throughout East Germany, was completed already in February 1946, indicating that material which survived the Second World War continued to be used in the postwar period.[134] Furthermore, political and ideological claims unique to East Germany were absent in the early exhibitions, but were the subject of subsequent campaigns.

The main political message of the three posters from 1946 in Figures 2.2a–2.2c, which were drawn in the style of the ones printed during the war, is a moralisation of sex and marriage, which was common throughout Europe in this era. This triptych tells two different stories. The focus is a woman who has two choices: either she refuses sex with a stranger and gets married, or she acquires an STD, after which she lies desperately on the bottom of the illustration – symbolic for the margins of society.

However, as the last poster shows, society gives her another chance: the doctor can cure her disease, and a future husband waits for her in the background to start a societally acceptable life. This theme raises awareness against casual sex

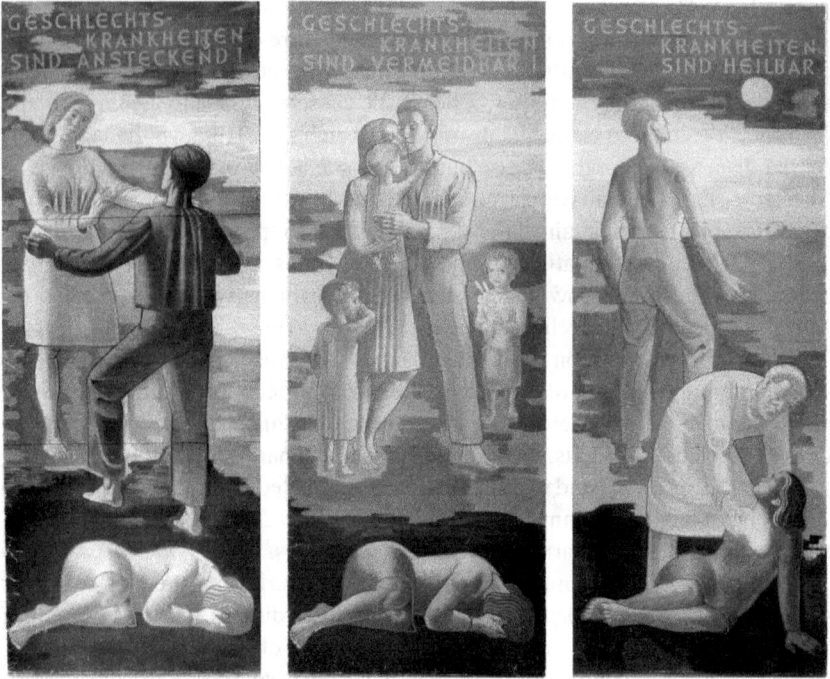

Figures 2.2a–c Exhibition posters, 1946

Transl.: "STDs are contagious!"; "STDs are avoidable!"; "STDs are curable" (from left to right).
Source: DHMD, 2013/483.1–483.3.

and promotes early marriage, and can be found in exhibitions until the beginning
of the 1950s (Figure 2.3). The notions of early marriage and protection against
STDs as being good for the state were also used in West Germany and the UK.[135]
In contrast, the GDR shifted attitudes away from enforcing early marriages in the
1950s because of its religious connotations, novel approaches in sexual education,
and the new roles of women in society.[136]

Furthermore, the exhibitions about STD prevention and treatment were supposed to contribute to the decrease of new infections by educating the population.
As the poster in Figure 2.4 of the small display exhibition from 1953 illustrates,
the creator of this material consciously aimed to prepare potential patients about
the procedures they faced in the *Ambulatorium*. Here, for example, it is clarified
to the audience that the STD patient has to reveal all of his sexual contacts – an
important element of the state's investigations into sources of infection.[137]

Figure 2.5 from 1953 demonstrates a similar style of education – it aimed to
remove silence, shame, fear, or concerns about prevention and treatment. These
ideas were utilised in order to stop patients from hiding their infections. The

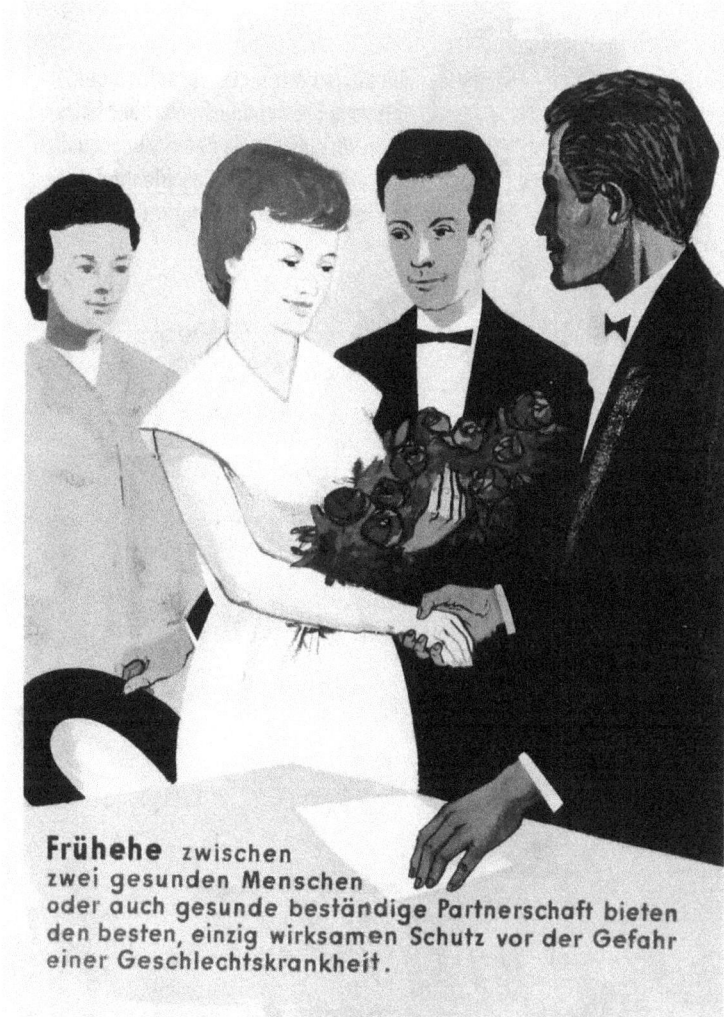

Figure 2.3 Exhibition poster, around 1954

Transl.: "Early marriage between two healthy human beings as well as healthy, consistent partnership offer the best, the only effective protection against the danger of an STD".

Source: DHMD, 2015/153.21.

poster shows a soldier who keeps a condom in his chest pocket to be prepared for any 'instances' – indicating the targeted audience.[138] Noteworthy is that the soldier is not a member of the Red Army, but an East German serviceman, probably from the newly founded *Kasernierte Volkspolizei* [Barracked People's Police – KVP], the predecessor of the NVA.

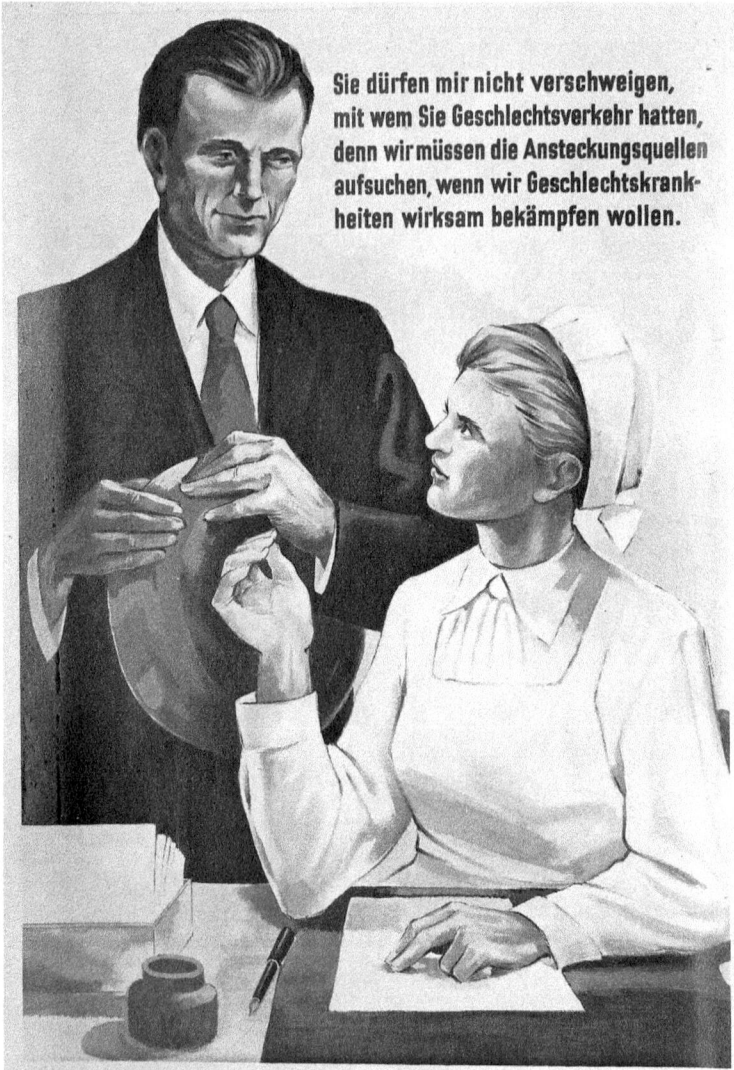

Figure 2.4 Exhibition poster, around 1953

Transl.: "You may not conceal from me with whom you had sex because we need to contact the source of infection, if we want to combat STDs effectively".

Source: DHMD, 2015/109.3.

Therefore, while in 1934 in Dresden the display of sexual hygienic articles was rejected because it was seen as "a violation of customs and decency", the postwar era saw a more open representation of contraceptives.[139] However, condom vending machines were a common feature of public toilets since the Weimar

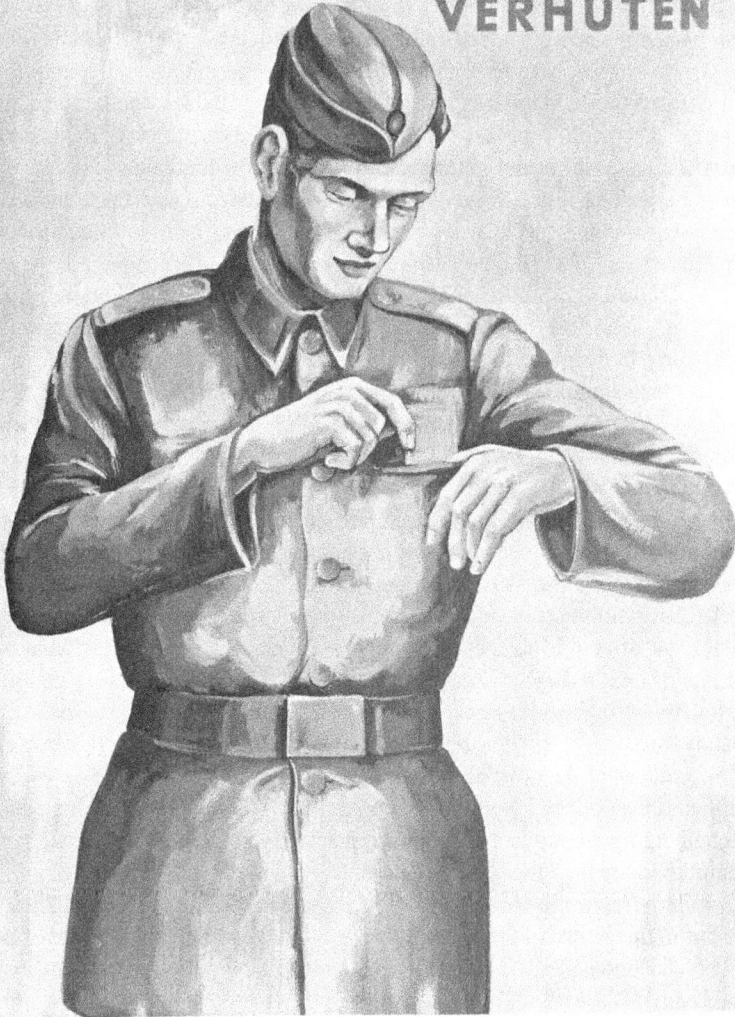

Figure 2.5 Exhibition poster, around 1953

Transl.: "Means of protection help to prevent STDs".
Source: DHMD, 2015/109.8.

Republic and – not without persistent dispute – continued to be available and considered an important aspect of STD prevention throughout the Third Reich and the GDR.[140] In contrast, the UK returned to silence over sexual matters in the 1950s and renewed the emphasis on marriage; therefore, condoms and other contraceptives became difficult to obtain again.[141]

In general, the opinion always existed that the availability of condoms acted as a stimulant and lowered people's inhibition to conduct casual sex. The so-called *Sittlichkeitsbewegung* [moralists or decency movement] emphasised the importance of an 'atmosphere of fear' and deterrence regarding sexual health to uphold their defined moral standards.[142] This view never fully disappeared and was used in the GDR as well, especially in the form of the state narrative against potential 'promiscuous', 'abnormal', and general 'socially deviant behaviour'.

The biggest problem for health officials, however, was the combination of these two so-called 'proletarian diseases': STDs and habitual alcohol consumption. Already in 1881, the Norwegian playwright Henrik Ibsen had connected in his play *Ghost* the troubling features of syphilis and alcohol addiction in his main character. Even if this man inherits the disease from his 'promiscuous' father, the social surroundings, personal ramifications, and his subsequent turn to alcohol are a typical theme for plays at the turn of the century.[143] However, Tennessee Williams' play *Sweet Bird of Youth* from 1959 demonstrates that the explosive combination of alcohol and STDs remained a common feature in plays beyond the first half of the twentieth century.[144]

Therefore, the exhibitions of the DHMD targeted the same issue, and thus it appeared in all subsequent educational campaigns (Figure 2.6, 2.8, and 2.9). All three posters have the same message: alcohol intake leads to loss of inhibition, lack of discrimination in selecting sexual partners, a higher libido, and, therefore, a high risk of acquiring STDs. In contrast, Figure 2.7 illustrates what a 'social and healthy gathering' is supposed to look like: depicting young people working together to rebuild and support East Germany on its way to Socialism. This 'healthy' relationship in combination with 'societal valuable' work was a common theme and part of the political and ideological re-education of the people. It was a significant part of East Germany's social didacticism and paternalistic approach. By challenging alcohol consumption and casual, indiscriminate sexual contacts, it attempted to create a new 'socialist citizen'.[145]

Furthermore, in the posters shown in Figure 2.2, 2.3, 2.6, 2.8, and 2.9 a woman was put in the centre of the illustration, and thus a significant amount of attention was placed upon her. Therefore, a gendered bias was also prevalent in DHDM exhibitions. The authors of this material perpetuated the idea that women were morally more responsible for sexual matters and thus the blame lay with her if an STD was transmitted.

The posters analysed are typical examples of the East German state narrative. They are carefully selected and implemented medical memories and experiences of authorities that were turned into public health policies. Medical expertise, stigmatisation, and social didacticism determined the layout of these posters. Moreover, two important elements from the illustrations are related to nineteenth-century

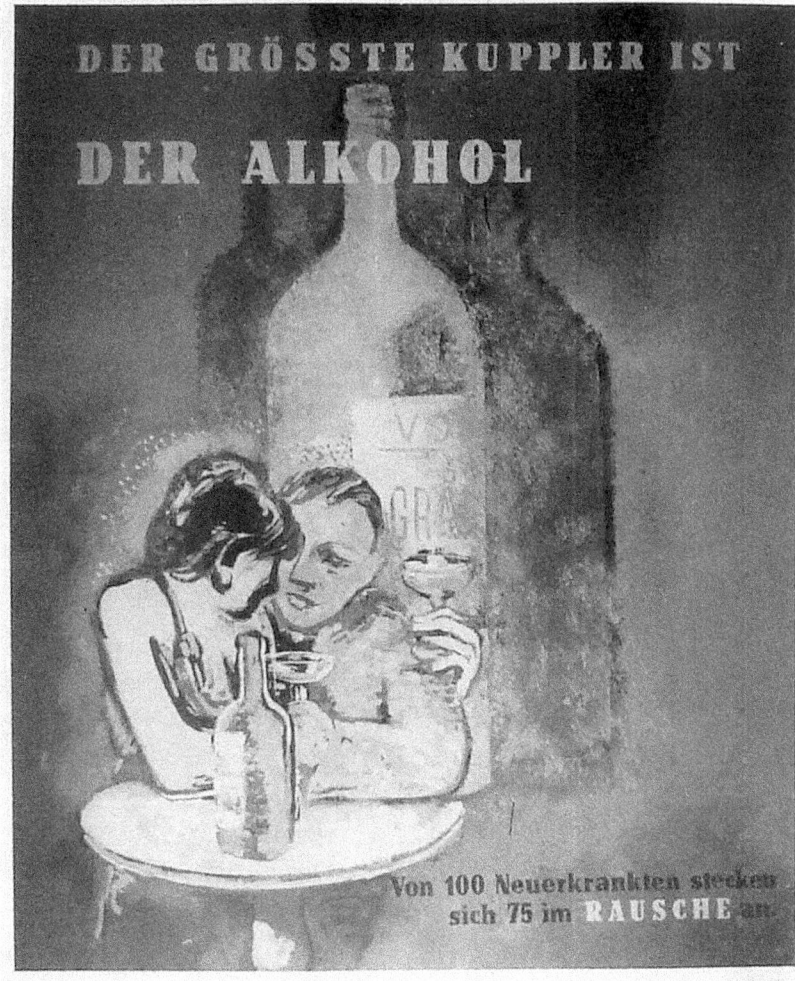

Figure 2.6 Exhibition poster, 1946

Transl.: "The biggest panderer is the alcohol. From 100 new patients, 75 have been infected while being intoxicated".

Source: DHMD, 2013/483.94.

medical concepts. Firstly, there is the notion of the three 'proletarian diseases' – Tbc, STDs and alcoholism[146] – which were perceived to be connected, and thus created the greatest concern for social welfare and health officials. Secondly, it was believed that people who drank too much alcohol, acquired STDs, or were unemployed or homeless must be 'asocial' or were listed as 'individuals with frequent promiscuous behaviour'. However, homelessness and unemployment were

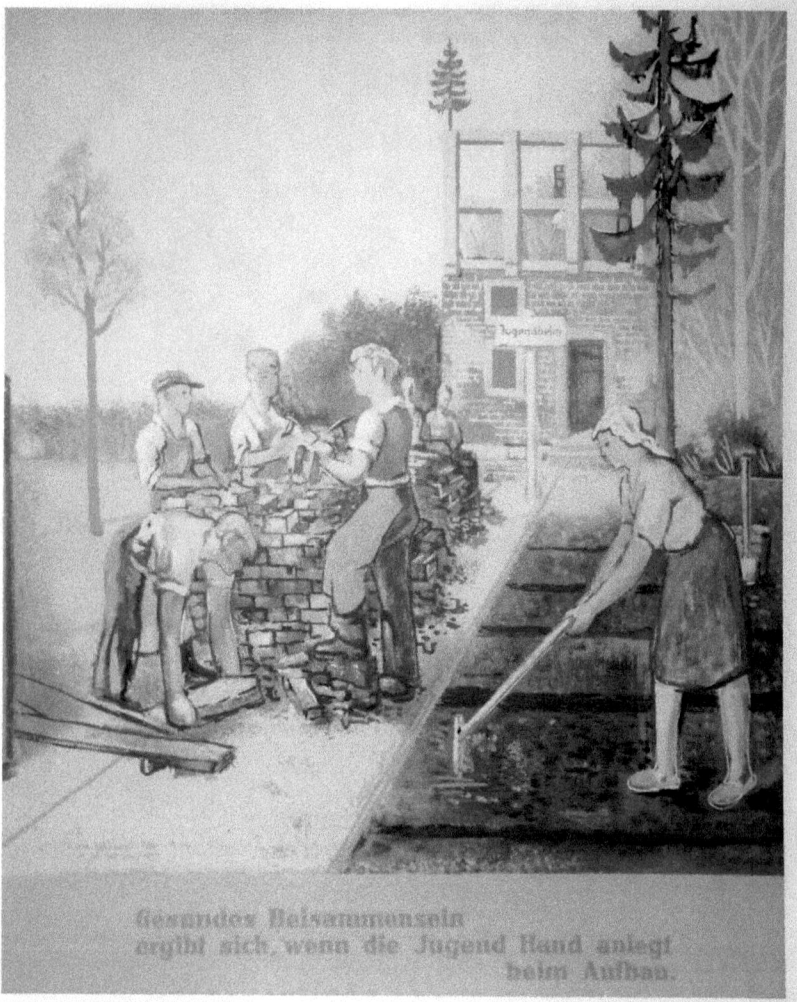

Figure 2.7 Exhibition poster, 1946

Transl.: "Healthy gathering arises when the youth lends a hand in the construction".
Source: DHMD, 2013/483.97.

hard to avoid for many people in the post–Second World War period as housing was limited due to bombing and the influx of refugees from the East. Nevertheless, addiction, health issues, and socially unacceptable behaviour were the main targets of health officials: the policies implemented and discussed thus show an increasing severity of the punishments of stigmatised people, not limited to hospitalisation, institutionalisation, and nightly raids in bars and clubs.

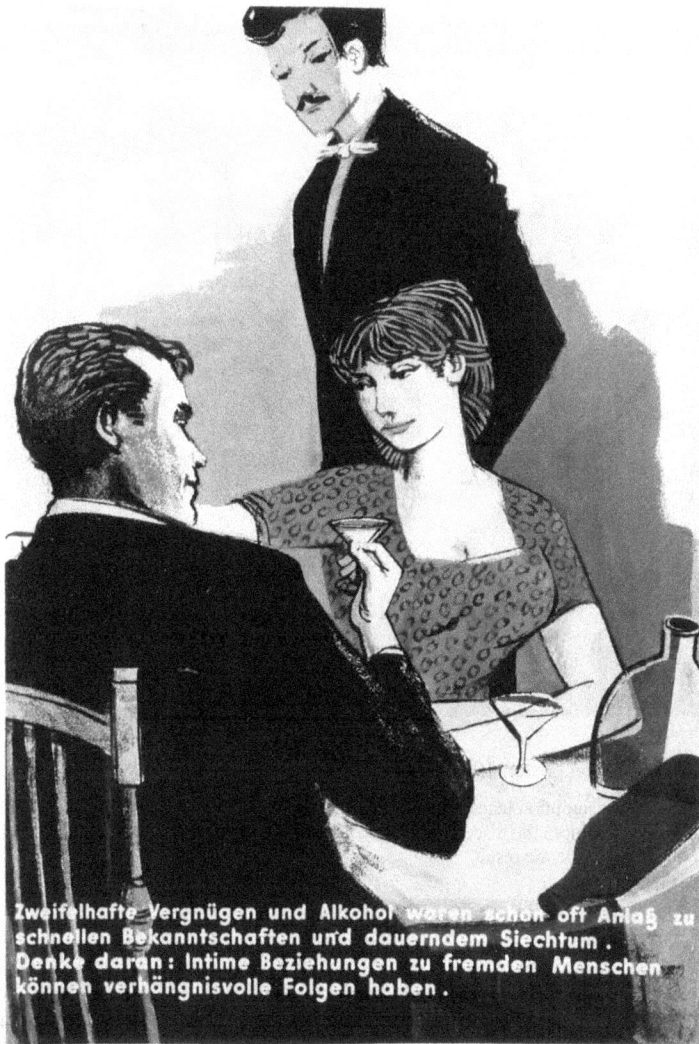

Figure 2.8 Exhibition poster, around 1954

Transl.: "Doubtful pleasure and alcohol were often the reason for quick acquaintances and lasting lingering illness. Remember: intimate relationships to strangers can have disastrous consequences".

Source: DHMD, 2015/153.16.

These exhibitions were educational, but they also functioned as a deterrent. On the one hand, they explained the diagnosis, symptoms, and treatment procedures through posters and models. On the other hand, in order to deter people from contracting sexual diseases, women were portrayed as 'promiscuous' or dangerous.

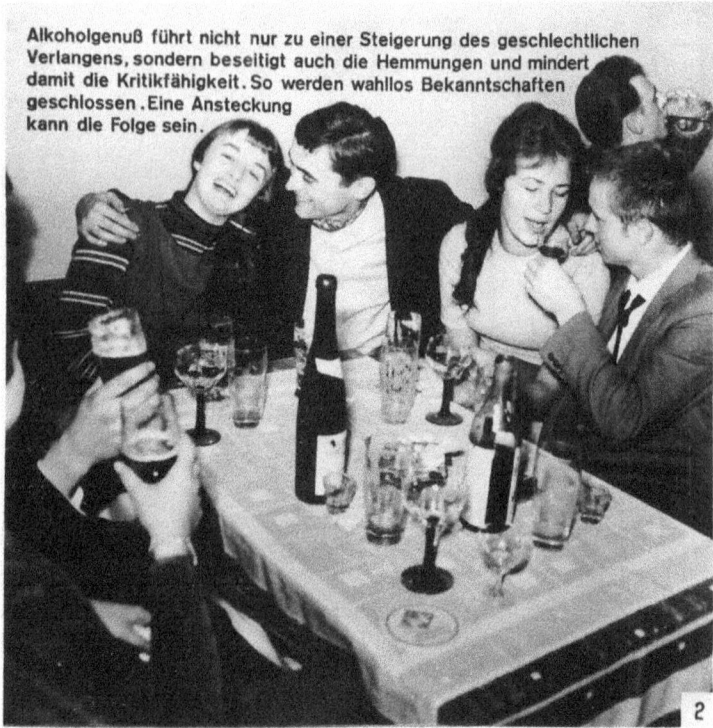

Figure 2.9 Exhibition poster, 1963

Transl.: "Alcohol consumption leads not only to an increase of sexual desire, but also eliminates the inhibitions and thus reduces the discerning ability. Subsequently, acquaintances are made indiscriminately. An infection can be the result".

Source: DHMD, 2015/174.3.

In Figure 2.10, a woman on the telephone was shown on four different occasions, with four different men – articulating sexualised gestures. This depiction suggested to the audience that she was a person with 'frequent promiscuous behaviour'. The intention of this poster was to stigmatise and thus prevent the exhibition visitors from behaving in a similar way.

However, Figure 2.11 went one step further: this poster not only showed that a person could be sentenced to one year in prison if she or he violated STD regulations and negligently spread the disease, but it also published the name, birthday, and residence of the woman accused in this openly accessible exhibition poster. The deterrent impact on the audience, apparently desired by the creator and the state alike, can be seen as a success. Neither woman nor man would want their name publicised in a nationwide travelling exhibition. Therefore, education and stigmatisation went hand in hand in East Germany because, as the poster in

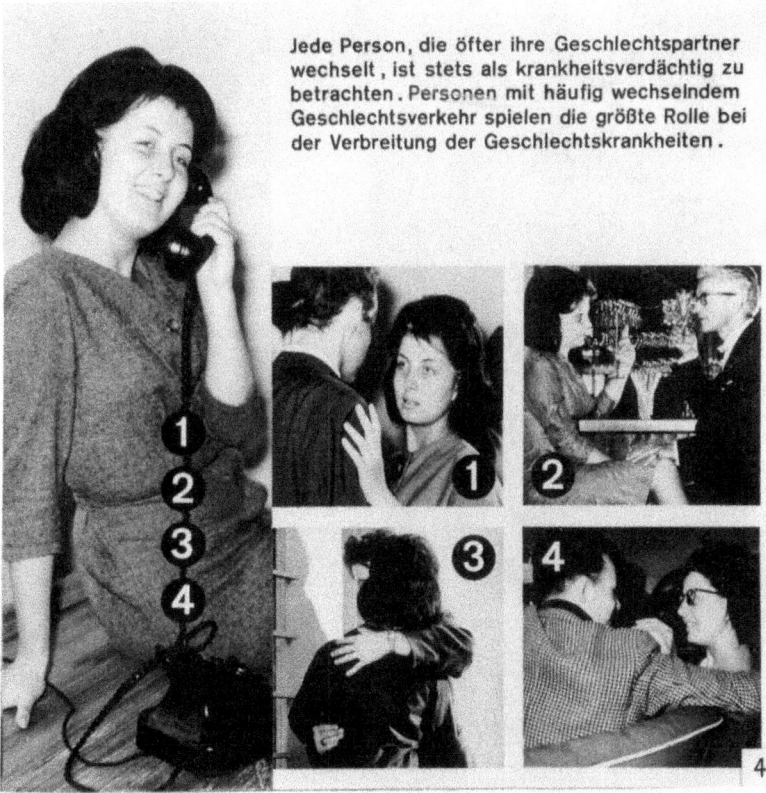

Jede Person, die öfter ihre Geschlechtspartner
wechselt, ist stets als krankheitsverdächtig zu
betrachten. Personen mit häufig wechselndem
Geschlechtsverkehr spielen die größte Rolle bei
der Verbreitung der Geschlechtskrankheiten.

Figure 2.10 Exhibition poster, 1963

Transl.: "Every person who often changes her sexual partners is always regarded as suspicious of suffering from a disease. People with frequent promiscuous behaviour play the biggest role in spreading STDs".

Source: DHMD, 2015/174.5.

Figure 2.11 summarised, "[t]he prevention and combat of STDs is the task of the whole society". Even in 1963, when STD statistics were far away from the peaks of the early postwar years, the GDR relied on targeting women, and thus employed this strategy throughout their campaigns.[147]

The last section has brought together all the themes discussed in this chapter. It has contributed to the socio-cultural approach towards the topic of sexual health, in this case for postwar East Germany. Elements of medicalisation and education, stigmatisation, and social didacticism could be found in the exhibitions of the DHMD and states' policies. Awareness campaigns, on the one hand, as well as raids, on the other, illustrated the dualism or ambivalent character of deterrence.

Die Verhütung und Bekämpfung der Geschlechtskrankheiten ist Angelegenheit der gesamten Gesellschaft.

Die Organe des staatlichen Gesundheitswesens arbeiten besonders eng
mit der deutschen Volkspolizei und
der Staatsanwaltschaft zusammen.

10

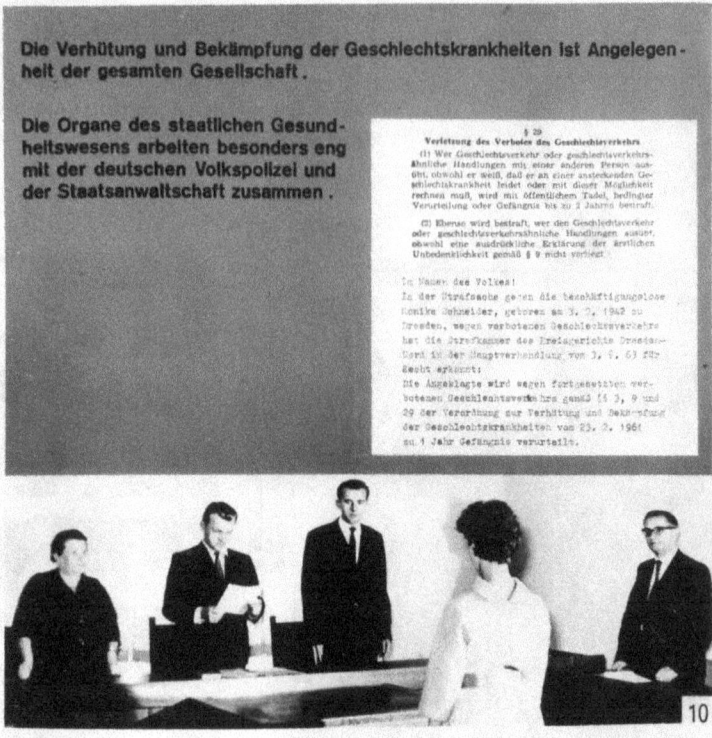

Figure 2.11 Exhibition poster, 1963

Transl.: "The prevention and combat of STDs is the task of the whole society. The organs of the state healthcare system closely work together especially with the People's Police and the public prosecution authority".

Source: DHMD, 2015/174.11.

This system resulted in individualised medical experiences that depended on a person's social status and judgement.

Especially, the local *Aktivausschuss* was an instrument for social control and disciplinary measures at the 'grassroots' of the new state. Similar to the de-Nazification committees in every district, these *Aktivausschüsse* heavily relied on the information received from neighbours and the reputation of the affected person in the community. Consequently, the committees were biased *a priori* in their judgements. In this way, however, the community worked for the state and supported the overall aim of creating a 'new' society with 'socialist personalities', all of whom would show morally correct behaviour and be reliable in their political consciousness – even in bed.

Furthermore, this chapter has expanded on Moser's and Harsch's concept of 'medicalised social hygiene' and proved that it is applicable for East Germany's

campaigns against STDs, if including the notion of 'positive demographic policies' as one of the main concepts behind the laws and regulations passed. Both
medical expertise and social hygienic agendas were part of the state narrative
and were implemented at the local level, which reveals the importance of medical memories of the individual, doctor, and health officials. Whether an authority
defined someone's sexual conduct, a person entered the premises of an *Ambulatorium*, or health workers carried out raids in bars, continuity was reflected not only
in policies and attitudes, but also in everyday situations. In addition, the medical
and social treatment of patients, the terminology used, and the prejudices they
faced demonstrate continuity with both the Weimar Republic and the Third Reich.

In conclusion, apart from some Soviet-directed influence in sexual health matters,
the Weimar Republic and its socialist and social hygienic movements, as well as
the longer traditions of sexual morals dating back to the nineteenth century, had the
strongest impact on the policy level, which East German state officials consciously
emphasised and utilised for their regulations. At the local level, however, a real
exchange of personnel, as seen in Chapter 1, and thus in language and medical concepts regarding sexuality and sexual health, did not occur. Therefore, doctors, health
authorities, and police officers remained often the same people as before 1945.

In one instance, according to Victoria Harris' study of prostitution in Germany
from 1915 to 1945, the result of this continuity was that one prostitute pursued
her business for 33 years undisturbed, despite multiple political changes.[148] This
finding exemplifies the stubbornness of mentalities and local conditions, in which
greater political alterations or an end of war could not cause a complete break
with the past.

The chapter has exposed these nuances, which have often been overlooked by
other historians who focussed only on state regulations.[149] With the help of the
concept of medical memories and experiences, the analysis of the treatment of,
and the attitude towards, STD patients has illustrated its dependency on locality,
officials and medical personnel in charge, reputation, and social surroundings.

Notes

1 Name was made anonymous due to public and archival restrictions. Therefore, the
   fictitious name of Susan Schneider will be used to enhance comprehensibility in the
   following.
2 'Protokoll, An hiesiger Amtsstelle erscheint auf Ladung durch das Ambulatorium
   [. . .], Fräulein [Schneider], 16. Januar 1950': StA DD, Dezernat Gesundheitswesen,
   4.1.12, Nr. 21, Bl. 217.
3 'Protokoll, An hiesiger Amtsstelle erscheint Herr Dr. Walter Korinek, 19. Januar 1950':
   StA DD, Dezernat Gesundheitswesen, 4.1.12, Nr. 21, Bl. 218.
4 "weil Sie in einem besonderen Falle einer Patientin Veranlassung hätten geben können,
   die Zuverlässigkeit städtischer Einrichtungen in Zweifel zu ziehen". 'Verwarnung des
   Korinek, 7. Februar 1950': StA DD, Dezernat Gesundheitswesen, 4.1.12, Nr. 21, Bl.
   217; Furthermore, see 'Protokoll, Auf Ladung erscheint an hiesiger Amtstelle Herr Dr.
   med. Walter Korinek, 19. Januar 1950': StA DD, Dezernat Gesundheitswesen, 4.1.12,
   Nr. 21, Bl. 218.
5 'Aktennotiz, 19. Januar 1950': StA DD, Dezernat Gesundheitswesen, 4.1.12, Nr. 21,
   Bl. 216.

6 Dagmar Herzog, 'East Germany's Sexual Evolution', in *Socialist Modern: East German Everyday Culture and Politics*, ed. by Katherine Pence and Paul Betts (Ann Arbor, MI: University of Michigan Press, 2008), pp. 71–95; Dagmar Herzog, *Sex After Fascism: Memory and Morality in Twentieth-Century Germany* (Princeton: Princeton University Press, 2005); Jennifer V. Evans, *Life Among the Ruins: Cityscape and Sexuality in Cold War Berlin* (Houndmills: Palgrave Macmillan, 2011).

7 Lesley A. Hall, *Sex, Gender, and Social Change in Britain Since 1880* (Houndmills: Macmillan Press, 2000); Lesley A. Hall, '"War Always Brings It on": War, STD's, the Military, and the Civilian Population in Britain, 1850–1950', in *Medicine and Modern Warfare*, ed. by Roger Cooter, Mark Harrison, and Steve Sturdy (Amsterdam: Rodopi, 1999), pp. 205–23; Paul Weindling, *Health, Race, and German Politics Between National Unification and Nazism, 1870–1945* (Cambridge: Cambridge University Press, 1989).

8 Edward Ross Dickinson, *Sex, Freedom, and Power in Imperial Germany, 1880–1914* (Cambridge: Cambridge University Press, 2014), pp. 304–5.

9 Herzog, *Sex after Fascism*, p. 8.

10 Donna Harsch, 'Medicalized Social Hygiene? Tuberculosis Policy in the German Democratic Republic', *Bulletin of the History of Medicine*, 86 (2012), 394–423.

11 Harsch, 'Medicalized Social Hygiene?', pp. 396, 402.

12 For this trend, see Richard Bessel, *Germany 1945: From War to Peace* (London: Simon & Schuster, 2009); Paul Betts, *Within Walls: Private Life in the German Democratic Republic* (Oxford: Oxford University Press, 2010); Evans, *Life Among the Ruins*; Donna Harsch, 'Socialism Fights the Proletarian Disease: East German Efforts to Overcome Tuberculosis in a Cold War Context', in *Becoming East German: Socialist Structures and Sensibilities After Hitler*, ed. by Mary Fulbrook and Andrew I. Port (New York: Berghahn Books, 2013), pp. 141–57; Herzog, *Sex after Fascism*.

13 Stadtpolizeidirektion Dresden, 'Gesundheitliche Gefährdung von Kindern durch umherliegende Schutzmittel im öffentlichen Verkehrsraum, 14. Dezember 1939': StA Dresden, Wohlfahrtspolizeiamt, 2.3.27, Nr. 31, Bl. 57.

14 Stadtpolizeidirektion Dresden, 'Gesundheitliche Gefährdung von Kindern durch umherliegende Schutzmittel im öffentlichen Verkehrsraum, 14. Dezember 1939': StA Dresden, Wohlfahrtspolizeiamt, 2.3.27, Nr. 31, Bl. 57.

15 Bessel; Jennifer V. Evans, 'Life Among the Ruins: Sex, Space, and Subculture in Zero Hour Berlin', in *Berlin: Divided City, 1945–1989*, ed. by Philip Broadbent and Sabine Hake (Oxford: Berghahn Books, 2012), pp. 11–22; Evans, *Life Among the Ruins*, p. 222; Herzog, *Sex after Fascism*, p. 1.

16 Michel Foucault, 'The Will to Knowledge', in *The History of Sexuality, Vol. 1*, trans. by Robert Hurley (London: Penguin, 1998), pp. 4, 36; Erving Goffman, *Behavior in Public Places: Notes on the Social Organization of Gatherings* (New York: The Free Press, 1985), p. 248; Erving Goffman, *Asylums: Essays on the Social Situation of Mental Patients and Other Inmates* (London: Penguin Books, 1991).

17 Wolfgang Höfs, 'Erfahrungen aus einer Ehe- und Sexual-Beratungsstelle für Männer', *Das Deutsche Gesundheitswesen*, 7 (1952), 571–5.

18 Höfs, p. 571.

19 Höfs, p. 571.

20 Herzog, *Sex after Fascism*, p. 189.

21 'Max Klesse, Über die Beurteilung der Geschlechtskrankheiten und die Maßnahmen zur ihrer Bekämpfung, 26. August 1946': BArch, DQ 1/1610, unpaginated.

22 For an example that this historical judgement continues to exist, see Elke Frietsch and Christina Herkommer, *Nationalsozialismus und Geschlecht: Zur Politisierung und Ästhetisierung von Körper, 'Rasse' und Sexualität im 'Dritten Reich' und nach 1945* (Bielefeld: Transcript, 2009).

23 Herzog, *Sex after Fascism*, p. 25.

24 For this notion, see Wolfgang König, *Das Kondom: Zur Geschichte der Sexualität von Kaiserreich bis in die Gegenwart* (Stuttgart: Steiner, 2016), p. 123; Dagmar Herzog, 'Hubris and Hypocrisy, Incitement and Disavowal: Sexuality and German Fascism', *Journal of the History of Sexuality*, 11 (2002), 3–21; Annette F. Timm, 'Sex with a Purpose: Prostitution, Venereal Disease, and Militarized Masculinity in the Third Reich', *Journal of the History of Sexuality*, 11 (2002), 223–55.

25 Herzog, *Sex after Fascism*, p. 31; Herzog, 'Hubris and Hypocrisy', p. 6; Foucault, pp. 44–5; Timm, pp. 224–5.

26 For an overview of this finding, see Mark Fenemore, 'The Recent Historiography of Sexuality in Twentieth-Century Germany', *The Historical Journal*, 52 (2009), 763–79.

27 'Max Klesse, Über die Beurteilung der Geschlechtskrankheiten und die Maßnahmen zur ihrer Bekämpfung, 26. August 1946': BArch, DQ 1/1610, unpaginated.

28 'Der Kommandeur der Sicherheitspolizei, 4. April 1945': StA Dresden, Krankenpflege- und Stiftamt, 2.3.24, Nachtrag 12, Bl. 3.

29 'Der Niedersächsische Minister für Arbeit, Aufbau und Gesundheit. Betr. Bekämpfung der Geschlechtskrankheiten (GK), 31. Juli 1948': BArch, DQ 1/292, unpaginated.

30 'Der Niedersächsische Minister für Arbeit, Aufbau und Gesundheit. Betr. Bekämpfung der Geschlechtskrankheiten (GK), 31. Juli 1948': BArch, DQ 1/292, unpaginated.

31 'Der Niedersächsische Minister für Arbeit, Aufbau und Gesundheit. Betr. Bekämpfung der Geschlechtskrankheiten (GK), 31. Juli 1948': BArch, DQ 1/292, unpaginated.

32 'Jahresbericht 1947': StA Dresden, Dezernat Gesundheitswesen, 4.1.12, Nr. 4, Bl. 13.

33 'Jahresbericht 1947': StA Dresden, Dezernat Gesundheitswesen, 4.1.12, Nr. 4, Bl. 13.; 'Erweiterte Vorstandssitzung vom 4. Juni 1946': BArch, DQ 1/139, Bl. 129; 'Unterbringung von etwa 40 geschlechtskranken Männern aus dem Behelfskrankenhaus Winterbergstraße im Fürsorgeheim Dresden-Leuben, 9. Februar 1948': StA Dresden, Fürsorgeamt, 2.3.25, AV I, Nr. 647, Bl. 134.

34 Hall, *Sex, Gender and Social Change*, p. 133.

35 For an overview of STD cases in Saxony during the postwar period and a comparison with the numbers of the West Zones, see BArch, DQ 1/292, unpaginated; BArch, DQ 1/1848, unpaginated; BArch, DQ 1/5440, Bl. 174–218; BArch, DQ 1/5855, unpaginated; Hans Philipp Pöhn and Gernot Rasch, *Statistik meldepflichtiger übertragbarer Krankheiten: Vom Beginn der Aufzeichnungen bis heute (Stand 31. Dezember 1989)* (Munich: MMW, 1994), pp. 177, 179.

36 'Jahresbericht über die Arbeit der Landeszentrale zur Bekämpfung der Geschlechtskrankheiten 1946': BArch, DQ 1/292, unpaginated, see especially *Anlage 3* with demographic statistics for Saxony in 1946.

37 The total number of new STD cases for people over the age of 18 was 14,204 in Saxony in 1948, which was used for the calculation in the text. BArch, DQ 1/5440, Bl. 174–218.

38 BArch, DQ 1/5440, Bl. 174–218.

39 BArch, DQ 1/5440, Bl. 174–218.

40 Evans, *Life Among the Ruins*, pp. 76–7.

41 Timm, pp. 227, 247. For further information, see Anna Maria Sigmund, *'Das Geschlechtsleben bestimmen wir': Sexualität im Dritten Reich* (Munich: Heyne, 2008), pp. 248–52.

42 'Parteivorstand SED an Herrn Staatssekretär Peschke, Ministerium für Arbeit und Gesundheitswesen, 7. Juli 1950': BArch, DP 1/7110, Bl. 13.

43 For a broader analysis of sex education in the nascent GDR, see Mark Fenemore, 'The Growing Pains of Sex Education in the German Democratic Republic (GDR), 1945–69', in *Shaping Sexual Knowledge: A Cultural History of Sex Education in Twentieth-Century Europe*, ed. by Lutz D H Sauerteig and Roger Davidson (London: Routledge, 2009), pp. 71–90.

44 'Max Klesse, Über die Beurteilung der Geschlechtskrankheiten und die Maßnahmen zur ihrer Bekämpfung, 26. August 1946': BArch, DQ 1/1610, unpaginated.

45 'Den Herren Kontrollärzten, die im Auftrage der Zentralverwaltung die Ambulatorien, Prophylaktorien, Geschlechtskrankenhäuser bezw. – Stationen sowie die zur Behandlung Geschlechtskranker zugelassenen Ärzte kontrollieren, hinsichtlich der Durchführung des Befehls Nr. 030, 30. Juli 1946': BArch, DQ 1/139, Bl. 49.

46 'Den Herren Kontrollärzten, die im Auftrage der Zentralverwaltung die Ambulatorien, Prophylaktorien, Geschlechtskrankenhäuser bezw. – Stationen sowie die zur Behandlung Geschlechtskranker zugelassenen Ärzte kontrollieren, hinsichtlich der Durchführung des Befehls Nr. 030, 30. Juli 1946': BArch, DQ 1/139, Bl. 49.

47 Günther Elste, 'Die SMAD-Befehle 25, 030 und 273: Ihre Bedeutung für die Verhütung und Bekämpfung der Geschlechtskrankheiten während des Aufbaus des antifaschistisch-demokratischen Gesundheitswesens von 1945 bis zur Gründung der Deutschen Demokratischen Republik', in *Die Bedeutung der Befehle der SMAD für den Aufbau des sozialistischen Gesundheitswesens der Deutschen Demokratischen Republik: Dokumentation aus Anlaß des 50. Jahrestages der Großen Sozialistischen Oktoberrevolution*, ed. by Hermann Redetzky (Berlin: Ministerrat der Deutschen Demokratischen Republik, Ministerium für Gesundheitswesen, 1967), pp. 61–5.

48 'Rundschreiben Nr. 6, 26. September 1945': StA Dresden, Dezernat Gesundheitswesen, 4.1.12, Nr. 1, Bl. 13.

49 'SMAD-Befehl Nr. 030, 12. Februar 1946': StA Dresden, Fürsorgeamt, 2.3.25, AV I, Nr. 647, Bl. 40.

50 'Jahresbericht 1946, 2. Januar 1947': StA Dresden, Dezernat Gesundheitswesen, 4.1.12, Nr. 3, Bl. 8.

51 Harsch also identified this pattern of continuity regarding the use of language for the treatment of Tbc patients. Harsch, 'Medicalized Social Hygiene?', pp. 399, 402.

52 'Verwaltung der SMA für das Bundesland Sachsen, Nr. 51, 21. Februar 1946': StA Dresden, Fürsorgeamt, 2.3.25, AV I, Nr. 647, Bl. 37.

53 'Verwaltung der SMA für das Bundesland Sachsen, Nr. 51, 21. Februar 1946': StA Dresden, Fürsorgeamt, 2.3.25, AV I, Nr. 647, Bl. 37–8; For a comparison with Command 030, see 'SMAD-Befehl Nr. 030, 12. Februar 1946': StA Dresden, Fürsorgeamt, 2.3.25, AV I, Nr. 647, Bl. 40.

54 'Rundverfügung Nr. 64. Anordnung zur Bekämpfung der Geschlechtskrankheiten im Bundesland Sachsen': StA Dresden, Fürsorgeamt, 2.3.25, AV I, Nr. 647, Bl. 33.

55 Anna-Sabine Ernst, *'Die beste Prophylaxe ist der Sozialismus': Ärzte und Hochschullehrer in der SBZ/DDR 1945–1961* (Münster: Waxmann, 1996), p. 145; Gerhard Naser, *Hausärzte in der DDR: Relikte des Kapitalismus oder Konkurrenz für die Polikliniken?* (Bergatreute: Eppe, 2000), pp. 54, 69. See Chapter 1.

56 In the single year of 1958, 927 doctors left the GDR for the West. Ernst, pp. 34, 55.Therefore, the doctors' communiqués from 1958 and 1960 granted far-reaching concessions as the state reaction to this high drainage. Many of these concessions, however, would be 'silently' repealed after 1961. 'Zu Fragen des Gesundheitswesens und der medizinischen Intelligenz, 16. September 1958', in *Dokumente der Sozialistischen Einheitspartei Deutschlands: Beschlüsse und Erklärungen des Zentralsekretariats und des Parteivorstandes, Band VII* (Berlin: Dietz, 1961), pp. 348–52; 'Kommuniqué des Politbüros des Zentralkomitees über Maßnahmen zur weiteren Entwicklung des Gesundheitswesens und zur Förderung der Arbeit der medizinischen Intelligenz, 16. Dezember 1960', in *Dokumente der Sozialistischen Einheitspartei Deutschlands: Beschlüsse und Erklärungen des Zentralsekretariats und des Parteivorstandes, Band VIII* (Berlin: Dietz, 1962), pp. 303–6.

57 'Rundverfügung Nr. 64. Anordnung zur Bekämpfung der Geschlechtskrankheiten im Bundesland Sachsen': StA Dresden, Fürsorgeamt, 2.3.25, AV I, Nr. 647, Bl. 33–4.

58 'Jahresbericht 1946, 2. Januar 1947': StA Dresden, Dezernat Gesundheitswesen, 4.1.12, Nr. 3, Bl. 8.
59 'Erweiterte Vorstandssitzung vom 4. Juni 1946': BArch, DQ 1/139, Bl. 130.
60 Ernst, pp. 32–3; *Bau von Ambulatorien und Polikliniken: 1. Mitteilung*, ed. by Kurt Liebknecht, Herbert Weinberger, and Kurt Winter ([n.p.]: Arbeitsgemeinschaft Medizinischer Verlag, 1949), pp. 5–6.
61 Weindling, p. 355; Evans, 'Life Among the Ruins', pp. 79–80.
62 For the discussions of a pure Stalinisation of East Germany, see Peter Grieder, *The East German Leadership, 1946–1973: Conflict and Crisis* (Manchester: Manchester University Press, 1999); Klaus Schroeder, *Der SED-Staat: Geschichte und Strukturen der DDR* (Munich: Bayrische Landeszentrale für politische Bildungsarbeit, 1998).
63 Weindling, p. 359.
64 'Entlassung von Fürsorgerinnen auf Grund der Direktive Nr. 24, 29. Januar 1947': StA Dresden, Dezernat Gesundheitswesen, 4.1.12, Nr. 1, Bl. 73. Susanne Hahn and Brigitte Rieske, *Das Arzt-Schwester-Patient-Verhältnis im Gesundheitswesen der DDR* (Jena: VEB Fischer, 1980).
65 'Ekelzulage, 9. Februar 1954': BArch, DQ 1/4436, unpaginated; 'Richtlinien für die Gewährung von Erschwerniszuschlägen für die Beschäftigten in den klinischen Einrichtungen für Haut- und Geschlechtskrankheiten für die dem Ministerium für Gesundheitswesen der DDR nachgeordneten Institute in Gross-Berlin': BArch, DQ 1/4910, unpaginated.
66 'Erweiterte Vorstandssitzung vom 4. Juni 1946': BArch, DQ 1/139, Bl. 130.
67 For a similar finding already for early-modern Spain, see Cristian Berco, *From Body to Community* (Toronto: University of Toronto Press, 2016).
68 'Abt. II/3 an die Landesregierung Sachsen, MfAuSF. Betr.: Ambulatorien für Haut-und Geschlechtskrankheiten, 28. Juni 1948': BArch, DQ 1/128, Bl. 289.
69 'Ministerium für Planung an Herrn Minister Steidle, 17. März 1950': BArch, DQ 1/2209, Bl. 101–2.
70 'MfG Sachsen an MfAuGW, HA GW, DDR. Betr.: Überführung der venerologischen Ambulatorien in die Polikliniken, 14. Juli 1950': BArch, DQ 1/2209, Bl. 169.
71 'Hauptgesundheitsamt, An die Ambulatorien I-VII, Infektionskrankenhaus Trachau, Behelfskrankenhaus Winterbergstraße und Fürsorgeheim Leuben, 30. September 1946': StA Dresden, Dezernat Gesundheitswesen, 4.1.12, Nr. 1, Bl. 54.
72 'Bericht über die am 7.3.1950 stattgefundene Besprechung betr. Bekämpfung der Geschlechtskrankheiten, 31. März 1950': BArch, DQ 1/2209, Bl. 344.
73 '17. Juli 1952': StA Dresden, Dezernat Gesundheitswesen, 4.1.12, Nr. 1, Bl. 253.
74 'Rundverfügung Nr. 64. Anordnung zur Bekämpfung der Geschlechtskrankheiten im Bundesland Sachsen': StA Dresden, Fürsorgeamt, 2.3.25, AV I, Nr. 647, Bl. 33; Ernst, p. 145; Naser, pp. 54, 69.
75 'Jahresbericht 1947 der Zentralstelle zur Bekämpfung der Geschlechtskrankheiten, 9. Januar 1948': StA Dresden, Dezernat Gesundheitswesen, 4.1.12, Nr. 4, Bl. 9.
76 Harsch's statement relies on a proposed lack of archival sources, which could also be due to the fact that she conducted research only in the Federal Archive. Harsch, 'Medicalized Social Hygiene?', p. 413.
77 'Jahresbericht 1947 der Zentralstelle zur Bekämpfung der Geschlechtskrankheiten, 9. Januar 1948': StA Dresden, Dezernat Gesundheitswesen, 4.1.12, Nr. 4, Bl. 9.
78 'Erläuterungsbericht Monat Januar 1947, 6. Februar 1947': BArch, DQ 1/128, Bl. 401.
79 Harsch, 'Medicalized Social Hygiene?', pp. 412–13.
80 'Ambulante Behandlung der Gonorrhoe mit Penicillin, 30. Mai 1951': BArch, DQ 1/2209, Bl. 128.
81 Doris Foitzik, '"Sittlich verwahrlost": Disziplinierung und Diskriminierung geschlechtskranker Mädchen in der Nachkriegszeit am Beispiel Hamburg', *Neunzehnhundertneunundneunzig*, 1 (1997), 68–82.

82 Melanie Arndt, *Gesundheitspolitik im geteilten Berlin, 1948 bis 1961* (Cologne: Böhlau, 2009), p. 201.
83 'Die augenblickliche Situation im Kampf gegen die Geschlechtskrankheiten – Grundsatzfragen in der Bekämpfung der Geschlechtskrankheiten. Gehalten vor den Kreisärzten des Bezirkes Dresden am 22. X. 1953 von Dr. Hörig, Bezirksvenereologe, Dresden': BArch, DQ 1/4436, unpaginated.
84 'Die augenblickliche Situation im Kampf gegen die Geschlechtskrankheiten – Grundsatzfragen in der Bekämpfung der Geschlechtskrankheiten. Gehalten vor den Kreisärzten des Bezirkes Dresden am 22. X. 1953 von Dr. Hörig, Bezirksvenereologe, Dresden': BArch, DQ 1/4436, unpaginated.
85 'Meldungen aus Sachsen-Anhalt, 20. September 1951': BArch, DQ 1/4672, unpaginated.
86 'Betr.: Eintägige Gonorrhoe-Behandlung mit Penicillin, 27. Januar 1950': StA Dresden, Dezernat Gesundheitswesen, 4.1.12, Nr. 1, Bl. 148; 'Antrag des Ministeriums für Gesundheitswesen des Landes Sachsen vom 2. April 1951, 18. Mai 1951': BArch, DQ 1/2209, Bl. 53.
87 Victoria Harris, *Selling Sex in the Reich: Prostitutes in German Society, 1914–1945* (Oxford: Oxford University Press, 2010), pp. 187–8; For further information, see Weindling, pp. 176–84, 357–9.
88 'Max Klesse, Über die Beurteilung der Geschlechtskrankheiten und die Maßnahmen zur ihrer Bekämpfung, 26. August 1946': BArch, DQ 1/1610, unpaginated.
89 Harris, pp. 186–9.
90 Foitzik shows that the language used and the categories established regarding women and female prostitutes as the main target were the same in Hamburg as in the SBZ or GDR. Foitzik, pp. 68–71, 80–1.
91 'Jahresbericht 1947 der Zentralstelle zur Bekämpfung der Geschlechtskrankheiten, 9. Januar 1948': StA Dresden, Dezernat Gesundheitswesen, 4.1.12, Nr. 4, Bl. 9.
92 Evans, *Life Among the Ruins*, p. 66.
93 'Einrichtung eines Sonderdienstes zur Erfassung von Unzüchtlerinnen, 14. Dezember 1938': StA Dresden, Wohlfahrtspolizeiamt, 2.3.27, Nr. 31, Bl. 54; Timm, pp. 242–3. For West Germany, see Foitzik.
94 For another exploration of the ambiguous category hwG and its history, see Timm, pp. 242–3.
95 'Bericht über die Tagung der Bezirksbeauftragten in der Landesverwaltung, Tiergartenstr., 1. Juni 1946': StA DD, Dezernat Gesundheitswesen, 4.1.12, Nr. 84, Bl. 2–3; 'Landes- u. Kreis-Aktionsausschüsse zur Bekämpfung der Geschlechtskrankheiten, 7. Mai 1949': BArch, DQ 1/4672, unpaginated.
96 'Btr.: HwG-Listen, 30. Dezember 1947': BArch, DQ 1/128, Bl. 336. See Chapter 5.
97 'Protokoll. Zusammenkunft des Activ-Auschusses am 8.7.1948. Beginn: 14 Uhr Ende: 16 Uhr': BArch, DQ 1/128, Bl. 287.
98 'Protokoll. Zusammenkunft des Activ-Auschusses am 8.7.1948. Beginn: 14 Uhr Ende: 16 Uhr': BArch, DQ 1/128, Bl. 287.
99 'Jahresbericht 1947 der Zentralstelle zur Bekämpfung der Geschlechtskrankheiten, 9. Januar 1948': StA Dresden, Dezernat Gesundheitswesen, 4.1.12, Nr. 3, Bl. 74; 'Rundschreiben Nr. 17, 13. November 1947': StA DD, Dezernat Gesundheitswesen, 4.1.12, Nr. 84, Bl. 70.
100 'Jahresbericht 1947 der Zentralstelle zur Bekämpfung der Geschlechtskrankheiten, 9. Januar 1948': StA Dresden, Dezernat Gesundheitswesen, 4.1.12, Nr. 3, Bl. 74; 'Auszug aus der Anordnung der Landesregierung – Gesundheitswesen – vom 16.12.46, 19. Dezember 1946': StA DD, Dezernat Gesundheitswesen, 4.1.12, Nr. 84, Bl. 16.
101 'Bericht über die Dienstreise nach Dresden am 18. – 20.1.49. Zusammenfassender Bericht über die Besichtigung, 24. Januar 1949': BArch, DQ 1/128, Bl. 33.
102 'Betr. Geschlechtskrankheiten. Erläuterungsbericht Monat Januar 1947, 6. Februar 1947': BArch, DQ 1/128, Bl. 401.

103 Foitzik also identifies that the perception of health officials was biased due to the distorted demography after the war, which meant also a potential higher rate of STDs among the female population. Foitzik, pp. 71–2; Evans, *Life Among the Ruins*, pp. 130–40.

104 'Vermerk, 21. März 1957': BArch, DP 1/1417, Bl. 126; 'Betr.: Neuregelung der Verordnung zur Bekämpfung der Geschlechtskrankheiten, 8. (22.) März 1957': BArch, DP 1/1417, Bl. 124.

105 'Jahresbericht über die Arbeit der Landeszentrale zur Bekämpfung der Geschlechtskrankheiten 1946': BArch, DQ 1/292, unpaginated.

106 However, it is important to note that West Germany and especially, as Foitzik shows, Hamburg used the same categories and public health methods. Foitzik, pp. 75–6, 79. For a recent study of the locked venereology wards in the GDR in the 1970s and beyond, see Florian Steger and Maximilian Schochow, *Traumatisierung durch politisierte Medizin: Geschlossene Venerologische Stationen in der DDR* (Berlin: MWV, 2015).

107 Foitzik, pp. 73–4; Evans, *Life Among the Ruins*, p. 79.

108 'Jahresbericht 1947 der Zentralstelle zur Bekämpfung der Geschlechtskrankheiten, 9. Januar 1948': StA Dresden, Dezernat Gesundheitswesen, 4.1.12, Nr. 4, Bl. 13.

109 'Betr.: Massnahmen zur Abstellung noch bestehender Mängel in der Durchführung des Befehls Nr. 030, 22. Juli 1946': BArch, DQ 1/139, Bl. 184.

110 'Entwurf: Zuständigkeit und Aufgabengebiet der Kriminalpolizei bei dem Delikt: Geschlechtskrankheitenverbreitung, 18. August 1947'. BArch, DQ 1/1010, unpaginated.

111 Foitzik, pp. 73–4.

112 'Aktenvermerk, 14. Februar 1948': BArch, DQ 1/128, Bl. 320.

113 'z.Hd. des Landesvenereologen Herrn Dr. Bettermann, 12. Februar 1948': BArch, DQ 1/128, Bl. 318.

114 'Razzien auf Geschlechtskranke, 9. März 1949': StA DD, Dezernat Gesundheitswesen, 4.1.12, Nr. 1, Bl. 137.

115 'DZVfGW and Landesregierung Sachsen, 7. November 1947': BArch, DQ 1/1010, unpaginated; 'Razzien auf Geschlechtskranke, 9. März 1949': StA DD, Dezernat Gesundheitswesen, 4.1.12, Nr. 1, Bl. 137. 'Entwurf: Zuständigkeit und Aufgabengebiet der Kriminalpolizei bei dem Delikt: Geschlechtskrankheitenverbreitung, 18. August 1947'. BArch, DQ 1/1010, unpaginated.

116 'Einrichtung eines Sonderdienstes zur Erfassung von Unzüchtlerinnen, 14. Dezember 1938': StA Dresden, Wohlfahrtspolizeiamt, 2.3.27, Nr. 31, Bl. 54.

117 'Bericht über die vor, während und nach der Frühjahrsmesse durchgeführten Massnahmen, 13. April 1955': StA Lpz, Stadtverwaltung und Rat, Nr. 7341, Bl. 177.

118 'Bericht über die vor, während und nach der Frühjahrsmesse durchgeführten Massnahmen, 13. April 1955': StA Lpz, Stadtverwaltung und Rat, Nr. 7341, Bl. 177.

119 Hall, *Sex, Gender and Social Change*, p. 94.

120 Betts, pp. 15, 162–72.

121 'Bericht über die vor, während und nach der Frühjahrsmesse durchgeführten Massnahmen, 13. April 1955': StA Lpz, Stadtverwaltung und Rat, Nr. 7341, Bl. 177.

122 'Bekämpfung der Geschlechtskrankheiten, Septemberberichtsauszug vom Lande Sachsen-Anhalt, 9. November 1951': BArch, DQ 1/4672, unpaginated.

123 Ilko-Sascha Kowalczuk, *17. Juni 1953* (Munich: Beck, 2013).

124 'Bericht über die vor, während und nach der Herbstmesse durchgeführten Massnahmen, 25. Oktober 1955': StA Lpz, Stadtverwaltung und Rat, Nr. 7341, Bl. 182.

125 'Betr.: Bekämpfung der Geschlechtskrankheiten': BArch, DQ 1/128, Bl. 500.

126 Betts, pp. 42–50. According to the recent study of Frank McDonough, 26 per cent of all Gestapo cases could be traced back to public and neighbour denunciations. Frank McDonough, *The Gestapo: The Myth and Reality of Hitler's Secret Police* (London: Coronet, 2015), chapter 5.

127 'Zeitungsausschnitt aus Die Tagespost, Nr. 56 vom 13.9.1946: Das Gericht im Krank-
    enhaus': BArch, DQ 1/347, Bl. 3.
128 'Die augenblickliche Situation im Kampf gegen die Geschlechtskrankheiten –
    Grundsatzfragen in der Bekämpfung der Geschlechtskrankheiten. Gehalten vor den
    Kreisärzten des Bezirkes Dresden am 22. X. 1953 von Dr. Hörig, Bezirksvenereo-
    loge, Dresden': BArch, DQ 1/4436, unpaginated.
129 Foitzik, pp. 80–1.
130 Lutz Sauerteig, *Krankheit, Sexualität, Gesellschaft: Geschlechtskrankheiten und
    Gesundheitspolitik in Deutschland im 19. und 20. Jahrhundert*, MedGG-Beihefte,
    12 (Stuttgart: Franz Steiner), pp. 89–125; Petra Ellenbrand, *Die Volksbewegung und
    Volksaufklärung gegen Geschlechtskrankheiten in Kaiserreich und Weimarer Repub-
    lik* (Marburg: Görich & Weiershäuser, 1999), pp. 50–68.
131 'DWK Berlin. Betrifft: Entlassung wegen Geschlechtskrankheit, 18. Feburar 1949':
    StA DD, Dezernat Gesundheitswesen, 4.1.12, Nr. 1, Bl. 136.
132 'DWK Berlin. Betrifft: Entlassung wegen Geschlechtskrankheit, 18. Feburar 1949':
    StA DD, Dezernat Gesundheitswesen, 4.1.12, Nr. 1, Bl. 136.
133 'DWK Berlin. Betrifft: Entlassung wegen Geschlechtskrankheit, 18. Feburar 1949':
    StA DD, Dezernat Gesundheitswesen, 4.1.12, Nr. 1, Bl. 136.
134 'Bericht des Deutschen Hygiene-Museums Dresden über die Durchführung der
    Wanderausstellungen zur Bekämpfung der Geschlechtskrankheiten im Jahre 1946':
    BArch, DQ 1/597, Teil 1, Bl. 448–9.
135 For the UK, see Hall, *Sex, Gender and Social Change*, p. 148. For West Germany, see
    Foitzik.
136 Fenemore, 'The Growing Pains of Sex Education', pp. 71–3, 85.
137 'Erläuterung zur Verordnung über ergänzende Strafbestimmungen zu dem Gesetz zur
    Bekämpfung der Geschlechtskrankheiten vom 18. Februar 1927 mit der Änderung
    vom 21. Oktober 1940, 20. Dezember 1945': BArch, DP 1/7109, Bl. 1.
138 For a broader study of the use of condoms in (West) Germany, see König.
139 'Ausstellung von sogenannten hygienischen Artikeln. Gegen die Verwendung von
    hygienischen Artikeln (Frauenduschen) für sexuelle Zwecke, 1. September 1934':
    StA Dresden, Wohlfahrtspolizeiamt, 2.3.27, Nr. 31, Bl. 52.
140 Timm, pp. 231–2.
141 Hall, *Sex, Gender and Social Change*, pp. 148, 152–60.
142 Ellenbrand, pp. 216, 218; König, chapter 1.
143 Henrik Ibsen, *Ghosts and Other Plays*, trans. by Peter Watts (London: Penguin
    Books, 1964).
144 Tennessee Williams, *Sweet Bird of Youth; A Streetcar Named Desire; The Glass
    Menagerie* (Harmondsworth: Penguin Books, 1979).
145 For the same approach towards alcohol, women, and STDs in Imperial Germany and
    the Weimar Republic, as well as in West Germany and the UK, see Hall, *Sex, Gender
    and Social Change*, p. 143; Weindling, pp. 9, 11–32, 184–6, 273–6, 353–7, 413–15,
    532.
146 Weindling, pp. 13, 19–20.
147 Pöhn and Rasch, pp. 177, 179.
148 Harris, pp. 187–8.
149 Grieder; Schroeder.

Bibliography

Primary sources

Unpublished

BUNDESARCHIV (BARCH)

Ministry of Healthcare

BArch, DQ 1/128 – Schriftwechsel mit Landes- und Provinzialverwaltungen; Sachsen, 1945–1949

BArch, DQ 1/139 – Bekämpfung von Geschlechtskrankheiten, Mitteilungen und Richtlinien der Deutschen Zentralverwaltung für Gesundheitswesen, Bd. 3, 1946–1947

BArch, DQ 1/292 – Rechtsvorschriften, Erarbeitung und Durchsetzung, Bd. 3, 1947–1949

BArch, DQ 1/347 – Gesundheitsfürsorge im Schulalter, Bd. 2, 1947–1949

BArch, DQ 1/597 – Haushaltspläne: Haushaltsjahr 1947, Bd. 1, 1946–1947

BArch, DQ 1/1010 – Bekämpfung von Geschlechtskrankheiten, Mitteilungen und Richtlinien der Deutschen Zentralverwaltung für Gesundheitswesen, Bd. 1, 1945–1949

BArch, DQ 1/1610 – Kampf gegen Geschlechtskrankheiten, Seuchen, Tuberkulose als Kriegsauswirkungen, 1945–1948

BArch, DQ 1/1848 – Bekämpfung der Geschlechtskrankheiten: Landes- bzw. Bezirkszusammenstellungen der statistischen Monatsberichte der Ambulatorien bzw. Behandlungsstellen: Berichtsjahre 1949 und 1950, 1949–1951

BArch, DQ 1/2209 – Bekämpfung der Geschlechtskrankheiten, 1948–1951

BArch, DQ 1/4436 – Monats- und Quartalsanalysen ("Wortberichte") der Bezirke und Schriftwechsel mit Räten der Bezirke, Bd. 1, 1953–1959

BArch, DQ 1/4672 – Bekämpfung der Geschlechtskrankheiten und Tuberkulose, 1949–1953

BArch, DQ 1/4910 – Lohn- und Gehaltsentwicklung im Gesundheitswesen, Bd. 2, 1953–1956

BArch, DQ 1/5440 – Lohn- und Gehaltsentwicklung im Gesundheitswesen, Bd. 2, 1953–1956

BArch, DQ 1/5855 – Bekämpfung der Geschlechtskrankheiten: Landes- bzw. Bezirkszusammenstellungen der statistischen Monatsberichte der Ambulatorien bzw. Behandlungsstellen: Berichtsjahr 1948, 1948–1949

Ministry of Justice

BArch, DP 1/1417 – Schutz vor Seuchen und Ansteckungskrankheiten, 1946–1949

BArch, DP 1/7109 – Vorschriften zur Bekämpfung von Geschlechtskrankheiten: Mitarbeit, Entwürfe, Durchführung, Bd. 1, 1945–1948

BArch, DP 1/7110 – Vorschriften zur Bekämpfung von Geschlechtskrankheiten: Mitarbeit, Entwürfe, Durchführung, Bd. 2, 1949–1955

DEUTSCHES HYGIENE MUSEUM, DRESDEN (DHMD)

Austellungstafeln (Exhibition posters)

DHMD, 2013/483.1
DHMD, 2013/483.2
DHMD, 2013/483.3
DHMD, 2013/483.94
DHMD, 2013/483.97

Kleintafelausstellungen (Small display exhibitions)

DHMD, 2015/109.3
DHMD, 2015/109.8
DHMD, 2015/153.16
DHMD, 2015/153.21
DHMD, 2015/174.3
DHMD, 2015/174.5
DHMD, 2015/174.11

DRESDEN, STADTARCHIV (STA DD)

StA DD, Dezernat Gesundheitswesen, 4.1.12, Nr. 1
StA DD, Dezernat Gesundheitswesen, 4.1.12, Nr. 3
StA DD, Dezernat Gesundheitswesen, 4.1.12, Nr. 4
StA DD, Dezernat Gesundheitswesen, 4.1.12, Nr. 21
StA DD, Dezernat Gesundheitswesen, 4.1.12, Nr. 84
StA DD, Fürsorgeamt, 2.3.15, AV I, Nr. 647
StA DD, Fürsorgeamt, 2.3.25, AV III Arbeitsanstalt, Rep. II: Anstaltsverwaltung, Section
    B: Die Organisation der Anstalt, Nr. 12
StA DD, Krankenpflege- und Stiftamt, 2.3.24, Nachtrag 12
StA DD, Wohlfahrtspolizeiamt, 2.3.27, Nr. 31

LEIPZIG, STADTARCHIV (STA LPZ)

StA Lpz, Stadtverwaltung und Rat, Nr. 7341

Published

Elste, Günther, 'Die SMAD-Befehle 25, 030 und 273: Ihre Bedeutung für die Verhütung
    und Bekämpfung der Geschlechtskrankheiten während des Aufbaus des antifaschistisch-
    demokratischen Gesundheitswesens von 1945 bis zur Gründung der Deutschen Demok-
    ratischen Republik', in *Die Bedeutung der Befehle der SMAD für den Aufbau des
    sozialistischen Gesundheitswesens der Deutschen Demokratischen Republik: Dokumen-
    tation aus Anlaß des 50. Jahrestages der Großen Sozialistischen Oktoberrevolution*, ed.
    by Hermann Redetzky (Berlin: Ministerrat der Deutschen Demokratischen Republik,
    Ministerium für Gesundheitswesen, 1967), pp. 61–5
Hahn, Susanne, and Brigitte Rieske, *Das Arzt-Schwester-Patient-Verhältnis im Gesund-
    heitswesen der DDR* (Jena: VEB Fischer, 1980)
Höfs, Wolfgang, 'Erfahrungen aus einer Ehe- und Sexual-Beratungsstelle für Männer',
    Das Deutsche Gesundheitswesen, 7 (1952), 571–5
'Kommuniqué des Politbüros des Zentralkomitees über Maßnahmen zur weiteren Entwick-
    lung des Gesundheitswesens und zur Förderung der Arbeit der medizinischen Intelligenz,
    16. Dezember 1960', in *Dokumente der Sozialistischen Einheitspartei Deutschlands:
    Beschlüsse und Erklärungen des Zentralsekretariats und des Parteivorstandes, Band
    VIII* (Berlin: Dietz, 1962), pp. 303–6
Liebknecht, Kurt, Herbert Weinberger, and Kurt Winter, eds., *Bau von Ambulatorien und
    Polikliniken: 1. Mitteilung* ([n.p.]: Arbeitsgemeinschaft Medizinischer Verlag, 1949)

'Zu Fragen des Gesundheitswesens und der medizinischen Intelligenz, 16. September 1958', in *Dokumente der Sozialistischen Einheitspartei Deutschlands: Beschlüsse und Erklärungen des Zentralsekretariats und des Parteivorstandes, Band VII* (Berlin: Dietz, 1961), pp. 348–52

Secondary sources

Arndt, Melanie, *Gesundheitspolitik im geteilten Berlin, 1948 bis 1961* (Cologne: Böhlau, 2009)

Berco, Cristian, *From Body to Community* (Toronto: University of Toronto Press, 2016)

Bessel, Richard, *Germany 1945: From War to Peace* (London: Simon & Schuster, 2009)

Betts, Paul, *Within Walls: Private Life in the German Democratic Republic* (Oxford: Oxford University Press, 2010)

Dickinson, Edward Ross, *Sex, Freedom, and Power in Imperial Germany, 1880–1914* (Cambridge: Cambridge University Press, 2014)

Ellenbrand, Petra, *Die Volksbewegung und Volksaufklärung gegen Geschlechtskrankheiten in Kaiserreich und Weimarer Republik* (Marburg: Görich & Weiershäuser, 1999)

Ernst, Anna-Sabine, *'Die beste Prophylaxe ist der Sozialismus': Ärzte und Hochschullehrer in der SBZ/DDR 1945–1961* (Münster: Waxmann, 1996)

Evans, Jennifer V., *Life Among the Ruins: Cityscape and Sexuality in Cold War Berlin* (Houndmills: Palgrave Macmillan, 2011)

———, 'Life Among the Ruins: Sex, Space, and Subculture in Zero Hour Berlin', in *Berlin: Divided City, 1945–1989*, ed. by Philip Broadbent and Sabine Hake (Oxford: Berghahn Books, 2012), pp. 11–22

Fenemore, Mark, 'The Growing Pains of Sex Education in the German Democratic Republic (GDR), 1945–69', in *Shaping Sexual Knowledge: A Cultural History of Sex Education in Twentieth-Century Europe*, ed. by Lutz D. H. Sauerteig and Roger Davidson (London: Routledge, 2009), pp. 71–90

———, 'The Recent Historiography of Sexuality in Twentieth-Century Germany', *The Historical Journal*, 52 (2009), 763–79

Foitzik, Doris, '"Sittlich verwahrlost": Disziplinierung und Diskriminierung geschlechtskranker Mädchen in der Nachkriegszeit am Beispiel Hamburg', *Neunzehnhundertneunundneunzig*, 1 (1997), 68–82

Foucault, Michel, 'The Will to Knowledge', in *The History of Sexuality, Vol. 1*, trans. by Robert Hurley (London: Penguin, 1998)

Frietsch, Elke, and Christina Herkommer, *Nationalsozialismus und Geschlecht: Zur Politisierung und Ästhetisierung von Körper, 'Rasse' und Sexualität im 'Dritten Reich' und nach 1945* (Bielefeld: Transcript, 2009)

Goffman, Erving, *Asylums: Essays on the Social Situation of Mental Patients and Other Inmates* (London: Penguin Books, 1991)

———, *Behavior in Public Places: Notes on the Social Organization of Gatherings* (New York: The Free Press, 1985)

Grieder, Peter, *The East German Leadership, 1946–1973: Conflict and Crisis* (Manchester: Manchester University Press, 1999)

Hall, Lesley A., *Sex, Gender, and Social Change in Britain Since 1880* (Houndmills: Macmillan Press, 2000)

———, ' "War Always Brings It on": War, STD's, the Military, and the Civilian Population in Britain, 1850–1950', in *Medicine and Modern Warfare*, ed. by Roger Cooter, Mark Harrison, and Steve Sturdy (Amsterdam: Rodopi, 1999), pp. 205–23

Harris, Victoria, *Selling Sex in the Reich: Prostitutes in German Society, 1914–1945* (Oxford: Oxford University Press, 2010)

Harsch, Donna, 'Medicalized Social Hygiene? Tuberculosis Policy in the German Democratic Republic', *Bulletin of the History of Medicine*, 86 (2012), 394–423

——, 'Socialism Fights the Proletarian Disease: East German Efforts to Overcome Tuberculosis in a Cold War Context', in *Becoming East German: Socialist Structures and Sensibilities After Hitler*, ed. by Mary Fulbrook and Andrew I. Port (New York: Berghahn Books, 2013), pp. 141–57

Herzog, Dagmar, 'East Germany's Sexual Evolution', in *Socialist Modern: East German Everyday Culture and Politics*, ed. by Katherine Pence and Paul Betts (Ann Arbor, MI: University of Michigan Press, 2008), pp. 71–95

——, 'Hubris and Hypocrisy, Incitement and Disavowal: Sexuality and German Fascism', *Journal of the History of Sexuality*, 11 (2002), 3–21

——, *Sex After Fascism: Memory and Morality in Twentieth-Century Germany* (Princeton: Princeton University Press, 2005)

Ibsen, Henrik, *Ghosts and Other Plays*, trans. by Peter Watts (London: Penguin Books, 1964)

König, Wolfgang, *Das Kondom: Zur Geschichte der Sexualität von Kaiserreich bis in die Gegenwart* (Stuttgart: Steiner, 2016)

Kowalczuk, Ilko-Sascha, *17. Juni 1953* (Munich: Beck, 2013)

McDonough, Frank, *The Gestapo: The Myth and Reality of Hitler's Secret Police* (London: Coronet, 2015)

Naser, Gerhard, *Hausärzte in der DDR: Relikte des Kapitalismus oder Konkurrenz für die Polikliniken?* (Bergatreute: Eppe, 2000)

Pöhn, Hans Philipp, and Gernot Rasch, *Statistik meldepflichtiger übertragbarer Krankheiten: Vom Beginn der Aufzeichnungen bis heute (Stand 31. Dezember 1989)* (Munich: MMW, 1994)

Sauerteig, Lutz, *Krankheit, Sexualität, Gesellschaft: Geschlechtskrankheiten und Gesundheitspolitik in Deutschland im 19. und 20. Jahrhundert, MedGG-Beihefte, 12* (Stuttgart: Franz Steiner)

Schroeder, Klaus, *Der SED-Staat: Geschichte und Strukturen der DDR* (Munich: Bayrische Landeszentrale für politische Bildungsarbeit, 1998)

Sigmund, Anna Maria, *'Das Geschlechtsleben bestimmen wir': Sexualität im Dritten Reich* (Munich: Heyne, 2008)

Steger, Florian, and Maximilian Schochow, *Traumatisierung durch politisierte Medizin: Geschlossene Venerologische Stationen in der DDR* (Berlin: MWV, 2015)

Timm, Annette F., 'Sex with a Purpose: Prostitution, Venereal Disease, and Militarized Masculinity in the Third Reich', *Journal of the History of Sexuality*, 11 (2002), 223–55

Weindling, Paul, *Health, Race, and German Politics Between National Unification and Nazism, 1870–1945* (Cambridge: Cambridge University Press, 1989)

Williams, Tennessee, *Sweet Bird of Youth; A Streetcar Named Desire; The Glass Menagerie* (Harmondsworth: Penguin Books, 1979)

3   Treatments for the past?

'War children' and the new state

Introduction

On 7 November 1946, a citizen appeared at Dresden's Head Health Administration to report upon the conditions in the house he lived in, and especially of one family and its 6-year-old son: "[t]he boy is frail, suffers from spinal polio and scabies. He already squeezes out the abscesses and is unclean. [. . .] The father of the child is very harsh; he beats the frail boy often without just cause".[1] Unfortunately, it was not possible to follow up the outcome of this report and to verify the claims of this citizen. However, assuming the description is correct, it shows the potential dangers and experiences which children faced during the war and postwar era. Here, a boy not only lived in a confined space among other families, which had to share one bathroom, but he also suffered from the unhygienic conditions, caught polio and scabies, as well as had to fear a violent father.[2]

This chapter discusses the complex medical memories and experiences of children, which included death, loss, malnourishment, disease, treatment, violence, and neglect, and the response by the state to their subsequent, perceived 'delinquent', behaviour in the postwar era. In general, children born before or during the Second World War were often robbed of their childhood. They had to take over adult responsibilities from an early age onwards, as older brothers or fathers were away or dead and thus unable to care for their families.[3] Nevertheless, there was a widespread belief that children were quite resilient to 'traumatic'[4] events: they were the first who conquered the rubble as their new playground.[5]

However, this view is widely refuted now, and current research claims that "children are the most jeopardised group" during and in the immediate aftermath of combat.[6] The understanding emerged that the scars of loss, violence, nights in bomb shelters, endless flights from battles, and famine with its subsequent diseases shaped the future of every child exposed to this dangerous situation.[7] The intensity and consequences of these scars are always highly diverse, and every individual is capable of coming to terms with his or her memories to a greater or lesser degree.

This chapter explores children's differentiated war experiences and their responses to the resultant medical memories and experiences in the microcosms of Dresden and Leipzig. Furthermore, it analyses the subsequent narratives created by the state and the medical profession that pathologised the behaviour of the youth in the transition from war to postwar.

Initially sparked by the publication of Günter Grass' novel *Im Krebsgang* [Crabwalk] as well as the book of the journalist Sabine Bode with the revealing title *Die Vergessene Generation* [The Forgotten Generation] a public discourse emerged about war children and their psychological wounds, which continues to this day.[8] The overall tone of this discussion has been that 'it is time to address' the sufferings and potential traumata of *German* children born in the period from circa 1930 to 1945 – thereby representing mainly the post-1929ers of Fulbrook's analysis.[9]

Most of the 'war children' are in retirement now and have started to document their memories and experiences. Psychologists – such as Hartmut Radebold – registered a rise of mental illnesses among the elderly, which they often attributed to childhood experiences, suppressed by the affected individuals during their working life.[10] Therefore, many psychologists, sociologists, and historians – each for different reasons – called for obtaining subjective narratives to preserve them for the future.[11] For example, Ulrike Jureit critically analyses in her article the creation of the 'war youth generation' as a retrospective endeavour, based on this age cohort's perceived shared 'war experiences' and thus the common starting point for commemoration. Despite the fallacies of generations as a concept, already discussed in Chapter 1, Jureit points out the necessity of this process – the engagement and self-reflection of the past – for German society.[12] However, other historians and survivors of the Holocaust have been targeting this endeavour, accusing the proponents of attempting to trivialise the victims of the Nazi regime.[13]

Therefore, the debate touches upon a sensitive issue that questions whether the children of potential perpetrators can also be 'victims' of the Second World War and the postwar era. This chapter cannot resolve this overarching problem of differentiating 'victimhood' appropriately. However, it provides another angle on the issue of 'war children', focussing on detectable behaviour, potentially caused by war experiences, and the state's reaction towards, as East Germany called them, the 'depraved youth'.[14]

Nevertheless, the difficulty of the topic is not only the politically motivated, public debate that surrounds the 'forgotten child' of the Second World War and the postwar era in East Germany, but also the shortage of sources addressing individual trauma experiences. This chapter circumvents the historiographical issue by utilising a considerable number of sources from the City Archives in Dresden and Leipzig, which include reports, petitions, statistics, and letters. The broad spectrum of sources prevents a biased approach as usually only extraordinary cases were recounted by state officials.

However, this study is not an attempt to diagnose any post-traumatic stress disorders [PTSD] retrospectively. The analysis shows that the whole debate, mentioned earlier, has shortcomings, and the diagnoses of PTSD and trauma are blurred, even in the realms of medicine and psychology.[15] Therefore, it can only provide a reference point to explain the 'up-rooted' youth in postwar East Germany.[16] Apart from the military context and the recognised psychological suffering of soldiers on the front line, described as 'shell-shock', trauma as a psychological impairment, caused by extreme events and situations, was hardly a medical concept in that era.[17]

Against this background, the chapter discusses the different experiences of children in the transition from war to postwar and examines the available archival sources for traces of war and postwar related experiences.[18] This analysis argues that children's war experiences are too complex to be described by using one 'medicalised' term, such as trauma. The loss of relatives, the witness of rapes, murder, or death, and the experience of abuse, illness, and torture had significant impacts upon children's socialisation. Medical memories of these experiences would influence their social 'performance', which leads to the next section: the aim to investigate the postwar behaviour of the so-called 'war youth', often caused by their war experiences, and the state's narrative.

Therefore, the second part of the chapter offers some insight into postwar realities and how the state authorities and the medical profession pathologised children's behaviour. In both East and West Germany, officials introduced paternalistic measures against the rise of criminality, delinquency, and 'sexual deviance'. This approach of the state authorities, medical personnel, and social environment, in general, represents another example of Erving Goffman's study of 'normal' and 'deviant' public behaviour.[19]

However, it needs to be stressed that only a minority was caught up in the so-called 'cycle of violence', meaning that violent experiences of the past resulted in violent or delinquent behaviour in the present.[20] The majority of the 'war youth' was able to suppress, or come to terms with, ferocious memories, and led – more or less – 'perfectly normal lives'.[21] This chapter raises the awareness of the complexity of individual responses and, vice versa, reveals the state's initiatives to reach out to the 'depraved youth', embracing and inducing them to be part of the socialist project: the hope for its future.

As mentioned earlier, the often invoked term of a 'traumatised generation' in current debates is misleading. Therefore, the conclusion of this chapter questions the rise in popularity of the 'forgotten war children' and the broad use of the term 'trauma' in Germany today. Without denying the long-term consequences of war experiences for the elderly and their sufferings today, this chapter, in line with Michael Heinlein's study, points towards the pitfall in these discussions: their 'apolitical' claim.[22] By using medical studies and terminology, the political agenda of the whole debate is disguised and invisible to its members.

The inherent issue is the arbitrary extension of trauma as a category to explain and to excuse social phenomena. This is not the first instance in history where medical concepts are used politically and to achieve the desired policies. Therefore, in exposing the bias in commemoration practices,[23] this study seeks to raise awareness of the subjectivity, ambiguous terminology, and problematic expansion of 'victimhood'.

After working through the framework of medical memories and experiences from the top of the East German state in the previous chapter, the structure of this analysis reveals more of a bottom-up approach by first discussing the individual and then moving towards the doctors, mnemonic communities, institutions, and state. It thereby offers another example of the use of medical memories as an analytical category, which allows approaching the issue from different angles. It exposes individual coping strategies, derived from the negotiation with past experiences, the present situation, and the future perspective, as well as with the social surroundings, the institutionalised practices, and the state narrative. Therefore, the concept encompasses not only social but also political, cultural, and medical methodologies combined under the framework of memory studies. In this regard, this approach contributes to the understanding of subjectivity and the fragility of remembrance, as well as the unpredictable behaviour of contemporaries for selfish reasons and self-justification in particular, and raises awareness of the limitation of historical research into the past in general.

'A youth exposed': experiences of East German children in the transition from war to postwar

The novelist Wolfgang Borchert was one of the most influential figures of postwar German literature. In his short story *Nachts schlafen die Ratten doch* [The Rats Do Sleep at Night], he introduced a young boy, Jürgen, who tries to guard his lost brother against small rodents:

> And then he said very quietly: My brother, he is down there. There. Jürgen pointed towards the collapsed walls with his stick. Our house got a bomb. Suddenly the light was gone in the cellar. And he was as well. We continued to call him. He was much smaller than me. Only four. He must be still there. He is so much smaller than me.[24]

It also features an old man who empathises with Jürgen's described situation. By offering him a rabbit and the explanation that rats go to sleep at night, the old man gives Jürgen the necessary relief from his fears, which have kept him watching the site since the day a bomb destroyed the home and buried his younger brother under the falling rubble. The outcome of this interaction, and whether Jürgen stops his guard during night time, though, remains open.[25]

In this short story, the multifaceted experiences of a child in the war and postwar era are captured by a fictional account. War can impose similar experiences of loss and grief on an individual, but the response and narrative of children can be highly diverse. More often than not, adolescents can come to terms with the event, especially, as in Jürgen's case, if they receive some social support, helping to cope with the event.

This section analyses youth experiences in the transition from war to postwar in East Germany, in particular in Dresden and Leipzig. During this process, the various, and often impenetrable, situations of children in these war-torn cities reveal a complexity which medicalised terms like 'collective trauma' or a 'traumatised society' fail to encompass.[26] Instead, this study follows Konrad Jarausch and Michael Geyer's argument that "[i]f there was something like a collective experience, it was the encounter with mass death, with irretrievable loss".[27] The ever-present end of lives represented one of the most decisive experiences for all people involved in the war.

However, adults, as well as children, were not only 'victims', even in the most dangerous and violent times. They also had agency to utilise, choices to make, and opportunities to seize, which often influenced decisions about life or death in the war context – a detail that is often overlooked in historical research. In this regard, methodological issues arise for the following interpretation from the fact that the sources utilised have an inherent bias that most of the officials' statements detailed negative and exceptional cases. However, other reports and statistics exist which address the general (medical) condition of Dresden's youth, offering a more differentiated insight into their war and postwar situation. From the vast amount of potential medical memories and experiences, this section limits its investigation to malnourishment and disease, negligence and homelessness, as well as adventure, violence, and sexual health. These seven often interrelated aspects provide the starting point for the discussion of the youth's behaviour that often had its origins in their war experiences and the state's reaction in the second section of this chapter.

Malnourishment and disease

"In front of the children's eyes a world undisguised and stripped of beauty unveiled itself", stated Elisabeth Pfeils in 1951, describing the situation of the youth among the refugees from the East. These experiences included, according to her, "perished animals, collapsing people, women who gave birth at the side of the road; people who were freezing to death, drowning, shot, run over".[28] The children, who were fleeing with their families from the advancing Red Army, had often lived through extremely violent and dangerous times that distinguished them from other adolescents who lived in Germany throughout the war.[29] In fact, some mainland German villages or smaller towns had no direct encounter with war until the very end.[30]

The one common experience shared by all, which was a threat to their health and wellbeing alike, was malnourishment. Since the beginning of the Second World War, food and other commodities were rationed, and the amount distributed to the people decreased continuously in the following years.[31] This deficit in basic foods extended into the postwar period, and rationing cards were not abolished until 1950 for West Germany and 1958 for East Germany.[32]

As shown in Figure 3.1, for pre-school and primary school children in Dresden – a city heavily bombed in February 1945 – the end of the war did not represent the end of hardships. In fact, the opposite was the case as nourishment worsened. A city like Dresden, for example, had to rely on the surrounding areas for food provision, which was insufficient due to food and stock confiscations by the occupying troops, the initial lack of a central administration for food distribution, and the war's impact on food suppliers in the immediate postwar era.[33] Therefore, city inhabitants across the country started to use parks, ruins, and any

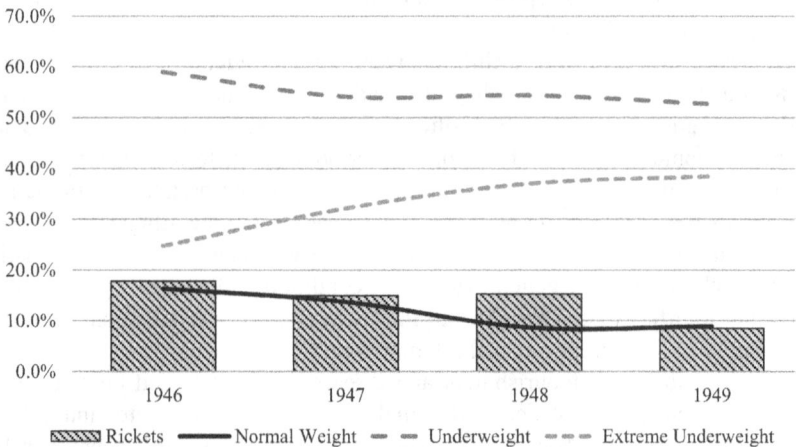

Figure 3.1 Weight and the appearance of rickets among pre-school and primary school children in Dresden between 1946 and 1949

Source: 'Jahresbericht 1946': StA DD, Dezernat Gesundheitswesen, 4.1.12, Nr. 3, Bl. 51, 53; 'Jahresbericht 1947': StA DD, Dezernat Gesundheitswesen, 4.1.12, Nr. 4, Bl. 203, 205; 'Jahresbericht 1948': StA DD, Dezernat Gesundheitswesen, 4.1.12, Nr. 5, Bl. 77, 79; 'Jahresbericht 1949': StA DD, Dezernat Gesundheitswesen, 4.1.12, Nr. 5, Bl. 98, 101. Percentages were calculated according to the overall number of children examined in each year. Unfortunately, the overall number of children varies greatly, and the sections of the forms are not always filled in sufficiently enough to draw broader conclusions.

other free space to grow vegetables, mostly potatoes.[34] Moreover, the statistics point towards a drastic decline in the number of children with normal weight and a subsequent increase in those who were underweight between 1946 and 1948. Not until 1949 does the number of underweight children seem to have stabilised itself, and the general tendency of the graph points towards better nourishment among the children.

The issue with the reports that are utilised for this analysis is that neither are they clear if all of Dresden's youth were included, nor do they provide a clear definition of what normal, under-, and extreme underweight constituted. However, the high percentage of underweight children, shown in Figure 3.1, was not limited to Dresden, but was valid for the rest of Germany.[35] This claim is corroborated by the 'Langeoog-Study', which examined children who had been selected and sent to the North Sea island of Langeoog for regeneration by the state of Lower Saxony in the British Occupied Zone of Germany between 1946 and 1950.[36] Doctors and psychologists involved in that study found that some of the adolescents weighed 20 per cent less than what was considered the 'norm' at the time and also lagged behind in their general growth – a situation that weakened their overall health condition and exposed them to the widespread diseases.[37]

The best indicator of malnourishment, especially relating to the deficit of proteins and vitamins, is rickets. In the postwar context, the deficiency of food led to an increase in rickets among Dresden's children. This development is shown in Figure 3.1, where an increase of this disease was accompanied by the drastic decline of adolescents with normal weight to under 10 per cent and the escalation of children suffering from extreme underweight to almost 40 per cent.[38] As a result, the condition of malnourishment was linked to the prevalence of diseases to an extent unknown in peacetime.[39] The unusual rise in 1948 – three years after the war had ended – was due to two successive strong, long winters across Europe, intensifying the scarcity of food and other resources, i.e. coal, urgently needed for heat.[40]

In Figure 3.2, this hardship is echoed in the progression of the diseases, where skin diseases and tuberculosis show a peak in 1948. However, as explained in Chapter 2, the renewed wave of infectious diseases was potentially due to the arrival of POWs and expellees from the East.[41] The sharp increase of detected skeleton malformation among Dresden's children suggests an influx from the outside rather than a development within this city because this category encompasses only deformations since birth and not as a result of rickets.[42]

As seen at the beginning of this chapter, medical memories and experiences of children regarding their health condition during the war could be much differentiated, depending on their food supply and living conditions. From the starting point of malnutrition and a subsequent weak immune system, the youth were exposed to various contagious diseases: not only tuberculosis or skin conditions,

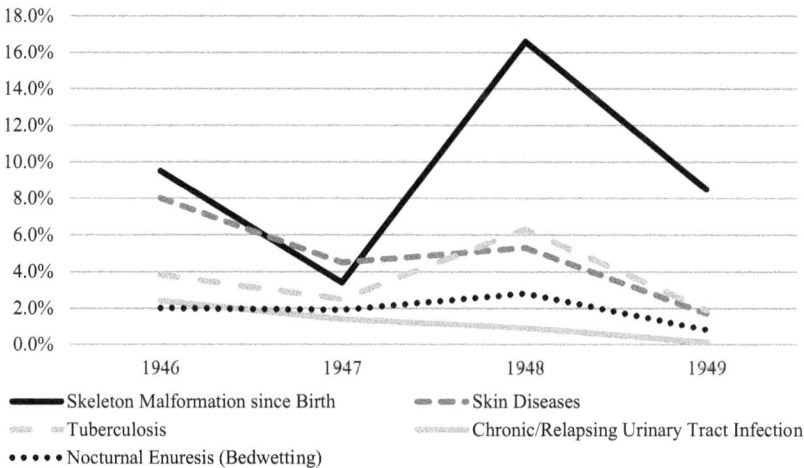

Figure 3.2 Occurrence of selected diseases or medical conditions among the pre-school and primary school children in Dresden between 1946 and 1949

Source: 'Jahresbericht 1946': StA DD, Dezernat Gesundheitswesen, 4.1.12, Nr. 3, Bl. 51, 53; 'Jahresbericht 1947': StA DD, Dezernat Gesundheitswesen, 4.1.12, Nr. 4, Bl. 203, 205; 'Jahresbericht 1948': StA DD, Dezernat Gesundheitswesen, 4.1.12, Nr. 5, Bl. 77, 79; 'Jahresbericht 1949': StA DD, Dezernat Gesundheitswesen, 4.1.12, Nr. 5, Bl. 98, 101. Percentages were calculated according to the overall number of children examined in each year. Unfortunately, the overall number of children varies greatly, and the sections of the forms are not always filled in sufficiently enough to draw broader conclusions.

but also diphtheria, scarlet fever, dysentery – which Reinisch describes as the typical disease of "social disorder and the lack of a functioning hygiene infrastructure"[43] – meningitis, and polio affected a considerable number of children.[44]

For children, infection with these diseases often meant a prolonged stay in a hospital, away from parents or their home.[45] They experienced the cruel realities of the hospital's deficits due to the destruction and general scarcity of, for example, coal and medical equipment.[46] The hardships of sickness and starvation were some of the most decisive aspects of the children's overall medical experiences after 1945, with potential consequences for their future quality of life.

Negligence and homelessness

According to Ackermann, the 'Langeoog-Study' came to the conclusion that the children "suffered due to the unhygienic living situations; they had no soap, their skin was dirty, encrusted, full of vermin, or infected with scabies".[47] In line with this statement, the high rate of skin diseases in Figure 3.2, including impetigo and microspores, points towards this section's second focus, which discusses the lack of hygiene, homelessness, and a potential negligence of children in the transition from war to postwar issues that were not limited to refugees.

To set the scene, Leipzig, for example, suffered through bombing an overall loss of 44,000 flats; 90,000 were heavily damaged. This situation determined that the whole of Leipzig's population could not be accommodated in the short term, leaving many of them living on the streets, in temporary shelters, or in confined spaces which they had to share with other families.[48] Due to these living conditions, the hygienic standard among the population suffered and increased their vulnerability to infections and diseases.

Dresden was similarly destroyed in the air raids of 13 and 14 February 1945. A report of the city's health officials from August 1948 about their visit to a city shelter for temporarily homeless people – those bombed out or refugees alike – illustrates the comparable circumstances. At this time, the institution housed 748 people, composed of 170 families and 238 children under the age of 14.[49] During their inspection, the health authorities scrutinised 12 flats within the city shelter, which they found in different conditions:

1   Married couple, 10 children, 17 years to 7 months old, 2 bed wetters, are bombed out, living there for 3 years already. Husband worker, salary RM 180 per month. Flat poor, meagre, but tidy. [. . .]
3   Married Couple, 9 children, 15 years to 9 months old, 2 bed wetters. Mother and 2 children with psoriasis. Living there for 3 years already. Husband worker, salary RM 40 up to RM 45. Uncleanliness in the flat. Husband keeps to himself, sleeps in the garden arbour.
4   Woman, 47 years old, receives public allowances. Moronic, sterilised, supposedly arranged by the husband. Husband still in captivity, 4 children, 17–13 years old, all pupils with special needs. All meagre, unclean, neglected.

5   Woman, 34 years old, Husband with one boy in the West. Here 2 boys, 13 and 14 years old, both had to repeat a year at school. Mother was not there. Mother has an affair with an 18-year-old. 2 rooms – Inventory: Kitchen: 1 old divan, 1 big table, 1 small table, 1 chair. Bedroom: 2 old beds, only one with mattress and blanket, everything neglected, woman profiteers and gives everything away for a smoke. [. . .]

8   Married couple, 5 children, 20–14 years old, all pupils with special needs, 2 bed wetters. The children are working, the oldest steals and exchanges everything, was in the mental asylum in Großschweidnitz already. Parents are imbecilic, mother sterilised. Mother has an affair with an asocial who also has intercourse with other women.[50]

Despite being written with a pejorative tone, these five examples from the total of 12 inspected flats shed light on the difficult circumstances that adults and children alike endured in adapting to the postwar period. Most of the families lived in cramped conditions, especially considering the high number of children they had to care for. They had to share their beds, which, according to the report, had mostly "inadequate, soiled [blankets and pillows]; bed linen was a rarity".[51] The report illustrates some subsequent diseases – like skin rashes – which most likely derived from the living conditions.[52]

In general, many of the descriptions in this report provide a glimpse into the complexity of medical memories and experiences that individuals faced in the postwar period. In these five examples alone, two females can be found who were sterilised before 1945 – in one case even initiated by the husband. Moreover, the often socially biased diagnosis of being 'moronic' or 'imbecilic', the stigma attached to marginalised individuals, endured the transition from war to postwar, proving the continuity of medical concepts particularly at the community level. These medical memories, inherent in the enforced health and social interventions, which were derived from socially constructed terminology, became the medical experiences of the stigmatised individuals. Both intervention and the subsequent experiences continued to shape people's real and perceived identity in the postwar period, and influenced their future.

In this institution, however, not only the flats were neglected, but also the children. In a couple of the cases mentioned in the preceding, the adult was, for different reasons, unable to take care of their sons or daughters. Their neglect resulted in a delay in their children's development.[53] For example, in three out of five families, two children suffered from nocturnal enuresis. Figure 3.2 shows that in the first years after the war around 2 to 3 per cent of the examined pre-school and primary school children suffered from bedwetting.[54] Despite being a natural process in a child's development, typically resolved by the age of 5, psychological stress – including diverse war experiences – could lead to a secondary nocturnal enuresis.[55] These renewed or prolonged phases of bedwetting are the only indications – if at all – of the impact war and bombing may have had on children's psyches.[56]

In the psychiatric sampling, carried out in this homeless shelter shortly after the city official's visit, the report stated that the inmates "for the most part are more or less imbeciles, who are socially fragile already in normal times and now show themselves to be particularly incapable of coping with the demands" of the postwar period.[57] With this argumentation, authorities denied not only the impact of war, bombing, and homelessness on people's psyches, but also the required psychological treatment.

This finding is in line with the general trend in child psychiatry at the time. In 1951, at the first meeting of the newly founded *Deutsche Vereinigung für Jugendpsychiatrie* [German Association for Youth Psychiatry – DVJ], Eckart Förster from the University of Marburg explained that "the experience of air raids had no pathogenetic influence on the later development of neuroses" in children.[58] In general, Förster rejected "the theory that neurosis would result from acute psychological childhood traumas" – a judgement which denied the impact of violent experiences on children.[59]

Furthermore, the controversial figure of Werner Villinger – who was also involved in the 'Euthanasia Programme' *Aktion-T4* – reported at the DVJ conference in 1954 about his experience in Dresden on 13 and 14 February 1945.[60] According to Villinger, the children that he encountered in the air-raid shelter showed only a "dull resignation", if anything.[61] He attributed their lack of reaction to their socialisation during the Third Reich and stated that the "psychological resilience" was apparently higher due to the Nazi regime's culture of heroism.[62] Despite the continuity of individuals and the corresponding persistence of medical attitudes from previous political systems – and, in the case of Villinger, even blatant Nazi ideology – he and Förster argued within the realm of contemporary psychological concepts. However, this view prevented children who had been affected by air raids from receiving treatment for their possible traumatic experience and its consequences.

In Dresden's annual reports, more mental diseases, such as epilepsy, 'imbecility', 'psychopathy', and 'moronism', can be found; most of them represent a socially defined diagnosis rather than a medical explanation. Moreover, only a handful of children were put in these problematic categories, and thus are not significant for the analysis of experiences in this section.[63] In general, mental disorders and subsequent treatment, employed in the event of a soldier's 'shell-shock', were usually absent in the civilian statistics utilised in this study. In West Germany, the diagnosis of 'dystrophy' was established for expellees who showed psychological disorders. It was the first explanation that analysed exogenous influences on mental health, here in the form of prolonged starvation.[64] In East Germany, this medical concept was, however, absent in the immediate postwar era. Only today, it has been established that trauma-related disorders could also be caused, for example, by bombing attacks on cities, the street fights at the war's end, and the death of close relatives – like Jürgen's younger brother in this section's opening quotation from Borchert's short story.[65]

This identified gap in the sources shows, however, that a public or medical platform for contemporaries who were haunted by the images of the past was non-existent; and if there was any treatment, then it was only for severe and 'socially deviant' cases. Section two of this chapter shows that the state's response towards children who potentially had psychological disorders was limited towards their contemporary behaviour, which often was the consequence of their past war experiences. Authorities, however, acted according to the leitmotif of 're-socialisation', instead of addressing the potential psychological causes inflicted upon children by war.

Adventure, violence, and sex

Homelessness, unhygienic conditions, mental distress within the social environment, and their possible neglect were part of children's everyday medical experiences in the postwar period. Families were often forced into poverty due to destruction, flight, and loss, which affected the children as much as the adults who were accustomed to certain wealth and status.[66] As mentioned before, however, children were not only passive subjects, but also had some agency during wartime, despite all the hardships listed earlier. Sometimes, the postwar period became, paradoxically, an adventure, a time of freedom and mischief: a typical phenomenon during periods of disorder and uncertainty.[67]

A compelling report from Dresden reveals that larger parts of the youth still roved around in Saxony as late as 1947. The social welfare department urged for state interventions, as "adolescents over 18 years appear daily in the youth department of the police, whom [officials] encountered without shelter".[68] However, the report continued that the Youth Office (*Jugendamt*) of the city – where the police transferred these young people to in most cases – also did not have space or resources to accommodate them. Therefore, officials were unable to intervene and were compelled to watch adolescents "hang around in disreputable pubs, involuntarily drifting more and more towards black market trading and *Schiebergeschäfte* [illegal profiteering]".[69] For officials in the West and the East of Germany, the scarcity of housing in war-damaged cities, the loss of parents, family, or other legal guardians, the experience of the Nazi dictatorship, and the accompanying lack of an 'orderly life' were seen as the causes for children and adolescents becoming 'strays' and being 'neglected' – not their personal war experiences as such.[70]

Authorities feared that roving teenagers – considered to be the future of the nation – would become 'asocial' and thus unfit for work. Furthermore, health and state authorities observed unrestrained sexual activity among them, which caused concerns about STDs and procreation, representing an urgent problem for the postwar society, as shown in Chapter 2. The last part of this section discusses children's agency regarding sexual awareness. However, their situation of being homeless and neglected also made them prone to physical and emotional violence, and sexual abuse by adults. Therefore, adolescents may have experienced a prolonged suffering from medical conditions, injuries, and diseases such as syphilis and gonorrhoea.

During the Second World War, especially due to the worsening housing situation, overnight stays in overcrowded air-raid shelters, long distances travelled on refugee routes, and not least experiencing or observing sexual violence, youth learned about sex and their sexuality at a much earlier age.[71] In her book about sexuality in the Third Reich, Anna Maria Sigmund cites a report of a mass STD screening at a school, which captured a glimpse into some forms of sexuality amongst young students. The report recounted five boys from the Hitler Youth who raped girls of the same age, of some girls 'experimenting' with soldiers, of boys and girls gathering for group sex after roll call, and one 'catamite [*Lust-knabe*]' offering himself for money.[72] According to Evans, the latter had been especially prevalent in the immediate postwar period. Both underage females and males discovered that prostitution was an easy way to make money in the fight for food and other 'luxury' goods – and sometimes just for 'fun'.[73]

In postwar Dresden the situation was similar. During their visit to the city's homeless shelter, officials were shocked about the conditions among the youth in this institution. They found 15 girls, between the ages of 16 and 21, suffering from STDs, and remarked that "adolescents [ranging in age from 14 to 18 years] had intercourse up to ten times a day" there.[74] However, they also stated that "sexual intercourse [amongst adults] had occurred in the presence of children, but is eliminated now".[75] How they stopped this from happening was not speci-fied. Nonetheless, this example suggests that learning about sex at a young age resulted in increased sexual activity among adolescents. The question to ask here is whether the adolescents only imitated the behaviour of adults, or whether it was a consequence of their war-inflicted traumatic memories. The latter might have contributed to widespread promiscuity as well as officials' perception of an 'uninhibited' sexual activity among children.

It can be argued that teenagers were more or less conscious about and utilised their sexuality. However, adults also recognised this 'early awakening'. Through-out the chaotic situation in the postwar era, adolescents and children were even more exposed to potential sexual abuse. The disclosure of this uneven relationship often occurred only when children acquired STDs. Evans, for example, refers to a case where a 4-year-old boy developed an STD after he was raped by American soldiers. However, the occupiers never faced prosecution – the boy and his par-ents had to live with this incidence, without official support.[76]

Figure 3.3 shows the distribution of STD cases among different age groups between 1947 and 1949. Unfortunately, the statistics lack the differentiation between infections by birth or due to sexual contact. Nevertheless, on the basis of the evidence, it is most likely that the high numbers of gonorrhoea cases among the 1- to 6- and 6- to 15-year-olds point towards either an early sexual activity or an abuse of children. As the experience of rape in its various forms – from touch-ing to actual sexual intercourse – impacts the memory, social behaviour, repro-duction, and medical condition of the child on multiple levels, it is an insightful example of the complexity that the concept of medical memories and experiences aims to encompass.

Already in December 1939, state officials were investigating the case of a 10-year-old child who was infected with gonorrhoea. However, their conclusion was that this boy possibly infected himself by playing with used condoms, which

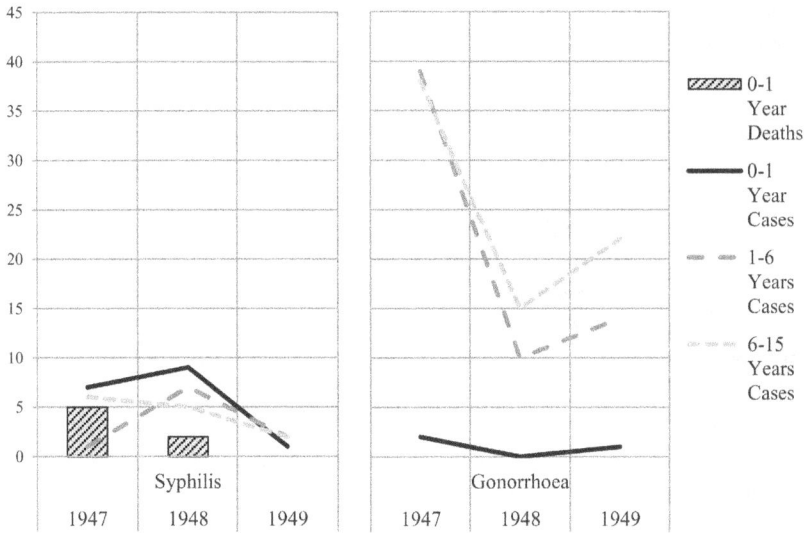

Figure 3.3 Infections with and death due to syphilis and gonorrhoea among the 0- to 1-, 1- to 6-, and 6- to 15-year-old children in Dresden between 1947 and 1949

Source: 'Jahresstatistik der anzeigepflichtigen übertragbaren Krankheiten in der sowjetischen Besat-zungszone für das Jahr 1947, 25. Februar 1948': StA DD, Dezernat Gesundheitswesen, 4.1.12, Nr. 4, Bl. 126–127; Jahresstatistik der anzeigepflichtigen übertragbaren Krankheiten in der sowjetischen Besatzungszone für das Jahr 1948, 24. Februar 1949': StA DD, Dezernat Gesundheitswesen, 4.1.12, Nr. 5, Bl. 1–2; Jahresstatistik der anzeigepflichtigen übertragbaren Krankheiten in der sowjetischen Besatzungszone für das Jahr 1949, 23. Dezember 1950': StA DD, Dezernat Gesundheitswesen, 4.1.12, Nr. 5, Bl. 83–84.

were apparently spread around the forest edges of the city, a situation which authorities strongly criticised.[77] This case illustrates that views on the transmission of STDs differed significantly compared to today's medical knowledge. Contemporaries ascribed the use of the same toilet, bed sheet, cup, or plate as possible sources of infection.[78] Even by acknowledging the poor hygienic standards in war and postwar times, a transmission of syphilis or gonorrhoea could hardly occur through these sources. For example, gonococci have a very specific, small-ranging temperature tolerance, resulting in the fact that any exposure to a different environment, like the toilet seat, would cause their immediate death. For both syphilis and gonorrhoea, a sexual-like interaction – a direct contact with mucosae for so-called 'smear infections' – is necessary.[79]

However, due to this different understanding, violent sexual experiences of children could be hidden and silenced – especially when official statements supported these beliefs. Therefore, the case of the 10-year-old child illustrates that children were not only exposed to rape by occupying powers but also – if not more so – molested by compatriots, who exploited the chaotic conditions of the war and postwar era. However, this aspect of sexual abuse during and after the Second World War has often been neglected in historiography. The violence exercised by the arriving Red Army in Germany – which had previously suffered dispropor-tionately at the hands of German forces – remained deeply engraved in the Ger-man consciousness. This finding also contradicts the recurring claims that sexual violence was a taboo topic in postwar and contemporary Germany.[80]

In conclusion, these examples indicate that minors often shared not only the traumatic experience of, but also a complicated suffering with, STDs, similar to their older contemporaries. Harmful medical memories and experiences should have inhibited children's development and thus inevitably put them under health and social authorities' strict monitoring systems. However, only the external, vis-ible scars of the war were treated; the internal, psychological scars in the form of (medical) memories were hardly addressed by health officials and doctors – repre-senting a continuity of views about traumatic experiences and their consequences from Wilhelmina Germany.[81] The consequences of this unevenly distributed treat-ment cannot be detected retrospectively. Nevertheless, the identified complex war experiences of children had an impact on their postwar behaviour, which was often perceived as 'social and sexual deviance' by authorities. Consequently, chil-dren became the target of the state and medical profession, who pathologised their social behaviour and put them into the social hygienic cycle of 're-education': they called them the 'depraved youth'.

'A youth depraved': the state and medical profession's response to the postwar youth's social behaviour

In the note about the visit of state health authorities in a Leipzig district in 1949, they wrote that

> [t]he low [moral] standard among these people is so significant that Miss [Meier] and all other people interested in the elimination of these conditions [. . .] expressed the urgent desire that this cancerous ulcer of society will be wiped out once and for all.[82]

This report bears witness to the persistence of eugenic terminology, and its inte-gration into social hygienic concepts after the Second World War. Health officials observed that, "already among teenagers, pronounced youth gangs are created. Sex offenders, people who are guilty of blood disgrace [incest], thieves, burglars, dealers, profiteers, slackers are living here together", and thus drew a dark picture of the moral attitudes among the families in this neighbourhood.[83] From these evaluations, authorities concluded that these families should be dissolved. The adults would be referred to workhouses and their children into orphanages or care homes, as "they are only endangered by such parents".[84] This suggestion ultimately meant a forceful separation of children from their families and thus represented an intrusion into the people's private sphere.

Nevertheless, postwar East Germany saw itself compelled to react with rather harsh measures to the rise of criminality, delinquency, and prostitution – especially among children – which was also prevalent in the West Zone.[85]

The quoted report from Leipzig is only one example of many, supporting the hypothesis that the state and the medical profession established a narrative which mainly targeted the consequences rather than the causes of delinquency and oppositional behaviour that potentially had its origins in children's war and postwar experiences.

On the one hand, the state saw delinquent behaviour as an 'abnormality' that needed to be corrected. On the other, however, the delinquent child was viewed as resisting the reconstruction of East Germany, and thus in opposition to the socialist idea. To explain children's misconduct, state authorities utilised and restored social hygienic, as well as eugenic, concepts and language to underpin their paternalistic approach towards youth deviance and defiance. The inherent legacy in these arguments is another questionable continuity of medical memories and experiences from the Third Reich and the Weimar Republic into postwar East Germany.

As in the previous section, a major methodological issue for this analysis is the prejudiced accounts about the youth's behaviour in the postwar era. Negative and extraordinary cases drew the attention of the state, whereas people's 'normal' and 'opportunistic' conduct was rarely reported. However, the utilisation of a vast number of archival sources, especially from the City Archives in Dresden and Leipzig, enables this study to qualify and to contextualise the reports.

In general, this book shows that children, after being exposed to the war and postwar situation, were also confronted with the subsequent medical memories and experiences inflicted on them by authorities and doctors. Both pathologised and stigmatised teenagers' behaviour and introduced corresponding policies and penalties. For the youth generation, however, it is important to acknowledge that, according to Michael Buddrus, 1945 already represented a significant rupture with their socialisation, childhood, and belief system, acquired during the Third Reich. The consequence was "a profound sense of shock, betrayal and uprooting" among adolescents, influencing their social behaviour, coping strategies, and conclusions for the future in the postwar era.[86] Therefore, the survival of children's pre-1945 medical memories and experiences in their minds, language, and actions embody another inherent continuity.

This section addresses this issue of continuity and rupture among adolescents, as well as analyses the subsequent narrative of the state and the medical profession, which was perpetuated as a reaction to the perceived 'depraved' or 'wayward' youth. The focus of the following is limited to the phenomena of 'social and sexual deviance', using the previously discussed war and postwar experiences of young people as the starting point of the analysis.

Genetics or socialisation? Eugenic and social hygienic explanations for social deviance among the youth

Max Klesse, the Head of the STD Department at the DZVGW, complained in August 1946 that "[i]n this area [referring to the youth], the twelve years of Nazi domination have thrown all psychological inhibitions overboard". He continued that "[o]nly gradually, the youth will be taught the fundamentals of hygiene, the respect of their fellow men, and the cultivation of their personality again, without which a cultural nation cannot fulfil its tasks".[87] According to Klesse's statement, 'social deviance' of the youth was the outcome of the Third Reich and its socialisation practices in HJ, BDM, and the drill towards the war. As a result, the 'depraved' youth, composed of children and adolescents roving around, parentless or homeless, was in danger of becoming delinquents and 'asocials' due to this criminal past. Therefore, they were seen as inhibiting the nation's goals, and thus became its target for reforms.[88] In the following, the state and medical profession's narrative about the causes for 'social deviance' among the youth is analysed and put in the context of the general development of psychological understanding in the postwar era in Germany.

In 1954, Gerhard Göllnitz, who later became an eminent GDR professor of child psychiatry at the University of Rostock, presented a paper at the – still pan-German – DVJ conference in Essen that dealt with the question: "Which children are especially affected by war and postwar damage?" During his talk, Göllnitz discussed the findings from his study of 600 children with 'abnormal' behaviour, which he compared with a control group of 300 'normal' ones. His conclusion was that the "crisis-related snowballing of negligence, criminality, and abnormal reactions [. . .] is almost restricted to such environmentally fragile and partly retarded children and adolescents, whose development has been impaired by early childhood damage to the brain".[89] Göllnitz's statement illustrates two important points for the postwar understanding of mental health: firstly, 'social deviance' had to have an organic cause and, secondly, was limited to children who were genetically prone to 'asocial' behaviour independent of war and postwar related experiences.

Additionally, the previously mentioned West German psychiatrist Förster claimed at the same conference that a "spontaneous improvement [of their mental health, M.W.] is absent only among a small part" of the youth.[90] In this regard, he continued, "no significant difference" was registered between war and non-war children.[91] With these assumptions, both Förster and Göllnitz denied the uniqueness of wartime for children's development from the psychological perspective. The mentality prevalent in these statements is in line with Goltermann's study, in which she revealed that the general doctrine in West Germany was that neuroses had purely endogenous causes, representing a continuity of eugenic scholarship within the medical profession across the occupied zones. Some psychiatrists started to question this purely endogenous model and to dedicate their studies to exogenous influences (for example, for the diagnosis dystrophy), including war, imprisonment, and the Holocaust. However, as Goltermann shows, a broader change in the common doctrine did not occur until the late 1950s and the beginning of the 1960s and was mostly driven by changes in the state and compensation law.[92]

In contrast to the view of the quoted psychiatrists, East German state and health officials' judgement about the causes of 'social deviance' appeared more differentiated. Like Klesse, authorities rather stressed the importance of the environment in which children were raised – an inherently social hygienic approach.[93] In this view, the milieu, the war situation, and "that many of these people grew up without any love" were decisive for their social conduct.[94] Even Erich Honecker, who with support from Soviet leader Leonid Brezhnev overthrew Walter Ulbricht as the First Secretary of the Central Committee of the SED in 1971, had declared in 1945 that the "German youth [went] through the criminal school of Adolf Hitler" and was "misused for acts of shame".[95] Between the lines of such an explanation, the narrative of victimhood can be identified. For a socialist state in the making, the clear demarcation from the previous political system was essential: a strategy for accommodating a society composed of nominal members and bystanders during the Third Reich, and ultimately turning them into an 'anti-Fascist' nation.[96]

Therefore, for the vast majority of cases of 'social deviance', the state often used the Nazi period as a scapegoat and implicitly denied people's agency. Therefore, as seen in Chapter 1, for the medical profession in particular, East Germany offered its population an alternative narrative, buying into their feelings, playing to their desire to 'forget the past', looking towards the future, and, simultaneously, underpinning its legitimacy as an 'anti-Fascist' state.[97] Below the surface of ideological claims, though, this model, driven by the predicaments, negotiation, and pragmatism of the postwar years, provided the precondition for the survival of xenophobia, Nationalism, and Fascism under the cloak of Socialism.[98]

In general, for both the state and medical profession, the most noteworthy influence on children's public behaviour was their home. Continuing the opening report about the quarter in Leipzig from 1949, health authorities observed that, after children were separated from their 'imbecilic' parents, they would "develop to their benefit significantly after only a little time".[99] The problem was, however, children's age. In their view, "the older the children are, the more difficult [the re-socialisation, M.W.] and the larger the characteristics of their environment loom".[100] Therefore, the state determined that to prevent delinquency the duration of negative socialisation needed to be minimised – and thus legitimised their socially intrusive actions with contemporary medical knowledge. According to the health officials, this issue was especially urgent, as the outcome of a 'wrong' upbringing endangered other adolescents if influenced by the 'deviant' child in school and kindergarten.[101]

The West German psychiatrist Villinger – who subscribed to the Nazi ideology – argued similarly, emphasising children's socialisation during the Third Reich as a cause for the observed "mass negligence [. . .] and the tremendous rise of youth criminality".[102] The West German paediatricians Bossert and Bleckmann followed Villinger and described "war as symptom and consequence of a general development" of society – and thus again denied a direct dependency between war experience and children's behaviour or mental disorder.[103]

Consequently, the state and medical profession laid blame on both parents and the social environment, which excused children's 'social deviance' in general: not least because they were seen as the future and hope of the new socialist nation. The logical result of these views was that the state took drastic measures to implement their social hygienic concepts by separating the child from negative influences, meaning in this case, from their parents and the accustomed environment.

The 'asocial' child

A health authority stated during a meeting in December 1949 that "[t]hese are no families [. . .] but criminal hideouts".[104] This evaluation shows that the official tone changed quickly as soon as somebody was seen not only as 'deviant', but also as 'asocial' – two very blurred and overused terms, which depended on the contemporary context and the writer's individual predisposition. Continuing the report from the meeting in 1949, health authorities followed the terminology and urged that "a clear distinction need to take place between criminal elements and people who are the product of societal development".[105] This expressed opinion indicates how the East German state denied 'asocials' the status of being human: these 'elements' of society were seen as unchangeable in their 'deviant behaviour', and thus a burden to the nation.

Authorities distinguished between individuals who were 'lost' – the 'incorrigibles'[106] – and people who, through intervention, could be educated and brought back to a 'normal life' – and for the most part, children were placed with the latter. This separation of the uprooted majority from the 'asocial' minority also features in the report about a district in Leipzig from 1949. Here, authorities underlined the notion of environmental influences, but also inherited, intergenerational characteristics, among the youth of 'asocials':

> The *Geburtenfreudigkeit* [avid procreation] amongst these people is extraordinary. [. . .] Their children are taught to beg and instructed to steal already at an early stage. Children's food ration cards are bartered away. Therefore, their abundance of children is a business for them. They are not aware of the responsibilities of having children. In this environment, these [children, M.W.] can only become criminals.[107]

This statement was written in a reproachful tone and shows no empathy with the situation of the people and their children in the postwar period. Authorities described childbearing as a business for the poor and 'asocial', which represents another continuity in language and narrative within the realm of medical memories and experiences, reaching back into the nineteenth century.[108] Moreover, it is recognisable that the state described the family situation among 'asocials' as a transgenerational cycle: genetics and socialisation transferred 'asocial' behaviour onto the children. This transmission of 'social deviance' underlined for authorities the necessity to break this causal chain with a paternalistic approach.

In summary, the state and medical profession's narrative had two explanations for 'social deviance' in the form of youth negligence and criminality. Firstly, the social environment was seen as a potentially negative influence on the socialisation of children – representing the social hygienic standpoint. Secondly, officials viewed 'asocial' adolescents not only as a product of their surroundings, but also that they inherited their 'spoiled' personality from their parents – the eugenic explanation of 'social deviance'. Both combined were a 'medicalised social hygiene', which was, according to Harsch and Moser, prevalent in East Germany during the late 1940s and 1950s.

However, this study underlines the continuation of eugenic and social definitions of deviance from the Third Reich.[109] In the social hygienic view, the solution was the creation of care homes, in which the neglected children of 'asocial'
parents and the 'asocial' youth itself should be gathered to be re-educated and
re-socialised, as well as taken off the streets and locked away from the public
sphere. Conversely, this meant that the state abandoned the parents, who were
seen as the main cause for 'social deviance', but irretrievably 'lost' for the new
society. Authorities directed all their policies towards children. Consequently, the
youth were the ones who faced separation from their parents and life in a care
home, and thus became the guinea pigs for the influencing and engineering of a
new personality, society, and socialist country.[110] The narrative of the state and the
medical profession had a direct impact on the medical memories and experiences
of children, which was limited to not only their social, but also their 'sexually
deviant and defiant behaviour'.

Policing sexual deviance among the youth

After utilising care homes as a solution, officials quickly complained that it was
inappropriate if "sexual *Haltlose* [promiscuous] are put together so closely –
regarding spatial environment – with the endangered youth who are in need of an
intensified education".[111] 'Socially and sexually deviant' people were often in one
and the same institution – a fact which faced constant criticism but was a necessity due to the housing situation in postwar Dresden.[112] Consequently, 'sexual
deviance' needs to be examined separately to capture more facets of children's
behaviour and agency during this period, as well as the state efforts to enforce
'normal' relationships. After a general introduction to children's 'promiscuity',
this section exemplifies this claim with the examples of homosexuality and prostitution among the youth in the postwar era.

For one case in the list of people who were under the scrutiny of Dresden's
Social Welfare Department, officials stated that "[t]he Patient [Maria Kunze],[113]
16 years old, divorced, one child, has itemised eleven [sexual] partners alone.
This [Maria Kunze] is, of course, without a job and was self-evidently put onto
the hwG list".[114] The exceptional nature of Maria Kunze's case should not obscure
the subliminal condemnation in the official statement that was applied to women
with 'frequent promiscuous behaviour' in general, as identified in Chapter 2. For
the East German state, an unemployed girl almost equalled a 'clandestine' prostitute, a potential transmitter of STDs, and thus an 'asocial'. Therefore, for sexual,
as well as for social, 'deviance', the 'asocial' definition was conflated with both
eugenic and social hygienic concepts of the past.[115]

This fact is proven by another report from 1957 which still used the Nazi terminology of *Blutschande* [blood disgrace] when describing a case of incest and transmission of gonorrhoea between a father and his daughter. However, officials were only
pointing towards the fact that the girl infected her father, proving her delinquency,
instead of questioning if the sexual intercourse was abusive or consensual.[116]

Nevertheless, according to the files, promiscuity – as defined by contemporary
officials – was a widespread phenomenon among the youth and was not limited

to female adolescents. The discovering of their sexual desire and its 'enjoyment' were thus a constant health and social target of both the East and West German state.[117] Their concerns were driven by the high rates of STDs, especially among teenagers, and the endangered image of femininity and masculinity in the postwar era, which led authorities to introduce harsh measures also in this field. In her article about *Bahnhof Boys*, Evans argues that these 'sexually deviant' boys were a "direct challenge to the reconstruction of a respectable German masculinity in the East as well as the West".[118]

Due to the renewed peak of diseases in general and STDs in particular during the influx of refugees from the East, the state Saxony introduced a law in 1947 which was supposed to contain the epidemic. They determined that men from 18 to 55 years and women from 16 to 45 years received their food ration cards for the second period only under one condition: they needed to provide the confirmation from an *Ambulatorium* that they had been tested for STDs.[119] This measure not only shows the gender bias again – as females were targeted at a younger age – but also represents an intrusion of the state into the most primal needs of postwar East Germans: the distribution of food. Conversely, apart from authorities' understandable intention to eliminate the high rates of STDs, it was also an open call for black market trading, profiteering, and prostitution among the youth, who evaded the test and, in general, tried to avoid being monitored by the state.[120]

In Leipzig in 1951, officials observed that "[a]mong the young people of rural communities [it is] an open secret that one can easily earn money by having [sexual] intercourse with homosexual men in the case of money shortage".[121] Health and social authorities were alarmed by the fact that the youth were seeking 'easy money' in the homosexual scene, thereby having their sexuality 'spoiled' and possibly contracting an STD.[122] The youth office representative welcomed the plan to intensify the investigations against men who seduce boys, as she was especially concerned "that this *Unsitte* [immorality] is proliferating more and more among the youth".[123] Therefore, places like known (gay) bars, parks, and especially train stations were targeted by the city authorities and faced frequent raids.[124]

As Evans illustrates for Berlin, the situation around train stations – inhabited by delinquent, criminal, and 'sexually deviant' people – represented for authorities the "index of the moral depravity brought about by defeat".[125] Therefore, the agency of Berlin and Leipzig's 'call-boys' and their female counterparts provoked greater state attention than their 'use' by adults. The underage prostitute – female or male[126] – faced monitoring by police, health officials, jurisdiction, or youth organisations and offices, whereas the 'John' was often released on the spot – depending on his societal status and reputation, as well as on previous convictions.[127]

Therefore, the previous finding regarding 'social deviance' is true for 'sexual delinquency' as well: the state was mostly policing the youth. In this case, the biased approach to sexual intercourse and sexuality, in general, aimed for societal transformation and simultaneously enforced the traditional image of a heterosexual relationship. In the same way, it was neglecting the agency of adults who potentially used postwar chaos and uprooted teenagers for their pleasure.[128]

Nevertheless, the state was concerned about neither the causes nor the past of 'sexual deviance', but directed all efforts to the present situation and the future – representing the essential teleological feature of the state narrative.

In both East and West Germany, child psychiatrists did not address the war experiences and rape of the youth, as well as their influence on 'sexual deviance'. Instead, the discussions questioned the veracity of children's testimonies about their sexual abuse – targeting the "dangerous witness" in the form of, for example, "degenerate cravers of recognition with infantile character" and "pathological liars and fantasists".[129] However, two findings of the psychiatrists are striking here. Firstly, the youth themselves rarely spoke about their rape experience, and, secondly, they sought psychological assistance rather than attempting to establish a lawsuit against the perpetrator.[130] In this context, the 'silence' around sex crimes can be identified and was sustained even by the victims themselves – whether out of fear of social stigmatisation or emotional exposure was tellingly not subject for discussion.

In conclusion, both the state and medical profession narrated the youth's behaviour from a future perspective, which legitimised their actions against children and the revival of medical concepts of the past. They saw in this new generation the hope for the new nation but simultaneously incarcerated any 'social and sexual deviance' that departed from the desired social engineering project. As delinquency potentially transgressed the borders of legal, health, and social systems, both 'socially and sexually deviant' children were put under the scrutiny of health, law, police, and youth office authorities. Subsequently, these various governmental bodies forced children into care homes for an indefinite period, where they faced medical and social treatment. Due to this procedure, the medical memories of children were disregarded, their current behaviour pathologised, and their future state directed – the biopolitics of the emerging East German state.[131]

In the end, it was the social hygienic cycle in which children were caught once they obtained the stigma of being 'asocial' or delinquent that inflicted new medical experiences on the already uprooted youth in the postwar era. The ultimate aim was the creation of 'valuable members of society with the right political consciousness towards the construction of Socialism'. However, the care home as such was not only a welcomed legacy of Weimar, but also a conscious continuation of Third Reich penal policies.[132] Furthermore, in this institution the survival and potential combination of eugenic and social hygienic concepts with a medicalised language is observable. This continuity, as well as the care home's purpose and questionable realisation of its aims in East Germany, where the medical personnel of pre-1945, the stigmatised woman, and the delinquent child were housed together, is exemplified on the basis of a case study in Dresden in the final chapter.

Conclusion: the recent hype of the 'forgotten war children' and 'trauma' questioned

"At the moment, the Second World War rampages in German retirement homes".[133] The frequently cited quotation from the journalist and author Katja Thimm at the Second 'War Children' Conference in Münster in 2013 suggests a heightened awareness about the Second World War and its consequences among today's elderly. Recent accounts speak of 'breaking the silence', or announce the 'end of a taboo topic' regarding the 'war youth' and their sufferings in the war and postwar era, and demand a 'collective *Aufarbeitung* [revision]' of this part of history.[134] Doctors and psychotherapists joined the interdisciplinary discussion with letters to the German medical journal *Deutsches Ärzteblatt*, in which one reader welcomed the debates and claimed:

> [T]his subject should have been scientifically revised a long time ago, albeit not politically, not ideologically, not historically, but initially only in the best sense medically, ethically, and in the exact (the scientific) meaning medically scientifically.[135]

Apart from best intentions, the journal reader shows predispositions regarding discourses outside of the realm of medicine, and thus his statement exemplifies the main bias in the popular debate around the 'traumatised war youth': the claim of an 'objective' science and of being 'apolitical'.[136]

In the conclusion of this chapter, the underestimation of subjective perception as well as the political use of terms, such as 'trauma' and the 'forgotten' war youth, are addressed. This finding is set in the context of the previous analysis of children's experiences and the state and medical profession's narrative in postwar East Germany.

The 'apolitical' claim and the search for the 'truth' of a 'traumatised generation' are misleading, but self-serving descriptions. Medical concepts were used to explain and to excuse social phenomena and behaviour. This represents a recurrence of historical processes in modern medical history, especially in Germany. Moreover, the analysis reveals how the (re-)constructed medical memories of the individual feed into the narrative of the state and vice versa: a mutual dependency, informing commemoration practices in the private and public realm in contemporary Germany.[137]

At an international conference in Frankfurt in 2005, psychoanalysts, doctors, witnesses, and other presenters claimed that the war youth is "overburdened in coping with this collective traumatisation alone".[138] Therefore, they argued, "collective traumata need a collective mourning, not only a coming to terms individually".[139] Without disputing the subliminal message and the importance of addressing the past of 'war children', these two statements alone exemplify the 'para-medicalised' language and nature of this debate. The term 'para-medicalised' describes the entanglement of politics with medical concepts and terminology to explain and pathologise social phenomena. The 'para-medicalised' debate consciously uses medical concepts to base its arguments in science, claiming to be 'apolitical', and thus is unaware of its own predisposition and the political implications of its statements.

Additionally, the use of 'collective' as a term is blurred and always has the tendency of homogenising the complexity of individual or group events, memories, and experiences. Therefore, this study refuted the utilisation of 'collective' in its analysis from the start because it has an inherent political motivation. The questionable character of these statements serves to accommodate the majority of people by offering them a narrative which gives them an identity, a sense of belonging to something greater.[140]

The feeling of 'finally breaking with a taboo' was another feature of the discussion that was most significant to the elderly 'war youth' today. It is often spoken of in terms of an emotional release and relief, the appreciation of being finally heard and understood.[141] The reason why German 'victimhood' became a silenced topic is not only the burden of Germany's guilt for causing the Second World War, but also the 1968 generation, which had not allowed any form of addressing the sufferings of their parents, or even their own as children during the war and postwar era.[142]

However, acknowledging the previous findings, the assumptions in this debate appear to be based on subjective perceptions and a political use of this past to stage commemoration. For postwar East Germany, this chapter revealed that there was not a total 'silence' in many ways. Especially for children, the emerging socialist state put effort into narrating their 'victimhood' and abuse by a criminal regime, thereby offering them a new start in a new state and political system. The long-term hope of the authorities was to achieve a generational change and break with the past, a process which they believed would create the idealised socialist citizens. This endeavour represents a typical social engineering project, which was conflated with social hygienic but also eugenic concepts in the medical and public realm.[143]

Nevertheless, the occurrence of rape was mostly excluded from this narrative. The health authorities were directed to erase all data of Soviet soldiers that involved the transmission of STDs in February 1946. In this process, the incidence of sexual violence inflicted by the occupation power was silenced.[144] However, Atina Grossmann has shown that initially there was a public understanding in this sensitive field in postwar East Germany that allowed otherwise illegal abortions for mostly raped women on the basis of 'social indication' – a term derived from eugenic and race concepts and applied for the 'inferior' babies from Russians even after 1945.[145]

In today's debates, women's rights organisations aim to establish rape as a "specific suffering of women", for which men would show no real interest, and raise awareness of the long-term psychological consequences for the victims.[146] Without mitigating this claim and the traumatic experience of rape, this study demonstrates that the limited focus on women and girls is untenable. Both female and male children faced sexual violence in the transition from war to postwar that, however, was often identifiable only if the child acquired an STD.

Moreover, it also became apparent that not only the occupying soldiers, but also compatriots, were a possible threat to youth's sexual and mental health. However, the state hardly addressed this issue, as contemporary medical knowledge often covered up and disregarded the abuse. In the postwar era, the understanding of gonorrhoea and syphilis provided the perpetrator with a narrative that the child probably infected themselves through cups, plates, or the common use of towels. Consequently, only the potential consequences in the form of 'social or sexual deviance' from this extreme, personality-invading medical experience became a concern of authorities. This bias represented an approach that often inflicted more negative medical memories on the children and protected the perpetrator of sexual violence from further investigations.

The postwar youth's – widely perceived – deviance and defiance in social and sexual affairs were a constant target of the East German state. The adolescents were viewed not only as 'abnormal' or 'asocial', but also as an opposition to the (re-)construction of the socialist country.[147] Therefore, the pathologising of experiences and behaviour, as well as their corresponding social and medical treatments, served political and social purposes. The state justified these interventions in the present by an idealised conception of the future: the future of Socialism and Communism. In this process, the medical memories and experiences of children were re-narrated and moulded to the state's interests to turn a nation of bystanders and nominal members into 'anti-Fascists'. In the light of the imminent Cold War, this approach was, firstly, a pragmatic one due to the postwar predicaments, but also, secondly, part of legitimising a minority pushing towards Socialism against the will of the majority of the population.[148]

In this sense, both the postwar era and the recent debate about children's war experience in Germany are 'para-medicalised' strategies to accommodate the 'war youth'. In the past, the state and its narrative were directed towards the future, using children's experiences during the Third Reich and the war and postwar eras to create a form of 'victimhood' that would explain, excuse, and treat the 'social deviance' of the masses. In the present, the debate about 'the forgotten war youth' and its narrative is directed towards the past, also using children's experiences during the Third Reich and the war and postwar eras to create a form of 'victimhood' that would offer an identity to the survivors as a 'traumatised generation'. In both cases, medical or psychological terminology, such as trauma and eugenic or social hygienic concepts, was used to explain social phenomena in political discussions.

Conversely, the outcome of these debates also influenced the medical profession and how doctors treated their patients socially or medically, who, for example, were 'labelled' as 'social deviants' in the past, or as 'traumatised elderly' people today. The biggest pitfall of these 'para-medicalised' discussions is their failure to address the biased nature of their diagnoses – 'asocial' and deviant, or trauma and PTSD – as they remain blurred, dependent on the subjective perception of the individual, and the contemporary medical knowledge.[149]

Nevertheless, the analysed narrative of trauma should not be understood as a top-down model because, as in the postwar era, the 'war youth' have agency that they use to reach their political goals: as Heinlein reveals, the elderly consciously utilise the 'para-medicalised' language in their biographies, and they attend conferences, make their voices heard by creating lobby groups, and thus form an enormous social network that influences the whole public narrative.[150] The inherent heterogeneity of narratives determines commemoration practices and thus, according to Heinlein, accommodates various life paths and provides the individual with "stability and historical depths" – they can locate themselves within something greater and establish their identity.[151] It is both the representation and reception as well as the consumption and expression of medical memories and experiences that are mutually dependent and trimmed into institutionalised narratives of the state, the mnemonic community, and the individual.

The problem with the current debate, however, is multifaceted. Firstly, it neglects the agency of children in the postwar era, which this chapter identified. Thereby, the current discussion has tendencies to establish the 'war youth' generation as a 'hero-victim' who had to cope with the situation without mourning and re-build the country, ultimately managing these tasks successfully.[152] Secondly, words such as 'silence', 'denial', 'loneliness', and 'taboo' frequently reoccur in the discussion and have been developed into politicised terminology.[153] Even if individual experiences have determined these descriptions, the problem arises when it becomes a 'collective' perception, which represents the third pitfall. If there was a common experience, it manifested itself in the ever-present death, malnourishment, and disease that affected almost all war children across geographical and social borders.[154] However, the term 'collective trauma', which is stressed in this debate, not only homogenises suffering, but also potentially trivialises 'victimhood' across nations and ethnicities. Despite the fact that this issue was addressed at the conferences about the 'war youth', it represents an inherent danger which should not be disregarded so easily and requires more scholarship in the future.[155]

A reader of the journal *Deutsches Ärzteblatt*, who is also a 'war child', and in vehement opposition to psychoanalysis, reacts to Thimm's claim, utilised as the opening quotation in this section, and states "[t]hat the Second World War rampages in German retirement homes [. . .] is utter nonsense".[156] Unlike this reader, the intention of the section was not to dispute subjective perception or individual war experiences and memories. However, it is important to raise awareness of the debate's nature. This study follows Heinlein's argument, which suggests a reconsideration of the terminology that until today has been biased and politically motivated.[157]

This chapter analysed children's war experiences and their consequences in postwar East Germany. In contrast to the other two main chapters, the third has approached the topic consistently from the local community to the state level. It has examined the complexity of 'war children's' medical memories and experiences and subsequently has explored the *treatment for their past* by the medical profession and the state in the form of their response and narration. These findings have been set in context with the current debates about the 'war youth' in the last section. In both cases, postwar and contemporary Germany, the analysis has shown that the children's past was not treated, in the medical and psychological sense, but utilised for political goals and a narrative that legitimised the state and its interventions.

Within these debates, a tendency towards simplification of past events and medical concepts, such as trauma, was recognised, which had a twofold purpose. On the one hand, it was supposed to offer a coping strategy for coming to terms with the past in the postwar era and today. On the other hand, in this process, an identity, as well as a connection of individuals to like-minded people, is created. Those people shared similar life stories, such as their perception that war experiences were a long-standing taboo topic, and thus established mnemonic communities of support and social power. Consequently, medical memories and experiences of individuals were 'collectivised' – 'trauma' became a shared identity.

In summary, this chapter has exemplified how the concept of medical memories and experiences captures the social interaction between the state and local level, the medical and political realm, as well as the individual and the community. To open up the framework for future research, the last chapter uses the case study of the Care Home Leuben in Dresden. This institution features the findings of all three main chapters and thus clarifies the concept behind the medical memories and experiences of the state, institution, mnemonic community, and individual.

Notes

1 'Niederschrift, 7. November 1946': StA DD, Dezernat Gesundheitswesen, 4.1.12, Nr. 2, Bl. 280.
2 'Niederschrift, 7. November 1946': StA DD, Dezernat Gesundheitswesen, 4.1.12, Nr. 2, Bl. 280.
3 For comparison, see Andreja Brajša-Žganec, 'The Long-Term Effects of War Experiences on Children's Depression in the Republic of Croatia', *Child Abuse & Neglect*, 29 (2005), 31–43; Atle Dyregrov and others, 'Grief and Traumatic Grief in Children in the Context of Mass Trauma', *Current Psychiatry Reports*, 17 (2015), 1–8.
4 The inverted commas are indicative of the author's awareness of the terms' ambiguity in regards to trauma, traumatic, traumatised, and similar medical descriptions or diagnoses. Throughout this chapter, the terminology is discussed and questioned. Therefore, in the following analysis, the chapter refrains from using inverted commas for trauma, as its biased character is implied. Only for cases of politically motivated word constructions, single quotation marks highlight their questionable nature.
5 The only case study of children during the Second World War was given by Dorothy Burlingham and Anna Freud, *Infants Without Families: The Case For and Against Residential Nurseries* (London: Allen & Unwin, 1964). For an exploration of this notion of youth resilience, see Volker Ackermann, 'Das Schweigen der Flüchtlingskinder: Psychische Folgen von Krieg, Flucht und Vertreibung bei den Deutschen nach 1945', *Geschichte und Gesellschaft*, 30 (2004), 434–64. For a critic of this view, see Dyregrov and others, p. 2.
6 Brajša-Žganec, p. 32.
7 Ackermann, p. 439. For examples of individual war experiences, see Sabine Bode, *Die vergessene Generation: Die Kriegskinder brechen ihr Schweigen*, 12th ed. (Munich: Piper, 2009), pp. 73–108.
8 Günther Grass, *Im Krebsgang* (Göttingen: Steidl, 2002); Bode.
9 Mary Fulbrook, *Dissonant Lives: Generations and Violence Through the German Dictatorships* (Oxford: Oxford University Press, 2011), chapters 6, 7 and 8.
10 For an overview about the psycho-social ramifications of war and trauma for the elderly, see Hartmut Radebold, ' "Kriegskinder" im Alter: Bei Diagnose historisch denken', *Deutsches Ärzteblatt*, 101 (2004), A1960–A1962; Hartmut Radebold, *Abwesende Väter und Kriegskindheit: Alte Verletzungen bewältigen* (Stuttgart: Klett-Cotta, 2010).
11 Petra Bühring, 'Die Generation der Kriegskinder: Kollektive Aufarbeitung notwendig', *Deutsches Ärzteblatt*, 102 (2005), A1190–A1193; Adelheid Jachertz and Norbert

Jachertz, 'Kriegskinder: Erst im Alter wird oft das Ausmaß der Traumatisierungen sichtbar', *Deutsches Ärzteblatt*, 110 (2013), A656–A658.

12 Ulrike Jureit, 'Generationen-Gedächtnis: Überlegungen zu einem Konzept kommunikativer Vergemeinschaftungen', in *Die 'Generation der Kriegskinder': Historische Hintergründe und Deutungen*, ed. by Lu Seegers and Jürgen Reulecke (Gießen: Psychosozial-Verlag, 2009), pp. 125–36.

13 For a critical analysis about the current debates, see Michael Heinlein, 'Das Trauma der deutschen Kriegskinder zwischen nationaler und europäischer Erinnerung: Kritische Anmerkungen zum gegenwärtigen Wandel der Erinnerungskultur', in *Narratives of Trauma: Discourses of German Wartime Suffering in National and International Perspective*, ed. by Helmut Schmitz and Annette Seidel-Arpacı (Amsterdam: Rodopi, 2011), pp. 111–28.

14 For this judgement, see 'Max Klesse, Über die Beurteilung der Geschlechtskrankheiten und die Maßnahmen zur ihrer Bekämpfung, 26. August 1946': BArch, DQ 1/1610, unpaginated.

15 Michael Heinlein, *Die Erfindung der Erinnerung: Deutsche Kriegskindheiten im Gedächtnis der Gegenwart* (Bielefeld: Transcript, 2010), p. 88.

16 For a critic of the use of trauma as a concept for historical investigations, see Svenja Goltermann, 'The Imagination of Disaster: Death and Survival in Postwar West Germany', in *Between Mass Death and Individual Loss: The Place of the Dead in Twentieth-Century Germany*, ed. by Alon Confino, Paul Betts, and Dirk Schumann (New York: Berghahn Books, 2008), pp. 261–74.

17 For more information about psychological concepts after the two world wars, see Svenja Goltermann, 'Psychisches Leid und herrschende Lehre: Der Wissenschaftswandel in der westdeutschen Psychiatrie der Nachkriegszeit', in *Akademische Vergangenheitspolitik: Beiträge zur Wissenschaftskultur der Nachkriegszeit*, ed. by Bernd Weisbrod (Göttingen: Wallstein, 2002), pp. 263–80; Paul Lerner, 'Psychiatry and Casualties of War in Germany, 1914–18', *Journal of Contemporary History*, 35 (2000), 13–28.

18 For an important exploration of children's Third Reich and war experiences, see Nicholas Stargardt, *Witnesses of War: Children's Lives Under the Nazis* (London: Pimlico, 2006).

19 Erving Goffman, *Behavior in Public Places: Notes on the Social Organization of Gatherings* (New York: The Free Press, 1985), p. 248.

20 Tobias Hecker and others, 'The Cycle of Violence: Associations Between Exposure to Violence, Trauma-Related Symptoms, and Aggression – Findings from Congolese Refugees in Uganda', *Journal of Traumatic Stress*, 28 (2015), 448–55.

21 This claim of leading 'perfectly normal lives' during the GDR has prominently been identified by Fulbrook and introduced into the overall historiography of East Germany, not without criticism. Fulbrook, *Dissonant Lives*, p. 478; Mary Fulbrook, *The People's State: East German Society from Hitler to Honecker* (London: Yale University Press, 2005), p. IX.

22 Heinlein, *Die Erfindung der Erinnerung*, pp. 86–7.

23 For more in-depth discussion of commemoration practices and their manifestations in society and politics as well as in historical research, see Aleida Assmann, 'History and Memory', *International Encyclopedia of the Social & Behavioral Sciences* (Elsevier, 2001), pp. 6822–29; Aleida Assmann, *Der lange Schatten der Vergangenheit: Erinnerungskultur und Geschichtspolitik* (Munich: Beck, 2006); *War and Remembrance in the Twentieth Century*, ed. by Jay Winter and Emmanuel Sivan (Cambridge: Cambridge University Press, 1999); Stefan Goebel, *The Great War and Medieval Memory: War, Remembrance, and Medievalism in Britain and Germany, 1914–1940* (Cambridge: Cambridge University Press, 2007).

24 Wolfgang Borchert, 'Nachts schlafen die Ratten doch', in *Das Gesamtwerk: Mit einem biographischen Nachwort von Bernhard Meyer-Marwitz* (Hamburg: Rowohlt, 1949), pp. 216–19.

25 Borchert, pp. 216–19.

26 For the problematic and extensive use of the term 'collective' in connection with trauma as reference in multiple forms, see, for example, Bode; Bühring, 'Die Generation der Kriegskinder', p. A1190.

27 Konrad H. Jarausch and Michael Geyer, *Shattered Past: Reconstructing German Histories* (Princeton: Princeton University Press, 2003), p. 353.

28 Elisabeth Pfeils, *Flüchtlingskinder in neuer Heimat* (Stuttgart: Klett, 1951), p. 11.

29 The difficulties of integrating refugees and expellees from the East in the GDR and FRG have been investigated by Patrice G. Poutrus, 'Zuflucht im Nachkriegsdeutschland: Politik und Praxis der Flüchtlingsaufnahme in Bundesrepublik und DDR von den späten 1940er bis zu den 1970er Jahren', *Geschichte und Gesellschaft*, 35 (2009), 135–75; Michael Schwartz, *Vertriebene und 'Umsiedlerpolitik': Integrationskonflikte in den deutschen Nachkriegs-Gesellschaften und die Assimilationsstrategien in der SBZ/DDR 1945–1961* (Munich: Oldenbourg, 2004).

30 Richard Bessel, *Germany 1945: From War to Peace* (London: Simon & Schuster, 2009), p. 332.

31 Christoph Buchheim, 'Der Mythos vom "Wohlleben": Der Lebensstandard der deutschen Zivilbevölkerung im Zweiten Weltkrieg', *Vierteljahreshefte für Zeitgeschichte*, 58 (2010), 299–328.

32 Dorothee Wierling, *Geboren im Jahr Eins: Der Jahrgang 1949 in der DDR: Versuch einer Kollektivbiographie* (Berlin: Links, 2002), p. 60.

33 Jessica Reinisch, *The Perils of Peace: The Public Health Crisis in Occupied Germany* (Oxford: Oxford University Press, 2013), pp. 6, 31, 37–9.

34 Bessel, pp. 343–53; Wierling, pp. 60–1.

35 Hermann Stutte and H. Reinecke, 'Wachstumsverhältnisse bei hessischen Schulkindern in den Jahren 1946–1949', *Kinderärztliche Praxis*, 19 (1951), 515–21. Bessel also identifies malnourishment as a pan-German issue. Bessel, p. 353.

36 Elisabeth Lippert and Claudia Keppel, 'Deutsche Kinder in den Jahren 1947 bis 1950: Beitrag zur biologischen und epochalpsychologischen Lebensalterforschung', *Schweizerische Zeitschrift für Psychologie und ihre Anwendungen*, 9 (1950), 212–322. A broader discussion about the foundation of and the people behind the 'Langoog-Study', see Ackermann, p. 442.

37 Ackermann, p. 445; Lippert and Keppel, p. 232.

38 Ackermann, p. 445.

39 Bessel, p. 352.

40 Wierling, p. 61. For the situation in 1945, see Bessel, pp. 353–4.

41 Reinisch, p. 228; Wierling, p. 68.

42 For the overview and description of diseases for the years 1946 to 1949, see 'Jahresbericht 1946': StA DD, Dezernat Gesundheitswesen, 4.1.12, Nr. 3, Bl. 51, 53; 'Jahresbericht 1947': StA DD, Dezernat Gesundheitswesen, 4.1.12, Nr. 4, Bl. 203, 205; 'Jahresbericht 1948': StA DD, Dezernat Gesundheitswesen, 4.1.12, Nr. 5, Bl. 77, 79; 'Jahresbericht 1949': StA DD, Dezernat Gesundheitswesen, 4.1.12, Nr. 5, Bl. 98, 101.

43 Reinisch, p. 295.

44 For an overview, see 'Jahresstatistik der anzeigepflichtigen übertragbaren Krankheiten in der sowjetischen Besatzungszone für das Jahr 1947, 25. Februar 1948': StA DD, Dezernat Gesundheitswesen, 4.1.12, Nr. 4, Bl. 126–7; 'Jahresstatistik der anzeigepflichtigen übertragbaren Krankheiten in der sowjetischen Besatzungszone für das Jahr 1948, 24. Februar 1949': StA DD, Dezernat Gesundheitswesen, 4.1.12, Nr. 5, Bl. 1–2; 'Jahresstatistik der anzeigepflichtigen übertragbaren Krankheiten in der sowjetischen Besatzungszone für das Jahr 1949, 23. Dezember 1950': StA DD, Dezernat Gesundheitswesen, 4.1.12, Nr. 5, Bl. 83–4.

45 Rolf Castell and others, *Geschichte der Kinder- und Jugendpsychiatrie in Deutschland in den Jahren 1937 bis 1961* (Göttingen: Vandenhoeck & Ruprecht, 2003), p. 146.

46 For example: 'Jahresbericht 1947 über das Stadtkrankenhaus Dresden-Plauen, 2. Januar 1948': StA DD, Dezernat Gesundheitswesen, 4.1.12, Nr. 4, Bl. 81–2; 'Urologische Klinik, StKh Plauen, Tätigkeitsbericht für das Jahr 1947, 29. Dezember 1947': StA DD, Dezernat Gesundheitswesen, 4.1.12, Nr. 4, Bl. 89. For the general situation of the healthcare system in postwar Germany, see Bessel, pp. 330–1.

47 Ackermann, p. 445; Lippert and Keppel, p. 232.

48 Bessel, p. 334; Wierling, p. 61.

49 'Niederschrift über die Besichtigung des Städtischen Obdachs, Dresden-N., Altpieschen 9, 16. August 1948': StA DD, Dezernat Sozial und Wohnungswesen, 4.1.10, Nr. 71, Bl. 71.

50 'Niederschrift über die Besichtigung des Städtischen Obdachs, Dresden-N., Altpieschen 9, 16. August 1948': StA DD, Dezernat Sozial und Wohnungswesen, 4.1.10, Nr. 71, Bl. 72–3.

51 'Niederschrift über die Besichtigung des Städtischen Obdachs, Dresden-N., Altpieschen 9, 16. August 1948': StA DD, Dezernat Sozial und Wohnungswesen, 4.1.10, Nr. 71, Bl. 73.

52 'Jahresbericht über die Arbeit der Landeszentrale zur Bekämpfung der Geschlechtskrankheiten 1946': BArch, DQ 1/292, unpaginated.

53 'Bestrafung der Eltern bei Vernachlässigung der geschlechtlichen Gesundheit der Schutzbefohlenen, 19. Januar 1946': BArch, DQ 1/139, Bl. 179. For a recent study, see Inka Wilhelm and Susanne Zank, 'Zweiter Weltkrieg und pflegerische Versorgung heute: Einfluss von Kriegstraumatisierungen auf professionelle Pflegesituationen', *Zeitschrift für Gerontologie und Geriatrie*, 5 (2014), 4–8.

54 See Figure 3.2; 'Jahresbericht 1946': StA DD, Dezernat Gesundheitswesen, 4.1.12, Nr. 3, Bl. 51, 53; 'Jahresbericht 1947': StA DD, Dezernat Gesundheitswesen, 4.1.12, Nr. 4, Bl. 203, 205; 'Jahresbericht 1948': StA DD, Dezernat Gesundheitswesen, 4.1.12, Nr. 5, Bl. 77, 79; 'Jahresbericht 1949': StA DD, Dezernat Gesundheitswesen, 4.1.12, Nr. 5, Bl. 98, 101.

55 Wm Lane M. Robson, 'Enuresis', *Medscape*, 2015 <http://emedicine.medscape.com/article/1014762-overview#a4> [accessed 30 January 2019]. Ackermann lists in his study nocturnal enuresis as one possible long-term consequence of war. Ackermann, p. 446.

56 Bode, pp. 48–50.

57 'Betr.: Psychiatrische Durchmusterung gefährdeter Familien im Obdachlosenasyl in Altpieschen, 18. August 1948': StA DD, Dezernat Sozial und Wohnungswesen, 4.1.10, Nr. 71, Bl. 74.

58 A Summary of Förster's paper was published in Castell and others, p. 104.

59 A Summary of Förster's paper was published in Castell and others, p. 104.

60 For a biography of Werner Villinger, see Castell and others, pp. 463–80.

61 Quotation of Villinger at the DVJ conference in 1954 is taken from Castell and others, p. 120.

62 Quotation of Villinger at the DVJ conference in 1954 is taken from Castell and others, p. 120.

63 'Jahresbericht 1946': StA DD, Dezernat Gesundheitswesen, 4.1.12, Nr. 3, Bl. 51, 53; 'Jahresbericht 1947': StA DD, Dezernat Gesundheitswesen, 4.1.12, Nr. 4, Bl. 203, 205; 'Jahresbericht 1948': StA DD, Dezernat Gesundheitswesen, 4.1.12, Nr. 5, Bl. 77, 79; 'Jahresbericht 1949': StA DD, Dezernat Gesundheitswesen, 4.1.12, Nr. 5, Bl. 98, 101.

64 For its use and contested definition, see Goltermann, 'Psychisches Leid und herrschende Lehre', pp. 272–5; Bode, pp. 48–50.

65 Alice Förster and Birgit Beck, 'Post-Traumatic Stress Disorder and World War II: Can a Psychiatric Concept Help Us Understand Postwar Society?', in *Life after Death: Approaches to a Cultural and Social History of Europe During the 1940s and 1950s*,

ed. by Richard Bessel and Dirk Schumann (Cambridge: Cambridge University Press, 2007), pp. 15–36.

66 As comparison, see the West German report from Hannover: 'Der Niedersächsische Minister für Arbeit, Aufbau und Gesundheit, betr. Bekämpfung der Geschlechts-krankheiten (GK), 31. Juli 1948': BArch, DQ 1/292, unpaginated.

67 Ackermann, p. 455; Jennifer V. Evans, *Life Among the Ruins: Cityscape and Sexuality in Cold War Berlin* (Houndmills: Palgrave Macmillan, 2011), p. 45.

68 'Fürsorgeheim Leuben, 10. Februar 1947': StA DD, Dezernat Sozial- und Wohnungs-wesen, 4.1.10, Nr. 71, Bl. 10.

69 'Fürsorgeheim Leuben, 10. Februar 1947': StA DD, Dezernat Sozial- und Wohnungs-wesen, 4.1.10, Nr. 71, Bl. 10.

70 Bessel, pp. 328–9.

71 Mark Fenemore, 'The Growing Pains of Sex Education in the German Democratic Republic (GDR), 1945–69', in *Shaping Sexual Knowledge: A Cultural History of Sex Education in Twentieth-Century Europe*, ed. by Lutz D H Sauerteig and Roger David-son (London: Routledge, 2009), pp. 71–90.

72 Anna Maria Sigmund, *'Das Geschlechtsleben bestimmen wir': Sexualität im Dritten Reich* (Munich: Heyne, 2008), p. 254.

73 Evans, *Life Among the Ruins*, p. 133; Jennifer V. Evans, 'Bahnhof Boys: Policing Male Prostitution in Post-Nazi Berlin', *Journal of the History of Sexuality*, 12 (2003), 605–36.

74 'Niederschrift über die Besichtigung des Städtischen Obdachs, 16. August 1948': StA DD, Dezernat Sozial- und Wohnungswesen, 4.1.10, Nr. 71, Bl. 71.

75 'Niederschrift über die Besichtigung des Städtischen Obdachs, 16. August 1948': StA DD, Dezernat Sozial- und Wohnungswesen, 4.1.10, Nr. 71, Bl. 71.

76 Evans, *Life Among the Ruins*, pp. 76–7.

77 'Stadtpolizeidirektion Dresden, Gesundheitliche Gefährdung von Kindern durch umherliegende Schutzmittel im öffentlichen Verkehrsraum, 14. Dezember 1939': StA DD, Wohlfahrtspolizeiamt, 2.3.27, Nr. 31, Bl. 57.

78 'Allgemeine Aufklärung über Geschlechtskrankheiten': BArch, DQ 1/292, unpaginated.

79 'Tripper (Gonorrhoe), [Without date]': BArch, DQ 1/991, Bl. 102. For a general over-view of how syphilis and gonorrhoea is spread, see 'Syphilis', *NHS*, 2016 <www.nhs.uk/conditions/Syphilis/Pages/Introduction.aspx> [accessed 30 January 2019]; 'Gon-orrhoea', *NHS*, 2016 <www.nhs.uk/Conditions/Gonorrhoea/Pages/Introduction.aspx> [accessed 30 January 2019].

80 Norman Naimark, *The Russians in Germany: A History of the Soviet Zone of Occupa-tion, 1945–1949* (Cambridge, MA: The Belknap Press, 1995), chapter 2; Atina Gross-mann, 'A Question of Silence: The Rape of German Women by Occupation Soldiers', *October*, 72 (1995), 42–63.

81 Lerner, p. 15.

82 'Aktenvermerk über die Dienstreise nach Dresden, Leipzig, Freiberg, Chemnitz (Land Sachsen) in der Zeit vom 12. bis einschließlich 16. Dezember 1949': BArch, DQ 1/20626, unpaginated.

83 'Aktenvermerk über die Dienstreise nach Dresden, Leipzig, Freiberg, Chemnitz (Land Sachsen) in der Zeit vom 12. bis einschließlich 16. Dezember 1949': BArch, DQ 1/20626, unpaginated.

84 'Aktenvermerk über die Dienstreise nach Dresden, Leipzig, Freiberg, Chemnitz (Land Sachsen) in der Zeit vom 12. bis einschließlich 16. Dezember 1949': BArch, DQ 1/20626, unpaginated.

85 For a comparison with the West Zone, see 'Der Niedersächsische Minister für Arbeit, Aufbau und Gesundheit, betr. Bekämpfung der Geschlechtskrankheiten (GK), 31. Juli 1948': BArch, DQ 1/292, unpaginated.

86 Michael Buddrus, 'A Generation Twice Betrayed: Youth Policy in the Transition from the Third Reich to the Soviet Zone of Occupation (1945–1946)', in *Generations in Conflict: Youth Revolt and Generation Formation in Germany 1770–1968*, ed. by Mark Roseman (Cambridge: Cambridge University Press, 1995), pp. 247–68. For another discussion of the HJ youth in the postwar era and its coping strategies in form of a 'community of silence', see Alexander von Plato, 'The Hitler Youth Generation and Its Role in the Two Post-War German States', in *Generations in Conflict: Youth Revolt and Generation Formation in Germany 1770–1968*, ed. by Mark Roseman (Cambridge: Cambridge University Press, 1995), pp. 210–26.

87 'Max Klesse, Über die Beurteilung der Geschlechtskrankheiten und die Maßnahmen zur ihrer Bekämpfung, 26. August 1946': BArch, DQ 1/1610, unpaginated.

88 For a report about the situation among the youth in Dresden, see 'Fürsorgeheim Leuben, 10. Februar 1947': StA DD, Dezernat Sozial- und Wohnungswesen, 4.1.10, Nr. 71, Bl. 10. Evans, *Life Among the Ruins*, p. 190.

89 Quotation taken from Castell and others, p. 126.

90 Castell and others, p. 118.

91 Castell and others, p. 118.

92 Goltermann, 'Psychisches Leid und herrschende Lehre', 2002, pp. 265–9.

93 Gabriele Moser, *'Im Interesse der Volksgesundheit . . .': Sozialhygiene und öffentliches Gesundheitswesen in der Weimarer Republik und der frühen SBZ/DDR. Ein Beitrag zur Sozialgeschichte des deutschen Gesundheitswesens im 20. Jahrhundert* (Frankfurt a.M.: VAS, 2002), pp. 42–67, 152, 154, 165, 207.

94 'Aktenvermerk über die Dienstreise nach Dresden, Leipzig, Freiberg, Chemnitz (Land Sachsen) in der Zeit vom 12. bis einschließlich 16. Dezember 1949': BArch, DQ 1/20626, unpaginated. Evans also identifies the continuity of mentalities and medical or social concepts regarding the youth from previous political systems. Evans, *Life Among the Ruins*, p. 145.

95 Quotation taken from Buddrus, p. 255.

96 Similar strategies can be identified in the narrative of the Dresden air raids, which the East German state quickly condemned as crimes against humanity, thereby serving the general mood among these cities and the general population for legitimization purposes. Important insights into the debates surrounding the bombing of German cities, especially of Dresden, as well as its narrative and commemoration in the past and present were given by Jörg Echterkamp, 'Von der Gewalterfahrung zu Kriegserinnerung: Über den Bombenkrieg als Thema einer Geschichte der deutschen Kriegsgesellschaft', in *Deutschland im Luftkrieg*, ed. by Dietmar Süß (Munich: Oldenbourg, 2007), pp. 13–25; Stefan Goebel, 'Coventry und Dresden: Transnationale Netzwerke der Erinnerung in den 1950er und 1960er Jahren', in *Deutschland im Luftkrieg*, ed. by Dietmar Süß (Munich: Oldenbourg, 2007), pp. 111–20; *Cities into Battlefields: Metropolitan Scenarios, Experiences, and Commemorations of Total War*, ed. by Stefan Goebel and Derek Keene (Farnham: Ashgate, 2011); Bill Niven, 'The GDR and Memory of the Bombing of Dresden', in *Germans as Victims: Remembering the Past in Contemporary Germany* (Houndmills: Palgrave Macmillan, 2006), pp. 109–29.

97 For further work on 'anti-Fascism' as legitimization strategy of the GDR, see Andrew H. Beattie, *Playing Politics with History: The Bundestag Inquiries into East Germany* (New York: Berghahn Books, 2008), chapters 3, 5; Siobhan Kattago, *Ambiguous Memory: The Nazi Past and German National Identity* (Westport, CT: Praeger, 2001), chapter 4; Ingo Loose, 'The Anti-Fascist Myth of the German Democratic Republic and Its Decline After 1989', in *Past in the Making: Historical Revisionism in Central Europe After 1989*, ed. by Michal Kopecek (Budapest: Central European University Press, 2008), pp. 59–71; Josie McLellan, *Antifascism and Memory in East Germany: Remembering the International Brigades 1945–1989* (Oxford: Clarendon, 2004).

98 For examples of studies that examine the survival and rise of xenophobia in East Germany in particular, see Jan C. Behrends and Patrice G. Poutrus, 'Xenophobia in the Former GDR: Explorations and Explanation from a Historical Perspective', in *Nationalisms Across the Globe: An Overview of Nationalisms in State-Endowed and Stateless Nations: Volume 1: Europe*, ed. by Wojciech Burszta, Tomasz Dominik Kamusella, and Sebastian Wojciechowski (Poznań: Wyższa Szkoła Nauk Humanistycznych i Dziennikarstwa, 2005), pp. 155–70; Anna Saunders, *Honecker's Children: Youth and Patriotism in East(Ern) Germany, 1979–2002* (Manchester: Manchester University Press, 2007), pp. 180–4; Jonathan R. Zatlin, 'Scarcity and Resentment: Economic Sources of Xenophobia in the GDR, 1971–1989', *Central European History*, 40 (2007), 683–720.

99 'Aktenvermerk über die Dienstreise nach Dresden, Leipzig, Freiberg, Chemnitz (Land Sachsen) in der Zeit vom 12. bis einschließlich 16. Dezember 1949': BArch, DQ 1/20626, unpaginated.

100 'Aktenvermerk über die Dienstreise nach Dresden, Leipzig, Freiberg, Chemnitz (Land Sachsen) in der Zeit vom 12. bis einschließlich 16. Dezember 1949': BArch, DQ 1/20626, unpaginated.

101 'Aktenvermerk über die Dienstreise nach Dresden, Leipzig, Freiberg, Chemnitz (Land Sachsen) in der Zeit vom 12. bis einschließlich 16. Dezember 1949': BArch, DQ 1/20626, unpaginated. For recent scholarship, see Ruth Seydlitz and Pamela Jenkins, 'The Influence of Families, Friends, Schools, and Community on Delinquent Behavior', in *Delinquent Violent Youth: Theory and Interventions*, ed. by Thomas P. Gullotta, Gerald R. Adams, and Raymond Montemayor (Thousand Oaks: Sage, 1998), pp. 53–97.

102 Castell and others, pp. 119–20, here 120.

103 Castell and others, pp. 121–2, here 122.

104 'Aktenvermerk über die Arbeitsbesprechung in Dresden – Leuben, 28. Dezember 1949': BArch, DQ 1/20626, unpaginated.

105 'Aktenvermerk über die Arbeitsbesprechung in Dresden – Leuben, 28. Dezember 1949': BArch, DQ 1/20626, unpaginated.

106 In his recent book, Greg Eghigian explores the treatment of convicts and sexual offenders – the 'corrigible' and the 'incorrigible' – in the Third Reich, GDR, and the FRG. Greg Eghigian, *The Corrigible and the Incorrigible: Science, Medicine, and the Convict in Twentieth-Century Germany* (Ann Arbor, MI: University of Michigan Press, 2015).

107 'Aktenvermerk über die Dienstreise nach Dresden, Leipzig, Freiberg, Chemnitz (Land Sachsen) in der Zeit vom 12. bis einschließlich 16. Dezember 1949': BArch, DQ 1/20626, unpaginated.

108 Moser, pp. 152, 154, 165, 207.

109 Donna Harsch, 'Medicalized Social Hygiene? Tuberculosis Policy in the German Democratic Republic', *Bulletin of the History of Medicine*, 86 (2012), 394–423; Moser, p. 207.

110 Buddrus, p. 252.

111 'An die Landesregierung, Ministerium für Arbeit und Sozialfürsorge, 17. Mai 1947': StA DD, Fürsorgeamt, 2.3.15, AV I/Nr. 647, Bl. 108.

112 For another complaint about the situation in the care home in Dresden, see 'Fürsorgeheim Leuben, 10. Februar 1947': StA DD, Dezernat Sozial- und Wohnungswesen, 4.1.10, Nr. 71, Bl. 10.

113 The name was made anonymous due to public and archival restrictions. Therefore, the fictitious name Maria Kunze will be used to enhance comprehension in the following.

114 'Protokoll über ein Besuch im Kreisambulatorium Zwickau/Sa., am 15. Dezember 1955': BArch, DQ 1/4436, unpaginated.

115 Evans also stresses the survival of eugenics in science and academia in the postwar period. Jennifer V. Evans, 'Decriminalization, Seduction, and "Unnatural Desire" in East Germany', *Feminist Studies*, 36 (2010), 553–77.

116 'Analyse zum Kurzbericht über g-Krankheiten für den Monat April 1957, 11. Mai 1957': BArch, DQ 1/4436, unpaginated.

117 For an insightful study, see Evans, *Life Among the Ruins*, pp. 13, 40, 72, 198–9, 222; Evans, 'Bahnhof Boys', pp. 608–9, 626–9, 634–6; Evans, 'Decriminalization, Seduction, and Unnatural Desire', p. 555.

118 Evans, 'Bahnhof Boys', p. 636.

119 'Rundverfügung Nr. 4, Landesregierung Sachsen, Ministerium für Arbeit und Sozialfürsorge, 16. Januar 1947': StA DD, Fürsorgeamt, 2.3.15, AV I/Nr. 647, Bl. 108.

120 Evans, 'Bahnhof Boys', pp. 619–20.

121 'Protokoll über die Sitzung des Beirates zur Bekämpfung der Geschlechtskrankheiten, am 28. Juni 1951': StA Leipzig, Stadtverwaltung und Rat, Nr. 7349, Bl. 252.

122 It was a prevalent view that sexuality of teenagers can be influenced by adults and their social environment. Evans, 'Decriminalization, Seduction, and Unnatural Desire', p. 560.

123 'Protokoll über die Sitzung des Beirates zur Bekämpfung der Geschlechtskrankheiten, am 28. Juni 1951': StA Lpz, Stadtverwaltung und Rat, Nr. 7349, Bl. 252.

124 'Protokoll über die Sitzung des Beirates zur Bekämpfung der Geschlechtskrankheiten, am 28. Juni 1951': StA Lpz, Stadtverwaltung und Rat, Nr. 7349, Bl. 252.

125 Evans, 'Bahnhof Boys', p. 609.

126 For the procedures against prostitutes and the gender bias regarding spreading STDs, see Evans, 'Bahnhof Boys', p. 619.

127 'Protokoll über die Sitzung des Beirates zur Bekämpfung der Geschlechtskrankheiten, am 28. Juni 1951': StA Leipzig, Stadtverwaltung und Rat, Nr. 7349, Bl. 252; Evans, 'Bahnhof Boys', pp. 624–8, 631–4.

128 For example, see Evans, *Life Among the Ruins*, pp. 76–7.

129 Quotation taken from Castell and others, p. 148.

130 These findings were presented by Erika Geisler at the third DVJ conference in Essen 1954. Castell and others, p. 117.

131 For the notion of biopolitics in East Germany, see also Evans, 'Decriminalization, Seduction, and Unnatural Desire', p. 572.

132 Also Evans identifies this twofold legacy of the juvenile homes in Berlin. Evans, 'Bahnhof Boys', p. 634.

133 Quotation taken from Jachertz and Jachertz, p. A658. For her recent book, see Katja Thimm, *Vatertage: Eine deutsche Geschichte* (Frankfurt a.M.: Fischer, 2011).

134 Bühring, 'Die Generation der Kriegskinder', p. A1190; Petra Bühring, 'Sexualisierte Gewalt: Das Schweigen brechen', *Deutsches Ärzteblatt*, 102 (2005), A1798.

135 H.W. Pollack, 'Aufarbeitung überfällig', *Deutsches Ärzteblatt*, 102 (2005), A1950.

136 For the discussion of the long-nineteenth century and the development of the political 'apolitical' doctor, see Tobias Weidner, *Die unpolitische Profession: Deutsche Mediziner im langen 19. Jahrhundert* (Frankfurt a.M.: Campus, 2012).

137 Heinlein, *Die Erfindung der Erinnerung*, p. 180.

138 Quotation taken from Bühring, 'Die Generation der Kriegskinder', p. A1190.

139 Quotation taken from Bühring, 'Die Generation der Kriegskinder', p. A1193.

140 Heinlein, *Die Erfindung der Erinnerung*, p. 182. Bode also identifies that survival, trauma, and its narrative create a sense of identity. Bode, p. 279.

141 For example, see Ackermann; Bode; Bühring, 'Die Generation der Kriegskinder'; Bühring, 'Sexualisierte Gewalt'; Jachertz and Jachertz.

142 Bode, pp. 27–9; Jachertz and Jachertz, p. A657. For a critic of this claim, see Heinlein, *Die Erfindung der Erinnerung*, p. 13.

143 Buddrus, pp. 252, 256–5.

144 For the classified orders, see 'Vertrauliche Mitteilung. Betr. Wochen- und Monatsmeldungen der Geschlechtskrankheiten, 21. Februar 1946': BArch, DQ 1/1010, unpaginated; 'Vertrauliche Mitteilung, 2. Mai 1946': BArch, DQ 1/1010, unpaginated; 'Betr. Vertrauliche Mitteilung v. 21. Febr. und 2. Mai 1946, 24. Mai 1946': BArch, DQ 1/1010, unpaginated.

145 Grossmann, pp. 53–61, here 55.
146 Bühring, 'Sexualisierte Gewalt', p. A1798.
147 For more information, see Evans, *Life Among the Ruins*, p. 215.
148 Buddrus, pp. 265–8; Plato, p. 224. Heinlein, *Die Erfindung der Erinnerung*, pp. 180–2.
149 For a critic of the use of trauma for historical investigations, see Goltermann, 'The Imagination of Disaster'.
150 Heinlein, *Die Erfindung der Erinnerung*, pp. 180–5. For examples for this development, see Bode; Radebold, *Abwesende Väter und Kriegskindheit*; Thimm.
151 Heinlein, *Die Erfindung der Erinnerung*, pp. 181–2, here 181. For another discussion of this issue, see Jureit, pp. 125–36.
152 Bühring, 'Die Generation der Kriegskinder', p. A1190.
153 For examples, see the discussion in the journal *Deutsches Ärzteblatt* about the article of Hartmut Radebold in 2004, Radebold, ' "Kriegskinder" im Alter'.
154 For a similar judgement, see Jarausch and Geyer, p. 353.
155 Bühring, 'Die Generation der Kriegskinder', p. A1190; Jachertz and Jachertz, p. A657. Here, this study distances itself from Jureit's conclusion that a trivialisation of the Holocaust victims would not occur in these debates, as a simplification of the issue. Jureit, p. 136.
156 F. Reimer, 'Wilde Konstruktionen', *Deutsches Ärzteblatt*, 110 (2013), A1197.
157 For the criticism and questioning of trauma as 'collective experience' in demarcation to an individual diagnosis, see Heinlein, *Die Erfindung der Erinnerung*, p. 184.

Bibliography

Primary sources

Unpublished

BUNDESARCHIV (BARCH)

Ministry of Healthcare

BArch, DQ 1/139 – Bekämpfung von Geschlechtskrankheiten, Mitteilungen und Richtlinien der Deutschen Zentralverwaltung für Gesundheitswesen, Bd. 3, 1946–1947
BArch, DQ 1/292 – Rechtsvorschriften, Erarbeitung und Durchsetzung, Bd. 3, 1947–1949
BArch, DQ 1/1010 – Bekämpfung von Geschlechtskrankheiten, Mitteilungen und Richtlinien der Deutschen Zentralverwaltung für Gesundheitswesen, Bd. 1, 1945–1949
BArch, DQ 1/1610 – Kampf gegen Geschlechtskrankheiten, Seuchen, Tuberkulose als Kriegsauswirkungen, 1945–1948
BArch, DQ 1/4436 – Monats- und Quartalsanalysen ("Wortberichte") der Bezirke und Schriftwechsel mit Räten der Bezirke, Bd. 1, 1953–1959
BArch, DQ 1/20626 – Heime für soziale Betreuung, Bd. 3, 1954–1960

DRESDEN, STADTARCHIV (STA DD)

StA DD, Dezernat Gesundheitswesen, 4.1.12, Nr. 2
StA DD, Dezernat Gesundheitswesen, 4.1.12, Nr. 3
StA DD, Dezernat Gesundheitswesen, 4.1.12, Nr. 4
StA DD, Dezernat Gesundheitswesen, 4.1.12, Nr. 5
StA DD, Dezernat Sozial- und Wohnungswesen, 4.1.10, Nr. 71

StA DD, Fürsorgeamt, 2.3.15, AV I/Nr. 647
StA DD, Wohlfahrtspolizeiamt, 2.3.27, Nr. 31

LEIPZIG, STADTARCHIV (STA LPZ)

StA Lpz, Stadtverwaltung und Rat, Nr. 7349

Published

Burlingham, Dorothy, and Anna Freud, *Infants Without Families: The Case For and Against Residential Nurseries* (London: George Allen & Unwin, 1964)
Lippert, Elisabeth, and Claudia Keppel, 'Deutsche Kinder in den Jahren 1947 bis 1950: Beitrag zur biologischen und epochalpsychologischen Lebensalterforschung', *Schweizerische Zeitschrift für Psychologie und ihre Anwendungen*, 9 (1950), 212–322
Pfeils, Elisabeth, *Flüchtlingskinder in neuer Heimat* (Stuttgart: Ernst Klett, 1951)
Stutte, Hermann, and H. Reinecke, 'Wachstumsverhältnisse bei hessischen Schulkindern in den Jahren 1946–1949', *Kinderärztliche Praxis*, 19 (1951), 515–21

Secondary sources

Ackermann, Volker, 'Das Schweigen der Flüchtlingskinder: Psychische Folgen von Krieg, Flucht und Vertreibung bei den Deutschen nach 1945', *Geschichte und Gesellschaft*, 30 (2004), 434–64
Assmann, Aleida, *Der lange Schatten der Vergangenheit: Erinnerungskultur und Geschichtspolitik* (Munich: Beck, 2006)
———, 'History and Memory', *International Encyclopedia of the Social & Behavioral Sciences* (Elsevier, 2001), pp. 6822–29
Beattie, Andrew H., *Playing Politics with History: The Bundestag Inquiries into East Germany* (New York: Berghahn Books, 2008)
Behrends, Jan C., and Patrice G. Poutrus, 'Xenophobia in the Former GDR: Explorations and Explanation from a Historical Perspective', in *Nationalisms Across the Globe: An Overview of Nationalisms in State-Endowed and Stateless Nations: Volume 1: Europe*, ed. by Wojciech Burszta, Tomasz Dominik Kamusella, and Sebastian Wojciechowski (Poznań: Wyższa Szkoła Nauk Humanistycznych i Dziennikarstwa, 2005), pp. 155–70
Bessel, Richard, *Germany 1945: From War to Peace* (London: Simon & Schuster, 2009)
Bode, Sabine, *Die vergessene Generation: Die Kriegskinder brechen ihr Schweigen*, 12th ed. (Munich: Piper, 2009)
Borchert, Wolfgang, 'Nachts schlafen die Ratten doch', in *Das Gesamtwerk: Mit einem biographischen Nachwort von Bernhard Meyer-Marwitz* (Hamburg: Rowohlt, 1949), pp. 216–19
Brajša-Žganec, Andreja, 'The Long-Term Effects of War Experiences on Children's Depression in the Republic of Croatia', *Child Abuse & Neglect*, 29 (2005), 31–43
Buchheim, Christoph, 'Der Mythos vom "Wohlleben": Der Lebensstandard der deutschen Zivilbevölkerung im Zweiten Weltkrieg', *Vierteljahreshefte für Zeitgeschichte*, 58 (2010), 299–328
Buddrus, Michael, 'A Generation Twice Betrayed: Youth Policy in the Transition from the Third Reich to the Soviet Zone of Occupation (1945–1946)', in *Generations in Conflict:*

Youth Revolt and Generation Formation in Germany 1770–1968, ed. by Mark Roseman (Cambridge: Cambridge University Press, 1995), pp. 247–68

Bühring, Petra, 'Die Generation der Kriegskinder: Kollektive Aufarbeitung notwendig', *Deutsches Ärzteblatt*, 102 (2005), A1190–A1193

———, 'Sexualisierte Gewalt: Das Schweigen brechen', *Deutsches Ärzteblatt*, 102 (2005), A1798

Castell, Rolf, Jan Nedoschill, Madeleine Rupps, and Dagmar Bussiek, *Geschichte der Kinder- und Jugendpsychiatrie in Deutschland in den Jahren 1937 bis 1961* (Göttingen: Vandenhoeck & Ruprecht, 2003)

Dyregrov, Atle, Alison Salloum, Pål Kristensen, and Kari Dyregrov, 'Grief and Traumatic Grief in Children in the Context of Mass Trauma', *Current Psychiatry Reports*, 17 (2015), 1–8

Echterkamp, Jörg, 'Von der Gewalterfahrung zu Kriegserinnerung: Über den Bombenkrieg als Thema einer Geschichte der deutschen Kriegsgesellschaft', in *Deutschland im Luftkrieg*, ed. by Dietmar Süß (Munich: Oldenbourg, 2007), pp. 13–25

Eghigian, Greg, *The Corrigible and the Incorrigible: Science, Medicine, and the Convict in Twentieth-Century Germany* (Ann Arbor, MI: University of Michigan Press, 2015)

Evans, Jennifer V., 'Bahnhof Boys: Policing Male Prostitution in Post-Nazi Berlin', *Journal of the History of Sexuality*, 12 (2003), 605–36

———, 'Decriminalization, Seduction, and "Unnatural Desire" in East Germany', *Feminist Studies*, 36 (2010), 553–77

———, *Life Among the Ruins: Cityscape and Sexuality in Cold War Berlin* (Houndmills: Palgrave Macmillan, 2011)

Fenemore, Mark, 'The Growing Pains of Sex Education in the German Democratic Republic (GDR), 1945–69', in *Shaping Sexual Knowledge: A Cultural History of Sex Education in Twentieth-Century Europe*, ed. by Lutz D. H. Sauerteig and Roger Davidson (London: Routledge, 2009), pp. 71–90

Förster, Alice, and Birgit Beck, 'Post-Traumatic Stress Disorder and World War II: Can a Psychiatric Concept Help Us Understand Postwar Society?' in *Life after Death: Approaches to a Cultural and Social History of Europe During the 1940s and 1950s*, ed. by Richard Bessel and Dirk Schumann (Cambridge: Cambridge University Press, 2007), pp. 15–36

Fulbrook, Mary, *Dissonant Lives: Generations and Violence Through the German Dictatorships* (Oxford: Oxford University Press, 2011)

———, *The People's State: East German Society from Hitler to Honecker* (London: Yale University Press, 2005)

Goebel, Stefan, 'Coventry und Dresden: Transnationale Netzwerke der Erinnerung in den 1950er und 1960er Jahren', in *Deutschland im Luftkrieg*, ed. by Dietmar Süß (Munich: Oldenbourg, 2007), pp. 111–20

———, *The Great War and Medieval Memory: War, Remembrance, and Medievalism in Britain and Germany, 1914–1940* (Cambridge: Cambridge University Press, 2007)

Goebel, Stefan, and Derek Keene, eds., *Cities into Battlefields: Metropolitan Scenarios, Experiences, and Commemorations of Total War* (Farnham: Ashgate, 2011)

Goffman, Erving, *Behavior in Public Places: Notes on the Social Organization of Gatherings* (New York: The Free Press, 1985)

Goltermann, Svenja, 'Psychisches Leid und herrschende Lehre: Der Wissenschaftswandel in der westdeutschen Psychiatrie der Nachkriegszeit', in *Akademische Vergangenheitspolitik: Beiträge zur Wissenschaftskultur der Nachkriegszeit*, ed. by Bernd Weisbrod (Göttingen: Wallstein, 2002), pp. 263–80

————, 'The Imagination of Disaster: Death and Survival in Postwar West Germany', in *Between Mass Death and Individual Loss: The Place of the Dead in Twentieth-Century Germany*, ed. by Alon Confino, Paul Betts, and Dirk Schumann (New York: Berghahn Books, 2008), pp. 261–74

'Gonorrhoea', *NHS*, 2016 <www.nhs.uk/Conditions/Gonorrhoea/Pages/Introduction.aspx> [accessed 30 January 2019]

Grass, Günther, *Im Krebsgang* (Göttingen: Steidl, 2002)

Grossmann, Atina, 'A Question of Silence: The Rape of German Women By Occupation Soldiers', *October*, 72 (1995), 42–63

Harsch, Donna, 'Medicalized Social Hygiene? Tuberculosis Policy in the German Democratic Republic', *Bulletin of the History of Medicine*, 86 (2012), 394–423

Hecker, Tobias, Simon Fetz, Herbert Ainamani, and Thomas Elbert, 'The Cycle of Violence: Associations Between Exposure to Violence, Trauma-Related Symptoms, and Aggression – Findings from Congolese Refugees in Uganda', *Journal of Traumatic Stress*, 28 (2015), 448–55

Heinlein, Michael, 'Das Trauma der deutschen Kriegskinder zwischen nationaler und europäischer Erinnerung: Kritische Anmerkungen zum gegenwärtigen Wandel der Erinnerungskultur', in *Narratives of Trauma: Discourses of German Wartime Suffering in National and International Perspective*, ed. by Helmut Schmitz and Annette Seidel-Arpacı (Amsterdam: Rodopi, 2011), pp. 111–28

————, *Die Erfindung der Erinnerung: Deutsche Kriegskindheiten im Gedächtnis der Gegenwart* (Bielefeld: Transcript, 2010)

Jachertz, Adelheid, and Norbert Jachertz, 'Kriegskinder: Erst im Alter wird oft das Ausmaß der Traumatisierungen sichtbar', *Deutsches Ärzteblatt*, 110 (2013), A656–A658

Jarausch, Konrad H., and Michael Geyer, *Shattered Past: Reconstructing German Histories* (Princeton: Princeton University Press, 2003)

Jureit, Ulrike, 'Generationen-Gedächtnis: Überlegungen zu einem Konzept kommunikativer Vergemeinschaftungen', in *Die 'Generation der Kriegskinder': Historische Hintergründe und Deutungen*, ed. by Lu Seegers and Jürgen Reulecke (Gießen: Psychosozial-Verlag, 2009)

Kattago, Siobhan, *Ambiguous Memory: The Nazi Past and German National Identity* (Westport, CT: Praeger, 2001)

Lerner, Paul, 'Psychiatry and Casualties of War in Germany, 1914–18', *Journal of Contemporary History*, 35 (2000), 13–28

Loose, Ingo, 'The Anti-Fascist Myth of the German Democratic Republic and Its Decline After 1989', in *Past in the Making: Historical Revisionism in Central Europe After 1989*, ed. by Michal Kopecek (Budapest: Central European University Press, 2008), pp. 59–71

McLellan, Josie, *Antifascism and Memory in East Germany: Remembering the International Brigades 1945–1989* (Oxford: Clarendon, 2004)

Moser, Gabriele, *'Im Interesse der Volksgesundheit. . .': Sozialhygiene und öffentliches Gesundheitswesen in der Weimarer Republik und der frühen SBZ/DDR: Ein Beitrag zur Sozialgeschichte des deutschen Gesundheitswesens im 20. Jahrhundert* (Frankfurt a.M.: VAS, 2002)

Naimark, Norman, *The Russians in Germany: A History of the Soviet Zone of Occupation, 1945–1949* (Cambridge, MA: The Belknap Press, 1995)

Niven, Bill, 'The GDR and Memory of the Bombing of Dresden', in *Germans as Victims: Remembering the Past in Contemporary Germany* (Houndmills: Palgrave Macmillan, 2006), pp. 109–29

Plato, Alexander von, 'The Hitler Youth Generation and Its Role in the Two Post-War German States', in *Generations in Conflict: Youth Revolt and Generation Formation in Germany 1770–1968*, ed. by Mark Roseman (Cambridge: Cambridge University Press, 1995), pp. 210–26

Pollack, H.W., 'Aufarbeitung überfällig', *Deutsches Ärzteblatt*, 102 (2005), A1950

Poutrus, Patrice G., 'Zuflucht im Nachkriegsdeutschland: Politik und Praxis der Flüchtlingsaufnahme in Bundesrepublik und DDR von den späten 1940er bis zu den 1970er Jahren', *Geschichte und Gesellschaft*, 35 (2009), 135–75

Radebold, Hartmut, *Abwesende Väter und Kriegskindheit: Alte Verletzungen bewältigen* (Stuttgart: Klett-Cotta, 2010)

———, ' "Kriegskinder" im Alter: Bei Diagnose historisch denken', *Deutsches Ärzteblatt*, 101 (2004), A1960–A1962

Reimer, F., 'Wilde Konstruktionen', *Deutsches Ärzteblatt*, 110 (2013), A1197

Reinisch, Jessica, *The Perils of Peace: The Public Health Crisis in Occupied Germany* (Oxford: Oxford University Press, 2013)

Robson, Wm Lane M., 'Enuresis', *Medscape*, 2015 <http://emedicine.medscape.com/article/1014762-overview#a4> [accessed 30 January 2019]

Saunders, Anna, *Honecker's Children: Youth and Patriotism in East(Ern) Germany, 1979–2002* (Manchester: Manchester University Press, 2007)

Schwartz, Michael, *Vertriebene und 'Umsiedlerpolitik': Integrationskonflikte in den deutschen Nachkriegs-Gesellschaften und die Assimilationsstrategien in der SBZ/DDR 1945–1961* (Munich: Oldenbourg, 2004)

Seydlitz, Ruth, and Pamela Jenkins, 'The Influence of Families, Friends, Schools, and Community on Delinquent Behavior', in *Delinquent Violent Youth: Theory and Interventions*, ed. by Thomas P. Gullotta, Gerald R. Adams, and Raymond Montemayor (Thousand Oaks: Sage, 1998), pp. 53–97

Sigmund, Anna Maria, *'Das Geschlechtsleben bestimmen wir': Sexualität im Dritten Reich* (Munich: Heyne, 2008)

Stargardt, Nicholas, *Witnesses of War: Children's Lives Under the Nazis* (London: Pimlico, 2006)

'Syphilis', *NHS*, 2016 <www.nhs.uk/conditions/Syphilis/Pages/Introduction.aspx> [accessed 30 January 2019]

Thimm, Katja, *Vatertage: Eine deutsche Geschichte* (Frankfurt a.M.: Fischer, 2011)

Weidner, Tobias, *Die unpolitische Profession: Deutsche Mediziner im langen 19. Jahrhundert* (Frankfurt a.M.: Campus, 2012)

Wierling, Dorothee, *Geboren im Jahr Eins: Der Jahrgang 1949 in der DDR: Versuch einer Kollektivbiographie* (Berlin: Links, 2002)

Wilhelm, Inka, and Susanne Zank, 'Zweiter Weltkrieg und pflegerische Versorgung heute: Einfluss von Kriegstraumatisierungen auf professionelle Pflegesituationen', *Zeitschrift für Gerontologie und Geriatrie*, 5 (2014), 4–8

Winter, Jay, and Emmanuel Sivan, eds., *War and Remembrance in the Twentieth Century* (Cambridge: Cambridge University Press, 1999)

Zatlin, Jonathan R., 'Scarcity and Resentment: Economic Sources of Xenophobia in the GDR, 1971–1989', *Central European History*, 40 (2007), 683–720

4 Institutionalised treatments of the past

The *Fürsorgeheim Leuben* in postwar Dresden

Introduction

In *Revolte im Erziehungshaus* [Mutiny in the Reformatory], the painter and author Peter Martin Lampel criticised the conditions of the youth reformatories in the Weimar Republic – a fictional account based on his own experiences in the juvenile welfare system. Despite his NSDAP and SA membership dating back to 1922, Lampel's social-critical works were banned during the Third Reich, and in 1936, he emigrated to Australia and later to the USA.[1] In his 1929 play *Revolte im Erziehungshaus*, one of the inmates, Fritz, complained to the new care worker that, after reaching the legal age of 21 years,

> [t]hen they send you to the outside, without a penny in your pocket. Where? No one of us knows that. No one wants former care children. Outside you are betrayed and sold. Then you go into the unknown – but your youth is gone.[2]

Lampel used in this play the inmates' voices to expose maltreatments and the failure to re-socialise the inmates in these institutions.[3] His critique shows that the failure of reformatories and similar institutions to reform people and their social conduct was publicly debated and known to authorities since at least the 1920s.[4] Nevertheless, the last chapters have revealed that people and authorities' mentality favoured those institutions locking away 'social disturbances', and thus postwar East Germany decided to continue this problematic legacy: medical and social *treatments of the past* for its 'sexual and social deviants'.

The most prominent example of this claim is the *Arbeitshaus*, the German version of the workhouse,[5] which was subject to re-labelling practices throughout its decades-long existence. It was called *Bezirksanstalt, Landesanstalt, Fürsorgeheim, Fürsorgeanstalt, Heim für soziale Betreuung*, and other, similarly vague, descriptions fitting of an institution with a multifunctional character.[6] Despite its recent problematic past that, as Sven Korzilius states, the workhouse had become a cog in the whole system of concentration and extermination camps during the Third Reich, German authorities in all four occupied zones were willing to continue the stigmatisation of adults and youths who transgressed the legal boundaries of social life and public health as 'asocial' and confine them into correctional institutions.[7] Only American officials instructed to dissolve the workhouses in their zone in February 1949 after an inspection revealed the unacceptable conditions in these institutions.[8] However, correctional facilities continued to exist in the West German state after 1949. Subsequently, German officials from the former American Occupied Zone still sent 'asocials' to workhouses in other areas. Until the *Verfassungsgericht* [Federal Constitutional Court] of West Germany in 1969 decided that the incarceration and claim to 'reform' citizens were unconstitutional, a total of 8,351 people were sentenced to workhouses.[9]

For this final chapter, the framework of medical memories and experiences is applied to the case study of the *Fürsorgeheim Leuben* [Care Home Leuben], as a continually challenged institution in a suburb of Dresden. This institution unites all three groups analysed in the preceding chapters and thus serves as a suitable 'litmus test' for the underlying concept.

The history of this form of a 'total institution', in the Goffmanian sense, is closely linked to the development of social care and poorhouses.[10] Since the nineteenth century and introduction of the Poor Laws in various European states, the official tone, perception, and legal, medical, and social treatment of people changed rapidly, with certain sections of society previously conceived of as 'deviant' and 'workshy' also becoming categorised as 'asocial'.[11] These terms are, of course, blurred and overused, and have always depended on the contemporary context and the writer's individual predisposition. In Germany, workhouses emerged from penitentiaries and similar institutions, were always driven by economic rather than social considerations,[12] and experienced a boom in the late-nineteenth century – largely due to increasing industrialisation and changes in patterns of labour.[13]

During this time, the *Bezirksanstalt Dresden-Leuben* [District Asylum Dresden-Leuben] was established (1 April 1883) in former farmhouses which had become obsolete through the increasing urbanisation of this peripheral area.[14] The use of abandoned buildings for social institutions, such as former monasteries after secularisation and castles, was common in Germany, as financial resources were often not sufficient to build new ones. More often than not, the buildings already housed penitentiaries or other 'total institutions' before they were converted into workhouses.[15] In contrast to new prisons and mental asylums built throughout the nineteenth century in the belief that architecture could generate a suitable environment that treats and reforms the human-being,[16] the workhouse often remained provisional in character, despite comprehensive conversion work on existing structures.[17]

Apart from these shortcomings, the workhouse represented a 'total institution': all aspects of a person's life occurred within a confined space; he or she was put under tight social and medical control among other individuals in a similar situation; and their daily routine was thoroughly managed by the staff of this institution.[18] Typically, it was a purposefully secluded institution – demonstrated by its walled-in design and remote location – which was supposed to prepare inmates for the outside world. However, further estrangement from external cultural and social developments occurred through this isolation.[19] The outcome of this 'frozen' image of society within the workhouse walls was that, after release, former inmates – who had experienced no cultural and social development since entering the institution – were even more unprepared for challenges on the outside and thus often returned to the 'total institution' quickly.[20]

As Ayaß has claimed, the principal aim of these institutions was to be a deterrent for broader society (general preventive effect) – to warn people not to become a 'social deviant' in any contemporarily defined form – rather than an actual reformatory for inmates (specific preventive effect).[21] As a result of this view, the conditions in workhouses were often worse than in prisons – not least due to the often new, modern architecture of the latter.[22] This perception was reflected in the fact that workhouses had a dreaded reputation among the population, which was the desired outcome for authorities and proponents of this form of social control.[23] For medical memories and experiences, it is here where a medical model was derived from contemporary definitions of social misconduct and its pathological manifestations in human beings: the continued existence of the institution already points towards the persistence of this concept throughout political upheavals and changes.[24]

In the following, the theoretical discussion of the framework of medical memories and experiences is grounded in the analysis of the *Fürsorgeheim Leuben* as a case study. The four levels of this concept defined in the introduction, including the state narrative, institutional memories, mnemonic community, and memories of the individual, are the guiding points through the final part of the book.

To demonstrate this concept, this chapter starts with the discussion of whether the workhouse was still appropriate in the postwar era and compatible with the 'new' political system and ideology. In the commission, which was set up to evaluate this issue, almost all members were trapped in their past, similar to the medical profession analysed in Chapter 1. Despite being lawyers and state officials, they utilised their medical memories and experiences to argue for the continuation of workhouses and established a suitable state narrative.

In the second section, the proposal of Leuben's Superintendent to the City Council of Dresden is analysed. This document confirms Rothman's finding that inside institutions, superintendents tried to implement their societal ideas and, as Yanni concludes, "create a microcosm of their vision of a proper society".[25] Therefore, medical memories and experiences shaped the conception as well as the layout and equipment of an institution, as shown for the *Ambulatorien* in Chapter 2. This process gives an important insight into the interdisciplinary connection between architecture, history, law, medicine, psychology, and sociology for the inquiry in this chapter.

Due to the common interest of multiple disciplines in one institution, however, there was a constant struggle between judicial, medical, and social welfare and other mnemonic communities over competencies, accountabilities, utilisation, and, most importantly, funding of this particular care home in Dresden. Section three of this chapter shows that none of these authorities wanted to take over full responsibility of this institution. This situation derived from their medical memories and experiences that the workhouse as an institution failed in the past.

The interpretation of the reasons which resulted in the inability of this institution to achieve its proposed aims and how to resolve the issue in the future was highly differentiated across departmental borders. However, no one questioned its general existence and necessity at the local level. Instead, authorities wanted to tighten laws for confining even more people within this institution. As identified in Chapters 2 and 3, they intended to broaden medical and social definitions of deviance and to extend the buildings to separate the inmates according to their legal, medical, and societal transgression.

With regards to the *Fürsorgeheim Leuben* itself, the fourth section discusses individual views, concepts, and narratives of inmates and staff regarding their medical memories and experiences inside and outside of this institution. For this final analysis, not only documents but also pictures and individual cases are utilised, offering a fresh look into the care home experience and exposing the gap between the proposed purpose and goals and their actual implementation and outcome in this institution.

Lastly, it has to be noted that all four sections of this chapter and thus all four levels of the concept are interrelated and intertwined with each other. On the one hand, individuals inform the state narrative, which subsequently influences the political strategies of local mnemonic communities. On the other hand, institutions and the perception of their past limit the implementation of both local and state policies. As a result, the framework of medical memories and experiences is developed to reveal the complexity of human behaviour, interactions, and legitimisation strategies rather than to simplify social conduct with an inherently limiting terminology.[26] Labels like 'collective' are misleading because societal memory is a cluster of highly heterogeneous reflections of the past: behind this term, many individuals with different narratives and memories can be found.

According to this concept, it is likely that only a few people develop a state narrative. However, this narrative is influenced by all other levels and has to be as incorporating and accommodating towards the majority of the population as is possible in order to be successful. This feature is essential to offer the opportunity to mnemonic communities and individuals to integrate their memories, political views, and narratives into the overarching framework, provided by the state. It needs to be a framework that is part – and enables them to make sense – of their lives in line with cultural and societal remembrance practices. In the case of the workhouse, this was an important step for selling the disreputable institution to the sceptical people of postwar East Germany and made it fit into the 'new socialist project'.

Medical memories of the state: the discussion of continuing correctional facilities in postwar East Germany

According to the protocol about the meeting of the commission about the future of workhouses in 1946, Ernst Scheidges, Senior Attorney at the Berlin Court of Appeal, stated that "if the workhouse did not exist, it would have to be invented".[27] This quotation bears witness to the general nature of the commission set up to assess the question of whether or not the workhouse could be viewed as an appropriate institution in postwar East Germany: it was a 'commission of the past'.

In the meeting held on 31 January 1946 and initiated by the *Deutsche Zentralverwaltung der Justitz* [German Central Administration of Justice – DZVJ], at least four out of the ten participants had a relevant Nazi past and were former members of Nazi organisations, but also occupied influential positions in the SBZ.[28] For example, the life paths of Karl Guski, Chief of the DZVJ Department V responsible for legislation and codification, and one of the directors of the DZVJ, Ernst Melsheimer, who was supposedly a friend of Roland Freisler, the notorious President of the *Volksgerichtshof* [People's Court] of the Third Reich, were determined by opportunistic behaviour.[29] Both can be described as 'turncoats': a valid categorisation for many doctors in postwar East Germany.[30]

The situation for Eduard Kohlrausch, a long-standing expert in criminal law since the days of the German Empire, was similar. Despite his involvement in the National Socialist penal system, both Americans and Soviets used his expertise regarding legal questions.[31] As Sven Korzilius concludes, Kohlrausch was the embodiment of past mentalities and beliefs.[32] Therefore, he stands for continuity after 1945. The SMAD even relied on his judgement that "forced sterilisations were not at all a particular National Socialist understanding", which exculpated doctors involved in this Nazi practice and potential medical crime in general.[33]

By contrast, Ernst Scheidges, quoted earlier, was director of the Workhouse Brauweiler, near Cologne, until 1933. After the Nazis had taken over the government, he was imprisoned due to allegations of corruption, which were initiated to replace him with an NSDAP member.[34] Despite this experience, Scheidges drew the conclusion from his medical memories that workhouses served the state's interests by reforming 'socially deviant' people. Therefore, he was strongly in favour of continuing this practice.[35]

From this starting point, the assessment of an institution like the workhouse had to be biased and blatantly linked to its questionable past. The medical memories and experiences of the people in charge – and here, in the commission – developed their views into a state narrative, which justified both the continuity of workhouses and the confinement of those deemed to be 'asocial' into correctional facilities in the postwar era.

The politics of medical memories and experiences[36] is an important category when analysing the motives, outcomes, and consequences of state narratives and their implications at the local level of society. As already shown in Chapter 3, the selection of memories, the creation of a 'para-medicalised' terminology, and the claims of 'breaking the silence' are highly political communication strategies, used to serve the ends of the addressed mnemonic community, such as the 'traumatised war children' or the 'forgotten generation'.

In the case of the workhouse, firstly, it suited the new state for cleansing postwar society of disturbing and so-called 'negative elements', as well as re-socialising the 'uprooted' people. It was furthermore a deterrence (a general preventive effect), encouraging its population to stay away from delinquency, promiscuity, and other criminal activities.

Secondly, the commission was very conscious of the history, the (medical) memory of the workhouse. The reflection was expressed, on the one hand, as a concern that the people would view the institution as a punishment and a home of the 'depraved' parts of society, which drew on their experiences and the form of treatment within the workhouse of the past. On the other hand, it was used as a justification for its continuous existence, as it would have proven itself a necessity.[37]

The questionable nature of the 'commission of the past' found its peak in Kohlrausch's statement which declared incarceration with indefinite duration in the case of a second confinement in the workhouse an "absolute progress" in the penal system.[38] The § 42 d, which regulates the confinement into workhouses according to the legal transgressions of § 361 No. 3–5, 6, 6a, and 8,[39] and § 42 f of the *Strafgesetzbuch* [German Penal Code – StGB], which specifies the length of the stay in this and similar social institutions, were introduced with the '*Gesetz gegen gefährliche Gewohnheitsverbrecher und über Maßregeln der Sicherung und Besserung* [Law Against Dangerous Habitual Offenders and Measures for Safeguarding and Bettering]' on 24 November 1933.[40] This timeframe exposes the fact that this law was created under the shadow of the recent *Ermächtigungsgesetze* [Enabling Acts] after the NSDAP took over the government in March 1933. The subsequent alterations to the criminal code meant a tightening of the penalties and an increased restriction of personal freedom.

Kohlrausch belittled the latter with the comment that a "classic *libertarian* evaluation [emphasis as in the original, M.W.]" of the law might consider it as undemocratic:

> However, one has to have the courage now, to admit, that our today's penalty law as a whole is not purely democratic, but largely designed according to socialist perspectives. It would mean a setback to abandon these socialist achievements.[41]

The effects of Kohlrausch's statement were twofold. Firstly, he used the 'old bourgeoisie' argument and the associated liberal views about personal liberty as a way of demarcating and simultaneously illustrating the deprivation of freedom by this penalty law as a socialist advancement superior to democratic principles. Secondly, he formed a justification and a fitting narrative that incorporated the law, evidently derived from a Third Reich background, into the socialist context. Kohlrausch embraced socialist ideas and tweaked the medical memories of the past into a suitable framework for transferring the workhouse into the postwar era and coming future.

Other members of the commission, such as the police and judicial representatives, also argued for the continuation of the law in its 1933 form. Moreover, some disguised the Nazi link by referring to its draft, already created in 1927.[42] In doing so, they tweaked the facts by presenting the law as being something derived from a Weimar Republic background more in keeping with socialist ideals.[43] This finding is also visible in the similar discussions surrounding the *Bewahrungsgesetz*

[Safekeeping Law], which started in the 1920s and continued after 1945 as a consciously selected legacy of Weimar.[44]

In the end, the DZVJ Department V concluded in its recommendation and final report of the commission that "the measure of the workhouse in its current form, not only contains no Nazi elements, but is also quite compatible with the democratic views of the time".[45] This statement is unsound and represents a clear contradiction of the previous analysis, including the denial of any Nazi legacy.[46] This finding is proven due to the fact that the report of the expert commission adopted the task description of the workhouse from the 1944 version of the '*Reichs-Strafgesetzbuch nach dem neuesten Stand der Gesetzgebung: Leipziger Kommentar* [German Reich Criminal Code According to Current State of Law: Leipzig Commentary]' by Johannes Nagler and Edmund Mezger almost word for word:

> The workhouse fulfils a twofold task: it is supposed to educate the workshy and parasitic social neurasthenics (idlers, beggars, vagabonds, prostitutes), through familiarisation with *Zucht* [discipline], obedience, and strict work, to an orderly life; however, if this is unsuccessful, [the workhouse] is supposed to defang this group of labile asocials through *Verwahrung* [safekeeping] with firm work discipline.[47]

The 'para-medicalised', almost militaristic language of this description reveals the continuity of the perception of workhouses and their inmates from the Third Reich and the eugenic standpoint into postwar East Germany. Therefore, the outcome of this 'commission of the past' was predictable from its assembling onwards.

Its problematic conclusion, however, led to issues between the 'real' socialists and the 'old elites' in the following years. While the latter group was pushing towards a broad application of the criminalised 'asociality' and stricter laws, the 'real' socialists put their trust in a 'bright future'. One year after the foundation of the GDR, the party leadership of the SED rejected the proposal of the new Ministry of Labour and Healthcare with the following: "[w]e need to see that the question of prostitution and begging will settle itself through our societal development to such an extent that it will not be a problem anymore".[48] This teleological explanation was always existent in the 'progressive circles' who also demanded, as identified in Chapter 2, to 'de-gender' the medical and social concept of STDs and promiscuity and to target both men and women.[49]

In the end, however, the 'old elites' won the struggle between the competing state narratives after it became apparent that the idealised views of the 'real' socialists were not achievable at the local level of society over a short period.[50] Nonetheless, immediately after the erection of the Berlin Wall in August 1961, the Ministry of Internal Affairs broadened the criminalisation of 'asocials' and declared 'social deviance' as an 'individual choice', as the societal conditions were viewed as ideal for the development of every citizen. This shift to individualising deviance not only justified increased incarceration, but also established a new state narrative denying the existence of social problems in GDR society as a whole.[51]

The section has demonstrated that the state narrative within the proposed concept depends on the people in charge and their medical memories: their past and experiences influenced the medical concepts of the present and future. However, a state narrative needed to respond to societal developments or, as in this case, continuity within influential mnemonic communities, local authorities, and the population. Even if some state officials with their ideals tried to overcome the old mentalities and stigmatisations, the local level often limited or hindered its implementation. Therefore, the state narrative had to be adapted to suit the majority of people in order to convince them of the socialist project. In this process, the state created an identity in defining 'social deviance' or what 'they' are not. Therefore, in the Goffmanian sense, inmates of the *Fürsorgeheim Leuben* and similar institutions served as the societal mirror for the state to demarcate the 'socialist identity' from the 'depraved' one.[52] In the end, a state narrative, also in the medical sense, is always written to legitimise the present state of affairs and broadly accepted definitions of 'normal' and 'abnormal' social conduct within a society.

Consequently, the state level does not exist on its own but requires the input of other levels and vice versa. For the workhouse, the state narrative relied on the enthusiasm of local authorities and the superintendents who, with the support of the upper echelons, implemented and developed this concept further. In the case of the *Fürsorgeheim Leuben*, it was in Director Hofmann that the state found a keen proponent for converting parts of the care home back into a workhouse in 1949.[53]

Medical memories of the institution: the history and use of the *Fürsorgeheim Leuben* in Dresden

The previous section has demonstrated how authorities often idealised the workhouse and its usefulness, viewing this institution as a welcome solution for the perceived widespread 'promiscuity' and 'social deviance' among the East German population after the Second World War. Therefore, in a report about the *Fürsorgeheim* in Dresden from 1952, health authorities proclaimed that

> [j]ust as the inmates in their variation reflect the extent of the collapse in 1945, then also gradually, the reduction of the occupancy of the institution, as well as the permanent structural improvement, reveals the steady rise of our German Democratic Republic by its own efforts.[54]

In this quotation, the *Fürsorgeheim Leuben* was described as a mirror of society, which, firstly, showed the disastrous situation in 1945, the widespread depravity and the general displacement of the people. Secondly, the author underlined how the socialist development had improved conditions, exemplified by the reduction of inmates and the general upgrading of facilities. By 1952, the institution was thus fully integrated into the political and ideological narrative of the GDR – either by the state or, in this case, by staff and superintendents, who reported to the Health Ministry and justified the existence of the workhouse by emphasising its successes.

This section examines how the state narrative was transferred onto an institutional level, and if and how this was reflected in its architecture and design. Moreover, the analysis illustrates the limitations of the state narrative being implemented at the local level. For example, it shows how local authorities established their vision of a successful reformatory along the ideological parameters of the state, as well as the necessities and situation on-site.

The *Fürsorgeheim Leuben* was created in 1883 and was since then subject to name changes, extensions, and the construction of new buildings designed to expand the numbers and the types of inmates. For example in the 1890s, Dresden city officials renamed the institution in Leuben to *Bezirks-Anstalt für Sieche, Versorgte, geistig Minderwertige und Korrektionäre* [District Asylum for the Sick, Beneficiaries, Intellectually Inferior and Corrigible] and split it into two sections: a care home for the sick, elderly, and 'inferior' and a workhouse for the 'corrigible' [*Pflege- und Arbeitsanstalt*].[55]

As mentioned, the legal basis for the forced confinement of people to the Leuben institution was, in particular, § 361 of the StGB, which was introduced with the foundation of the German Empire in 1871 and based on the former Prussian penal code.[56] This law targeted, inter alia, 'vagabonds', 'beggars', 'workshy' people, gamblers, and prostitutes to institutionalise and educate them through work. In the Weimar Republic, § 20 of the *Reichsfürsorgepflichtverordnung* [Empire Welfare Duty Decree] from 1924 expanded the regulations to confine people. It determined that beneficiaries who refused to work, neglected the obligation to support their relatives, or caused their poverty through 'immoral behaviour' could also be sent to workhouses by the welfare office.[57] The heterogeneous composition of inhabitants in Leuben – comprising of not only adults, but also children branded as beggars, vagabonds, orphans, prostitutes, and 'moronic' or 'imbecilic' – reveals that city councillors also consciously created a multifunctional institute, taking full advantage of the outlined legal framework, to 'sanitise the streets' of Dresden.[58]

The medical memories embedded in this institution, however, were composed of problematic events: in 1916, decreased food rations caused by the First World War led to 46 deaths through malnourishment among prisoners.[59] In the late 1920s, inmates scornfully called the food received in the *Fürsorgeheim* "cow pats", indicating that the living situation in this institution was harsh and a danger to their health. The disregarding of their criticism by staff eventually led to a mutiny in this care home in 1929, in which a few buildings were set on fire. In the end, the rebellion was fended off, and its leaders sentenced to incarceration in penitentiaries.[60]

After the NSDAP gained power in 1933, they passed the already mentioned 'Law Against Dangerous Habitual Offenders and Measures for Safeguarding and Bettering' on 24 November of the same year. This law introduced, inter alia, § 42 d and f of the StGB, extending the legal opportunities to institutionalise and keep 'asocials' in workhouses for an infinite period.[61] The mentality inherent in this law towards the people branded as 'asocial' or 'mentally deficient', namely the denial of being valuable members of society on the grounds of eugenic reasons, had also an impact on Leuben. For example, following an inspection – "according to political aspects" – by the *Arbeitsgauobmann* of the *Reichsarbeitsdienst* (Regional Leader of the Reich Labour Service), criticism was levelled at the Leuben staff for their lenient treatment of inmates.[62] The Regional Leader demanded from the superintendent the recruitment of more guards, the arming of guards with fire-arms, the introduction of a "militaristic drill" alongside more severe punishments, and that a "greater value be put on the German salute".[63]

Regarding the latter point, however, the superintendent prohibited its perfor-mance by 'asocials', as "thereby the salute would be degraded".[64] His view of the inmates' inferiority for German society was enshrined not least in the '*Gesetz zur Verhütung erbkranken Nachwuchses* [Law for the Prevention of Genetically Diseased Offspring]' from 14 July 1933 (effective since January 1934), which resulted in the abolishment of holidays for people "capable of reproduction" in Leuben to prevent a passing on of their "deficient genetics".[65] In this way, as Korzilius pointed out, workhouses and multifunctional institutions became part of the racist custodial system in the Third Reich that included concentration and extermination camps – thus, the inmates in Leuben also had to fear deportation and potential death.[66] Due to the association with these medical memories, the reputation of the Leuben workhouse was poor among inmates and the local popu-lation.[67] Postwar East Germany would need to re-brand and re-define the institu-tion if it wanted to continue to use it as a reformatory within the ever-growing suburb of Dresden.

A report from September 1945 stated that "[w]hen someone knows the con-ditions in the barrack [camp]s, then the infirm in Leuben lead, and *it is truly welcomed*, an idyllic existence [emphasis as in the original, M.W.]".[68] The euphe-mistic description of this home by local authorities clarifies that the *Fürsorgeheim* rested on a status quo in the immediate postwar period. As in the Western Zones, it appears that the occupying power initially released inmates out of suspicion that they were held there for political reasons. Subsequently, the future of the institute remained initially uncertain.[69]

In autumn 1945, Leuben was described as a nursing home and hospital and thus housed only the elderly and infirm. However, several women still incarcerated under the former workhouse regulations were also in this institution.[70] Consider-ing that Leuben would have had up to 310 inmates in the following years, the *Für-sorgeheim* with its 99 inhabitants in September 1945, the surrounding condition of a bombed-out city, and the completely intact institution could give the impression of an 'idyllic' island amidst the chaos.

Nevertheless, the composition of inmates changed quickly: soon after this report, the Social Welfare Department of Dresden seized Leuben to accommodate the 'endangered youth', who otherwise would have been homeless and neglected in the streets of Dresden – a group explored in Chapter 3.[71] As a result, the *Für-sorgeheim* became a reformatory again at the end of 1945.

Nevertheless, 'uprooted' adolescents were not the only group of inmates that have been discussed in this study. As shown in Chapter 2, the Soviet and East German authorities implemented strict medical monitoring to curb the spread of

STDs after 1945. In their directives, they also decided that people displaying 'frequent promiscuous behaviour' – so-called hwG-people – who were declared as 'workshy', 'imbeciles', and potential sources of infection could be sentenced to incarceration in workhouses following an initial stay in prison.[72] Therefore, state authorities instructed that all East German regions had to create suitable institutions for this procedure in the suburbs of their cities. From the perspective of the available archival files, this development was independent of the DZVJ decision to continue the institution, as discussed in section one. Instead, as Korzillius recognises as well, it was SMAD Command 030 that was ultimately decisive in re-introducing the workhouse into the SBZ in 1946.[73] German and Soviet authorities shared similar legal views and the same understanding regarding 'promiscuous' people, especially women, who would represent a danger to the health of society and thus should not only be treated medically, but also be educated.[74] In both countries, medicine served as deterrence for 'socially and sexually deviant behaviour'.

In Dresden, local health authorities seized the *Fürsorgeheim Leuben* for this purpose of medical and social control. This decision was made not only due to the general lack of housing, but also because Leuben was also seen as the only available 'total institution' in Dresden after the Second World War again.[75] After the announcement of SMAD Command 030 of 12 February 1946 and the subsequent Directive 64 of the SMAS, released on 4 March 1946, the re-instated *Fürsorgeanstalt Leuben* [Care Asylum Leuben] was again split into two departments: one 'common' and one 'special'. The former was still used by Dresden's Social Welfare Department for the 'troubled youth', whereas the 'special department' was "an institution for safekeeping, compulsory treatment, and education through work for STD cases".[76] The institution's House H was utilised for these social and medical monitoring procedures. House H had been purpose-built as an infirmary in 1894, extended in 1907, and had contained an STD ward since June 1932.[77]

This local compromise shows that, on the one hand, officials had the leeway to alter the central regulations to their necessities on-site. On the other hand, it also supports the assumption that, based on a common understanding of various public health issues, Soviet authorities were willing and, in some cases, had to rely on German expertise. This process is not unprecedented for this matter, but has only recently been investigated for various internal affairs.[78]

Analysing the plan of the *Fürsorgeheim Leuben* in Figure 4.1, it is visible that its layout was not ideal for this dual-purpose. Houses A, B, and E, which consisted of dormitories, common rooms, and some functional spaces, inhabited 'uprooted', 'depraved', and difficult adolescents in 1947. As a result, Dresden's Social Welfare Mayor Martin Richter[79] complained to the city council and Saxony's Ministry of Labour and Social Welfare, criticising the confiscation of the entire House H as an STD lock ward for allegedly 'promiscuous' women. He stated that "[t]he danger of communal living [in this institution] between troubled boys, and girls who are riddled with STDs and more or less declining into prostitution, does not need any further explanations".[80] However, the mayor's concerns and reference to

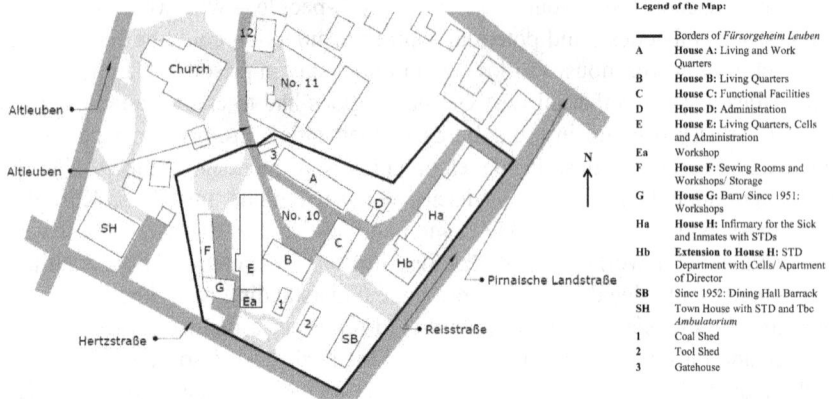

Figure 4.1 Plan of the *Fürsorgeheim Leuben* and its surroundings with street names in Dresden in its state around 1952

Note: The plan is only an approximation to the actual scale and was created with SketchUp, using Google Maps and the information from the following archival source.

Source: StA DD, 8.22, Bauamt, Nr. 1205, unpaginated; StA DD, 8.22, Bauamt, Nr. 1206, unpaginated; StA DD, 10, Bau- und Grundstücksakten, Nr. 37116.

the promise that the use of Leuben according to Command 030 would be only a 'temporary solution' were not acted upon.

Instead, Leuben increased its binary character, not least due to some strong proponents in the local government and the enactment of the SMAD Command 273 from 1948, which tightened the laws against denounced 'promiscuous' women. The Director of the *Fürsorgeheim Leuben*, Hofmann, approached the City Council of Dresden with his '*Gedanken zur Errichtung eines Arbeitshauses* [Thoughts regarding the Establishment of a Workhouse]' in June 1949. Unfortunately, his forename, background, and personal history are lost. His paper, however, is the best example of Rothman and Yanni's observation that superintendents tried to implement their vision of society inside their own institutions and bears witness to the medical memories, engraved in these buildings and in the minds of the people in charge.[81]

In his proposal, Hofmann presented himself as a reformer who invented new methods of re-socialisation, in line with socialist principles, to overcome the past failed attempts to re-integrate workhouse inmates into society.[82] While discussing the circle of individuals who would be confined in this 'new' workhouse, and the potential reasons for their social negligence, Hofmann strikingly pointed towards a continuity: "the women and girls who will be admitted, are probably even personally known to us due to our activity during the time of the hospital [in House H] and thus the personnel is familiar with their peculiarities".[83] The description points towards not only the on-going existence of the 'special' section in Leuben under a new name and supposedly new strategy, but also the tendency in postwar East

Germany to tighten laws and increase the time of custody. The targets of this, such as the 'promiscuous' woman, however, remained the same.

The legal basis for this extended incarceration of mainly 'promiscuous' women was, as mentioned, the new SMAD Command 273 regarding STDs and prostitution. The directive that came into force at the beginning of 1948 represented an increase of punishments despite the drastic decline of STDs, shown in Chapter 2.[84] This command was drafted by Karl Linser – already introduced in Chapter 1 – who became a leading venereologist in Dresden during the Weimar Republic and in 1947 the head of the DZVGW.[85] As such, Command 273 was more a German than a Soviet construct, once again showing how selected German officials within the central administration were able to weigh their views into the immediate postwar laws alongside the socialist determinants, defined by Moscow.

At the local level, Hofmann and his proposal are an example of this situation: he took the initiative to express and implement his views about the workhouse, potentially derived from his past experiences, political predisposition, and knowledge of the ideological requirements of the time. Notwithstanding Richter's complaints, Hofmann planned to make House A the main building of the new workhouse, meaning another loss in capacity for the 'troubled boys'.[86] In his view, this move inside the premises was necessary "as the behaviour of the inmates is not always impeccable" and House H was next to a street.[87] In the end, the director's expectations were exceeded by city officials. He proposed to house 80 inmates, but a note from August 1949, shortly after the workhouse was established, spoke of "200 beds [. . .] for roving girls".[88] Leuben was thus a multifunctional institution for social and medical control, while its initially desired specialisation was ultimately abandoned in 1949.

The plan of the *Fürsorgeheim Leuben* in Figure 4.1 reveals that this institution was not a typical workhouse; rather, due to its former use as a farm, it was more a decentralised complex of buildings.[89] As a result, it was a difficult undertaking to establish a 'total institution' here, not least because its surroundings and layout could not prevent escapes: a report from August 1947 noted that ten inmates had disappeared from Leuben in a single month.[90] Furthermore, this situation continued beyond 1949 and the (re-)establishment of the workhouse section. Soviet military authorities complained in 1951 that their soldiers would be able to come to Leuben at night and 'call out their girls', who could easily escape due to the insufficient height of the fences. To counter this, they established a Soviet Task Force that was put in action in case of this form of 'mischief'.[91] These shortcomings of the premises in Leuben point towards the general failure of this institution to fulfil its proposed aims by Hofmann, city authorities, and state officials of East Germany.

Inside the buildings, however, the *Fürsorgeheim* was fully equipped to function as the desired institution. Alongside basic facilities like kitchen, bathrooms, administration rooms, and dormitories,[92] ancillary buildings offered workshops and sewing rooms for implementing regulated workdays for inmates, separate day rooms for different leisure activities, dishwashing and potato peeling rooms, and cells for those who contravened house rules. Provision for the latter was increased during the years of its existence, and in House H individual cells were created for offenders suffering from STDs.[93]

The continuity of the arrangements inside and outside of the buildings through-out the decades of its existence and into the postwar period is also reflected in Superintendent Hofmann's proposals. In his vision, re-education through work and the familiarisation of inmates to a regulated daily life were his highest aims – as it had been the proclaimed purpose of workhouses in the past.[94]

"Not punishment and revenge, but re-education and prevention" proclaimed Hofmann as the leitmotif of this institution, thereby emphasising his attempt to demarcate his proposal from the use of the workhouse between 1933 and 1945.[95] For example, his educational and political programmes suggest that he tried to ini-tiate a new period of 'socialist humanism' in Leuben that was in line with the ideas of Anton Makarenko, relying on the self-management and positive peer pressure within the 'collective' of inmates, as well as work therapy.[96]

However, Hofmann was trapped in the medical memories and perception of this institution.[97] As a 'new' educational scheme, he envisioned a system of dif-ferent levels of freedom in Leuben, within which the inmates were promoted or relegated according to their behaviour and work ethics, "whereas the best group should have the nicest recreation rooms and the greatest freedoms".[98] His pro-posed reward system for obedient inmates was, however, not unique to the postwar period, having existed in various forms throughout the history of reformatories, workhouses, and asylums.[99]

Nevertheless, one of the new features was the growing political influence over the workhouse. Hofmann not only planned political education, but also intended to establish branches of GDR political organisations, such as the FDGB, FDJ, and *Demokratischer Frauenbund Deutschlands* [Democratic Women Association of Germany – DFD] within the walls of the *Fürsorgeheim Leuben*. His attempt, as well as the previous analysis, reveals two important insights into his views: firstly, Hofmann rejected any monotonous or meaningless work for inmates, which was the problem of workhouses of the past.[100] Instead, he demanded their involvement in the real economy of the GDR. Furthermore, the inclusion of the political and societal environment in this institution proves the hypothesis that he, as the super-intendent, wanted to create a microcosm of socialist society within Leuben.[101]

Secondly, Hofmann, with the previous aim in mind, also wanted to import the outside world inside the institution. He was aware of the danger of inmates' estrangement from the reality of society, which was subject to Goffman's analy-sis of patients in asylums.[102] Therefore, he urged the extension of aftercare for inmates so as to successfully integrate them back into society and avoid their return to Leuben.[103]

However, a report of the Social Welfare Department of Dresden from 1951 reveals that Hofmann's suggestions remained an idealised vision. Despite the creation of the workhouse on 1 July 1949, problems of re-education and re-integration remained the same, and the largest contingent of inmates were so-called 'regulars' – a fact which is investigated in more detail in the fourth sec-tion of this chapter.[104]

In general, the medical memories and experiences associated with Leuben as a workhouse were seen as detrimental to its goals, the superintendent's vision, the inmates' future, and the state's reputation among the local population. Therefore, two months after re-establishing a workhouse in the *Fürsorgeheim Leuben*, it was re-branded as *Heim für soziale Betreuung* [Home for Social Care].[105] The new name was a disguise for the actual continuity of institutionalised medical memories in the form of its arrangement, medical concepts, purposes, and the confined groups of people, analysed in this section.

In summary, using the *Fürsorgeheim Leuben* as a case study for this level of the concept of medical memories and experiences clarified that buildings have 'memories', which affected their present use and prospects. Nevertheless, the desire to confine people deemed to be 'socially deviant' into workhouses was not limited to the medical profession, but also involved judicial, police, and social departments – of which all had different expectations and memories of this institution. As a result, the interdisciplinary cooperation caused a struggle over competencies, funding, and responsibilities regarding Leuben: a competition of mnemonic communities over medical memories and the official narrative at the local level.

Medical memories of mnemonic communities: the competence struggle between the departments of health, justice, police, and social welfare over Leuben

One aspect united all departments involved in the setup and maintenance of the workhouse: those deemed to be unfit for society had to be confined to a 'total institution' because "this group of people does not belong to the public sphere, without them being thoroughly educated first".[106] Apart from this common ground, the health, judicial, police, and social authorities often disagreed about the practical implementation of state policies at the local level, determined by diverse views on, and medical memories of, this institution. Therefore, each of these professions can be described as a mnemonic community similar to a village:[107] they were composed of heterogeneous individuals who shared a similar life path and were socialised within a certain bureau, and thus (medical) memories were part of the social bond among colleagues. With this basis of a constructed common identity, they achieved an internal closure and a common narrative that protected members from outside attacks and enabled them to pursue a potentially unambiguous (political) strategy, as identified in Chapter 3 for the mnemonic community of the 'forgotten war children' today.

In this section, I examine how all four departments stressed the functionality of the *Fürsorgeheim Leuben* in their political strategy and narrative. However, none of these professions initially wanted to take over full responsibility and funding for this institution.[108] In theory for this particular case, Dresden's Justice Department was responsible for confining people to the institution, and the police for guarding them. Dresden's Health Department was in charge of providing medical services and the Social Welfare Department of educating and organising work for inmates.[109] This description alone indicates that overlapping competencies could potentially create conflicts at the local level.

Therefore, the following reveals how the state narrative and institutional memories discussed in previous sections affected mnemonic communities at the local level, especially regarding their aims for this particular institution, and the integration of both other levels into the local narrative in order to justify the use of the *Fürsorgeheim Leuben* for official purposes. To reach this understanding with the concept of medical memories, two examples are given, in which the perceptions of different professions conflicted with each other: the question of the Leuben's utilisation after the war and the debate about the dissolution of this institution in the mid-1950s.

After the *Fürsorgeheim Leuben* had been selected for imprisoning 'promiscuous' people in 1946, Saxony's Department of Justice made clear that they refused to fund this form of workhouse as it was seen as an extra-judicial institution. They stated that it *"was never covered by the budget of the judicial administration* [emphasis as in the original, M.W.]" and thus represented an extra financial expenditure, which they declined to take on.[110] The department of social welfare and the department of health also came into conflict with each other over the demarcation of competencies and, especially, the question over which department had to pay the costs of an in-patient's stay.[111]

All three agreed that this institution was a necessity, but none claimed sole responsibility for an endeavour, wherein the medical memories were conflated with the negative connotations of penitentiaries and asylums of the past.[112] The resulting contest over competencies, in particular between Dresden's Social Welfare and Health Departments, was reflected in the organisation of Leuben itself: they established a dual-leadership, shared between the superintendent and the medical director.[113] This condition caused persistent problems inside and outside of the *Fürsorgeheim* in the form of struggles between social and medical superintendents: the on-site embodiments of two competing local departments and their narratives.

As previously mentioned, Richter, the Social Welfare Mayor in Dresden, complained to Saxony's State Government in May 1947 that they had promised that the *Fürsorgeheim Leuben* would be seized only temporarily by the health department. The decision to continue and even extend its use for imprisoning 'promiscuous' women hampered, according to Richter, the education of the 'difficult' youth, for whom his social welfare department was responsible.[114] However, the Head Department of Healthcare at Saxony's Ministry of Labour and Social Welfare disregarded his complaint, referring to the persistent lack of appropriate housing.[115]

The refusal by governmental bodies caused frustration and protest at the local level, and, one year later in February 1948, the revenge of the social welfare department followed, as described by Hering, the Medical Director of Leuben:

> After my return from holiday on the 2.2.48, I was confronted with accomplished facts [. . .] From the *Fürsorgeheim Leuben*, which serves the curbing of STDs and is subject to the SMAD Command 030, half of the rooms and

beds [. . .] were seized by social welfare without authorisation during my holiday. [. . .] For this reason, I, as the Medical Director, cannot take responsibility for the non-implementation of Command 030.[116]

The exact circumstances of this dispute remain unclear, and the analysis is based on the potentially biased reports of competing departments. However, the description of Hering alone reveals the deep divide between the healthcare and social welfare departments. The latter in the person of Director Hofmann responded promptly, stating that "Dr Hering based his statement on the erroneous assumption that he, as the Medical Director [of Leuben], carries sole responsibility for the implementation of Command 030".[117] The superintendent claimed that the social welfare department was the institution's main authority, as the central task was ministering to the education and reform of 'socially deviant' people.

While emphasising that the 300 beds for 'promiscuous' women were never fully used, Hofmann criticised the fact that the 50 inmates of the reformatory department of Leuben – the 'uprooted' youth – worked in the fields and garden, cooked food, and washed or repaired the clothes of the people with STDs: "[t]his, however, cannot be the task of a reformatory, to carry out the *Schmutzarbeiten* [dirty work] [. . .] for the people with STDs, who are subject to Command 030".[118] Therefore, he demanded that only House H should be used by the health department for 'promiscuous' people and the rest of the *Fürsorgeheim Leuben* utilised for the 'difficult' youth.[119]

The competing narratives of two mnemonic communities came into conflict over the functionality of Leuben. The health department's interest was to increase the capacity of the *Fürsorgeheim* for their purposes, firstly, because they wanted to 'purge' their other medical institutions of the hwG-people, as required by Command 030. Secondly, according to the health department's medical memories and experiences, the medical treatment of patients who acquired STDs multiple times due to their 'deviant' lifestyles was not alone sufficient, and a subsequent deterrent lesson should be applied.[120] For this educational standpoint, the health department needed, in the case of Dresden, the *Fürsorgeheim Leuben*.

Nevertheless, the social welfare department had similar interests but for a broader spectrum of people: the criminal, 'uprooted', neglected, and homeless youth. For them, these adolescents represented the more urgent issue; the widespread STDs were only part of a grander problem. Therefore, their medicalised concepts of 'social deviance' required the reformatory to educate the 'new generation'; otherwise, they argued, the confinement of these people was "an eternal cycle, which cannot be combated with medicine but only with education".[121]

The seizure of large parts of Leuben by the health department without an actual utilisation was seen as hampering the aims of the social welfare department. One year later, however, Superintendent Hofmann and Medical Director Hering appeared to have reached an agreement, as was discussed in the previous section: the re-establishment of the workhouse within the *Fürsorgeheim Leuben*, or later *Heim für soziale Betreuung* for 'promiscuous' women, combining medical and social control and the goals of both departments.

The putative unity among healthcare and social welfare authorities was tightened due to an external threat: at the end of 1952, the state level approached Saxony with the demand to dissolve *Heime für soziale Betreuung* due to the criticised standard within these institutions and the overstretched laws for confining 'promiscuous' people in this state.[122] The ensuing response of Dresden's Social Welfare and Housing Department reveals a local alliance among the police, social, and healthcare officials caused by the state intervention.[123]

The four-page long document is the best proof for two significant findings of this study: firstly, the implementation of new policies was never a complete top-down procedure, but rather experienced severe limitations at the local level of society. Historiographical accounts of the past have underestimated the agency at the local sphere and emphasised the overruling power of the centralised state and the SED.[124] However, especially immediately after the war, the chaos and unclear structure of new state bodies in the SBZ provided the opportunity to interpret state policies, thus allowing local officials to implement their own visions of society. Later on, these deviations were centralised and often altered. Nonetheless, local authorities maintained their sovereignty for the circumstances on-site – if only in a defined and narrow state-controlled frame of the socialist ideology.[125]

Secondly, the city officials' reply regarding the dissolution of Leuben shows how intelligently the mnemonic communities utilised the state narrative to justify their views, derived from their medical memories. In a self-serving endeavour, they accomplished the integration of the *Fürsorgeheim* or *Heim für soziale Betreuung Dresden-Leuben* in the overall ideological narrative of the SED, thereby ultimately securing the existence of this institution for another three years.[126]

Dresden's officials argued in their letter to the state that "[i]n the area of education and care for endangered people, we cannot hurry ahead of the development because the required preconditions are not met yet".[127] As authorities on the state level for the conflict between the hardliner and idealists in the SED, shown in the first section of this chapter, city officials argued that the local situation was an unsuitable environment for 'uprooted' people outside of the institution. The population, they continued, was not ready to take over responsibility at the workplace and in the leisure time to support the 'endangered' person.

City authorities were also eager to re-brand the institution once again, this time to *Heim für gesellschaftliche Erziehung* [Home for Societal Education]. As such, they intended to stress the educational aim of the home – returning the inmates back into society – as opposed to simply the safekeeping and caring for the 'social deviant'.[128] Whether the supposedly reformed institution could achieve this goal by simply re-branding is questionable. Especially after analysing the proposed changes of Leuben in this final chapter and the general character of 'total institutions', which, according to Goffman, always 'deculturate' the inmate, the *Fürsorgeheim* was predestined to remain a place of incarceration and safekeeping rather than educating and re-socialising the 'social deviant'.[129]

In the end, the letter – which incorporated the views of the local *Volkspolizei* [People's Police – VP], the Social Welfare, and the Healthcare Department of Dresden – utilised elements of Walter Ulbricht's speech at the II. Party Conference of the SED. According to city officials, the First Secretary of the Central Committee of the SED, Ulbricht, claimed at this meeting that "[s]abotage and espionage are waged with the most criminal means against the peaceful development of Socialism in the GDR".[130] From this starting point, the authors of the letter drew upon the importance of the *Heim für soziale Betreuung Dresden-Leuben*. They argued that 'promiscuous' women, who were confined in the workhouse, were:

> not only a threat to public health, but also a threat to our further development [. . .] The girls without work, without shelter, without money are points for attacks against our state.[131]

In this quotation, city authorities politicised 'sexual and social deviance' along the lines of the state narrative. Consequently, the inmates of Leuben became subjects of competing ideologies in the nascent Cold War. This reasoning justified the goals of mnemonic communities, their views of the workhouse as an institution with medical memories, and its purpose for the present and the future, with which they apparently convinced the state level: the city departments involved successfully saved Leuben's disreputable workhouse for another three years.[132]

In summary, the level of mnemonic communities within the concept of medical memories has shown the complexity of interactions between the state, local officials, and the institution in question. Consequently, mnemonic communities in the form of professions or bureaus, such as police and the health department, derive their contemporary views, for example, about the use of the workhouse from their medical memories and experiences with this institution and from the agreed narrative of their working communities. In the case of Leuben, the legacies evoked to justify the use, as well as the stated aims of the workhouse in the contemporary situation, differed among these communities of shared values and memories. The following struggle among them resulted in the dual-leadership of the *Fürsorgeheim Leuben*, as, initially, neither the social welfare nor the health department wanted to take over the full responsibility for, or costs incurred by, the institution. As soon as the state intervened, local mnemonic communities formed a bond through a shared understanding that they wanted to preserve the workhouse and fend off interventions from the state into what they considered their business.

The best example of differing views in the case of Leuben are the previously mentioned overstretched practices of confinement in Saxony. The local officials were eager to increase legal competencies, and complained to the state after Leuben was transformed into a workhouse:

> that there are several dozen girls in Dresden alone, who again and again are treated for newly acquired gonorrhoea, without the legal opportunity to confine them in the workhouse [Leuben], which currently only has three inmates.[133]

The following rejection by state authorities – who criticised the tendency in Saxony to ease legal regulations, which had the problematic outcome that a woman was confined in a workhouse if only one sexual encounter could be verified – reveals the local agency and the continued existence of a biased and potentially arbitrary procedure in reducing cases of STDs. Saxony's authorities were still caught in the past, believing that deterrence was the best means to prevent 'promiscuity' and the spread of these diseases.[134]

As a report from 1951 reveals, the criticism of GDR authorities about the proposed procedure had no effect. By contrast, Saxony's Police continued to confine people to workhouses who were arrested in the name of eliminating the STD epidemic, but without any legal basis or court ruling.[135] Consequently, the last section of this chapter examines the people who were sent to the *Fürsorgheim Leuben* by the police, local, and state authorities and offers insight into the daily routine of this 'total institution'.

Medical memories of individuals: the inmates and staff of the *Fürsorgeheim Leuben*

In his report from 1951, the Chief of the Head Department III at the Ministry of Justice, Werner Gentz – who was also a member of the workhouse commission, analysed in the first part of this chapter – expressed his dismay about the information he received from Müller, his Justice's Senior Advisor, regarding the situation in the workhouses in Saxony. According to him, "Müller found at his inspection of Dresden-Altleuben that these people were lying around in the bushes and getting up to mischief in broad daylight".[136] Therefore, he continued, that especially for Dresden, "Senior Advisor Müller describes the conditions in these institutions as catastrophic".[137]

Throughout the Saxon state, around 750 people were incarcerated in workhouses at the end of 1951, one-third of them in the *Heim für soziale Betreuung Dresden-Leuben* alone. However, Gentz's criticism was not targeted against the large number of people confined; his concerns were rather directed towards the lack of differentiation between the inmates:

> Men and women are housed in the same institutions. They sit around for days without work. [. . .] Especially unpleasant would be [according to Müller] the fact that there are also many mentally retarded people in these institutions; half-idiots, for whom [their grade of illness] does not suffice to be transferred to a mental asylum.[138]

The described composition of inmates reflected the multifunctional character of Leuben and similar workhouses across Saxony, which was due to overlapping laws and competencies revealed in previous sections.

Regarding the question of who and on which legal basis was confined in the *Fürsorgeheim Leuben*, this study showed that, on the one hand, the social welfare department sent the 'uprooted' youth to the reformatory part of this institution. The health department, on the other hand, used Leuben as a deterrence lesson and confined women who were deemed to be 'promiscuous'.[139] This dual use, however, was viewed by authorities as an unbearable situation and inhibitor to the institution's goals. In particular, the undesired co-existence of female and male inmates (Figures 4.2a–b, 4.3a–b, 4.5a–b, and 4.6a–b) in one and the same institution was seen as the main inhibitor for any re-socialising efforts, especially by Richter.[140]

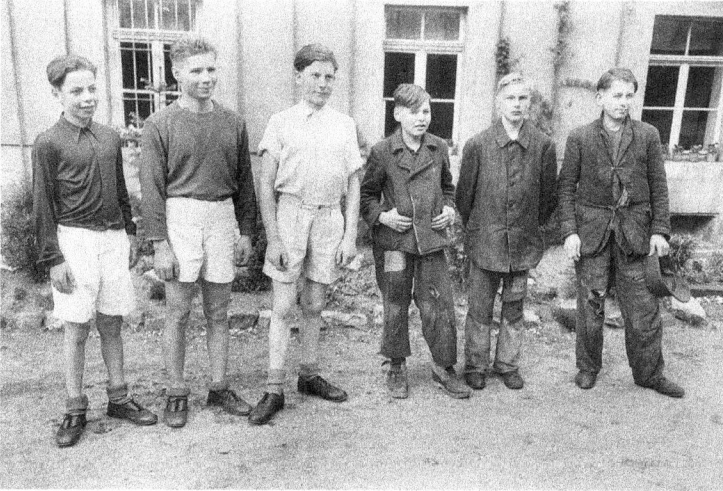

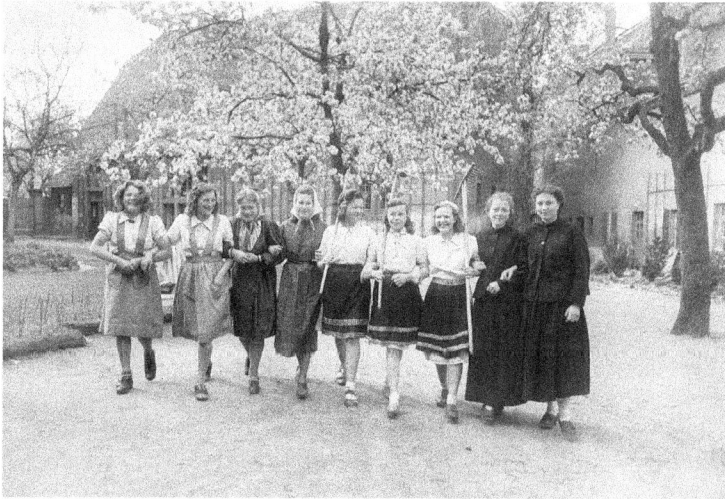

Figures 4.2a–b Two images of the inmates in the *Fürsorgeheim Leuben* in 1949

Note: (a) Boys who assumingly are confined as 'difficult' adolescents; (b) a couple of wardens (on the right in black) with girls who probably are incarcerated on the basis of SMAD Command 273.

Source: SLUB Dresden/Deutsche Fotothek/Erich Höhne und Erich Pohl: Dresden, Leuben. Fürsorgeheim Leuben, 1949, Aufn.-Nr. df_hp_0022793_007; SLUB Dresden/Deutsche Fotothek/Erich Höhne und Erich Pohl: Dresden, Leuben. Fürsorgeheim Leuben, 1949, Aufn.-Nr. df_hp_0022795_014.

By using the description of the conditions in this institution as the starting point, the section shifts the approach towards the local level of society: the individual and his or her medical memories and experiences. The specific aim is to analyse staff and inmates of the *Fürsorgeheim Leuben* as far as sources allow, and expose what it meant for a person to be incarcerated or employed in this particular institution. Therefore, the last part of the final chapter investigates the impact of the state, institutional, and mnemonic community level discussed in the previous sections on the lives inside Leuben and vice versa. The following analysis reveals that many of the narratives, established by upper levels – either locally or nationally – remained idealised and consciously utilised to justify the existence of the institution, both of which were far removed from the actual conditions within the walls of the *Fürsorgeheim Leuben*.

Methodologically, this section represents the most problematic part of this chapter. Due to the nature of the topic, archives are highly restrictive in granting access to files of inmates of this institution. The view is additionally limited, as personal accounts of former staff or patients of Leuben are not yet available. Therefore, the following investigation relies on case histories written by the social welfare department of 12 women who were confined to the *Fürsorgeheim* for different periods of time, and on reports about the situation within Leuben.[141]

An unusual addition to these sources is photographs from the Digital Archive of the *Sächsische Landesbibliothek, Staats- und Universitätsbibliothek Dresden* [Saxon State and University Library in Dresden – SLUB]. The images on the following pages are a selection from the collection of two famous Dresden photographers, Erich Höhne (*1912–†1999) and Erich Pohl (*1904–†1968). Both were freelancers who documented the reconstruction of this city after the Second World War. They joined the SED and worked for the Dresden City Council, local newspapers, and the *Zentralbild Berlin* [Central Images Berlin], the central organisation for photography for GDR media.[142]

Despite the potential political bias inherent in their photographs, this section can offer valuable insights into Leuben via these media, serving as a starting point for future research. Theoretically, the following engages with Goffman, as he provided a critique of 'total institutions' in general, by discussing the conditions and lives of their inmates in particular.[143] It is the purpose of this final part to explore the available sources within the theoretical framework and, subsequently, to define the individual level for the concept of medical memories and experiences.

According to Goffman, 'total institutions' have a 'binary character': a chasm between the group of people who are watched and controlled – the inmates – and the group who watches and controls – the staff.[144] The biggest difference between these two groups is that, firstly, inmates live, work, and sleep within the walls of the workhouse, whereas staff spend only their working hours inside the institution, also having lives on the outside.[145] Furthermore, there is usually a high turnover of inmates, whereas staff tend to change less frequently. Staff are an embodiment of continuity, especially with regard to medical memories, as shown for the postwar medical personnel in general.[146]

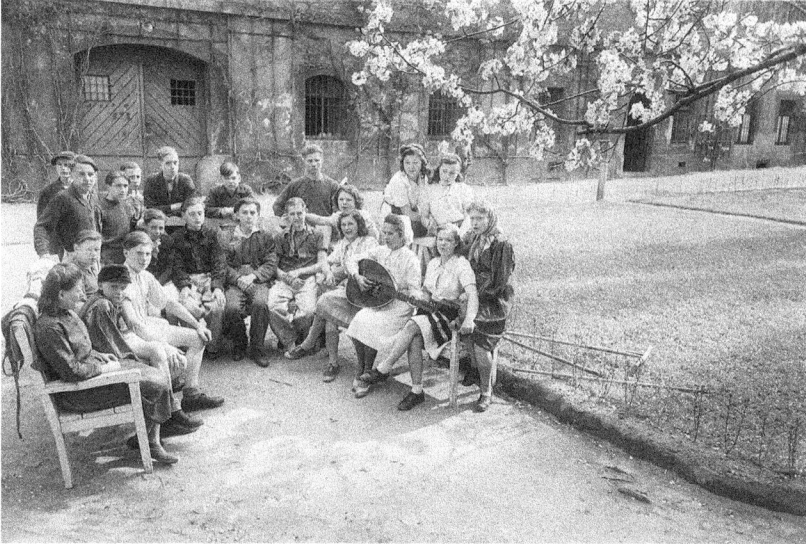

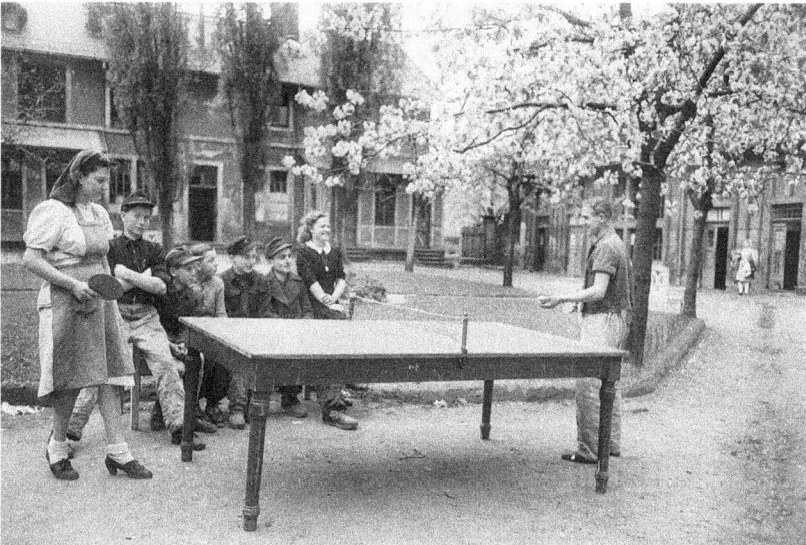

Figures 4.3a–b Two images of possible leisure activities with inmates and staff in the *Fürsorgeheim Leuben* in 1949

Note: (a) Girls and boys are gathered to sing along with the warden playing the guitar; (b) both female and male inmates play table tennis in the main courtyard.

Source: SLUB Dresden/Deutsche Fotothek/Erich Höhne und Erich Pohl: Dresden, Leuben. Fürsorgeheim Leuben, 1949, Aufn.-Nr. df_hp_0022794_009 SLUB Dresden/Deutsche Fotothek/Erich Höhne und Erich Pohl: Dresden, Leuben. Fürsorgeheim Leuben, 1949, Aufn.-Nr. df_hp_0022796_038.

Secondly, due to the 'house rules',[147] scheduled daily life, and medical as well as social treatment, the 'binary character' is institutionalised as inmates and staff are diametrically opposed to each other. Both established "narrow hostile stereotypes" of the other group, constituting a ritual or precondition for ensuring the social distance between the controlled and the controllers.[148]

In the case of the *Fürsorgeheim Leuben*, this separation and distance was initially implemented by official instructions for the department for 'promiscuous' people. The regulations determined that "the staff is only allowed to have a conversation with [the inmates] thus far, as the service requires it".[149] This strict rule, however, is not reflected in the pictures, for example, in Figures 4.2b and 4.3a; the photographs of Höhne and Pohl suggest an intimate relationship between inmates and staff and an apparent family-like atmosphere in this institute.

Unfortunately, the purpose of these photographs remains unclear from the descriptions. However, considering that the photographers worked for newspapers, documenting the reconstruction of Dresden and socialist achievements in general, the assumption must be that the pictures were supposed to show the *Fürsorgeheim* in its best possible light. Consequently, they are themselves a political and cultural construction of the desired reality in the new state. They show, as Betts points out, a new form of 'socialist realism' – not least for legitimacy purposes to demarcate itself from the West.[150]

Despite this hypothesis derived from the images, a report from 1952 illustrated that the desired boundaries and thus the social distance between the inmates and the staff were non-existent in Dresden, and demanded that:

> [t]here must be a clear demarcation between the educator and the educated. The girls develop an uncanny activity in sharing out the educational work, which they find inconvenient. They are indeed not voluntarily in the home. They continuously play off one staff member against the other with the experience that in the case of disagreements among the staff they can have their wishes easily fulfilled. These [wishes] are, of course, not compatible with the educational aim [of Leuben].[151]

The breakdown of social distance within Leuben, as described in this quotation, partly validates the nature of the pictures in this section. The rules which the upper levels of the state tried to enforce were not implemented in this unrelenting form inside the *Fürsorgeheim*. The responsibility for this limitation at the local level lies, according to the report, with Superintendent Hofmann. His views, discussed previously, did not conform to the demands of the state, which ultimately resulted in his replacement with a female superintendent in 1952.[152]

Hofmann's attempt to create a microcosm of society in accordance with his beliefs in this care home is also visible in these photographs – thus forming a part of the everyday experiences of the confined people. Both female and male inmates had to work on a regular basis, such as sewing, cooking, farming, and manufacturing (Figures 4.4a–b), for which they were often sent to companies outside of the institutional premises. After work, the inmates also enjoyed some limited

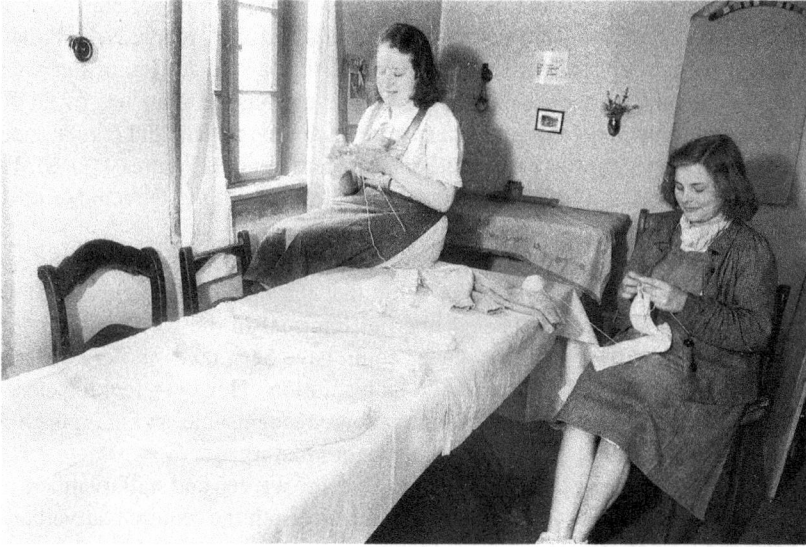

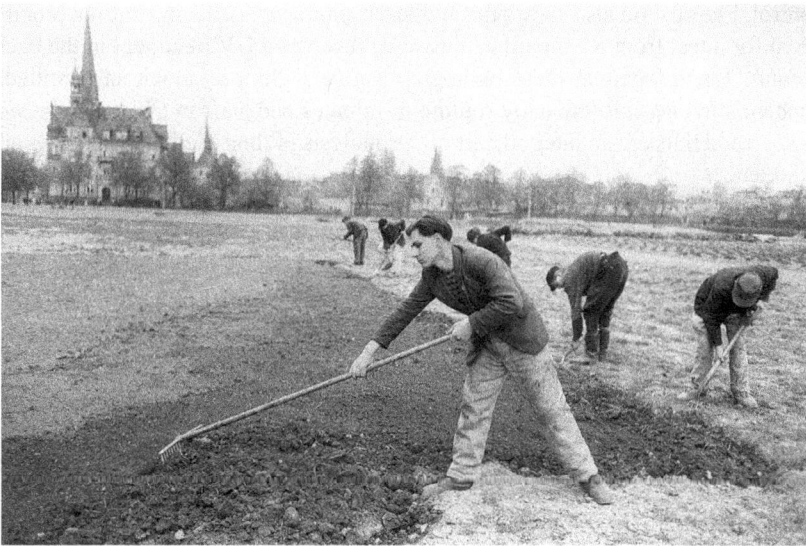

Figures 4.4a–b Two images of possible work which inmates had to carry out during their stay in the *Fürsorgeheim Leuben* in 1949

Note: (a) Girls who knit clothes; (b) boys who work on the field, south of the *Fürsorgeheim* (visible in the background on the middle right).

Source: SLUB Dresden/Deutsche Fotothek/Erich Höhne und Erich Pohl: Dresden, Leuben. Fürsorgeheim Leuben, 1949, Aufn.-Nr. df_hp_0022797_001; SLUB Dresden/Deutsche Fotothek/Erich Höhne und Erich Pohl: Dresden, Leuben. Fürsorgeheim Leuben, 1949, Aufn.-Nr. df_hp_0022797_042.

leisure activities such as singing and table tennis (Figures 4.3a–b). The problem, however, was that the institution lacked an appropriate number of staff, thereby inhibiting the creation of more sport and cultural interest groups. Nevertheless, Hofmann particularly emphasised, as shown in the second section of this chapter, the political education in Leuben and thus established branches of GDR's political and societal organisations inside the institution which held regular meetings, book reviews of progressive authors, and conferences (Figures 4.5a–b). The inmates even elected a 'mayor', who worked closely with the Directorate of the institution.[153]

Consequently, the pictures and the criticisms of the upper levels about the conditions in the *Fürsorgeheim Leuben* show that the medical experiences of the inmates included some unexpected liberties, unusual to the workhouses of the past. On first sight, many of the images could have been taken in very different places and occasions, not limited to a 'total institution'. However, looking closely at these pictures, the iron bars in the windows are recognisable, and in Figure 4.5b the subtitle of the mural indicates that it is a reformatory.

Furthermore, even if not immediately visible, the warden and staff members are often among them in the photographs – indicating both the required surveillance but also the lack of social distance (Figures 4.2b and 4.3a). Apart from this social control, Figure 4.6b also shows the medical monitoring in this institution: blood is taken for a test from a woman, while a man receives a UV treatment in the background. Taken together, these photographs give a glimpse, albeit an admittedly euphemistic one, into the daily routine of inmates and staff in the *Fürsorgeheim Leuben* and thus are an integral part of the analysis of their medical memories and experiences.

Another 'binary' exists in the form of the differing narratives within 'total institutions'. On the one side, the staff create a (medical and social) case history of the inmate, whereas, on the other, the inmate develops a narrative for themselves and their social environment.[154] Both narratives are derived from different medical memories and thus serve as justifications for the individual's confinement in a 'total institution' from at least two different angles.[155]

Unfortunately, as mentioned before, this analysis has only one side of this narrative: case histories of several inmates of Leuben, provided by the Social Welfare Department of Dresden. These individual reports described 12 women between the age of 19 and 27. For most of them, the report initially discussed the potential reasons for becoming 'uprooted' and 'promiscuous': some women were daughters out of wedlock, refugees, orphans, 'spoiled' children, or had other general upbringing difficulties.[156] Apart from traditional mentalities and stigmas, all of these girls and women had troublesome medical memories, and thus were part of those 'uprooted' children with complex war and personal experiences, discussed in Chapter 3.

For example, the report stated for Petra,[157] born in 1927, that her foster parents caused her 'socially deviant behaviour' "because they supported [her] dissolute moral conduct".[158] From such a starting point – a pathologised living situation and

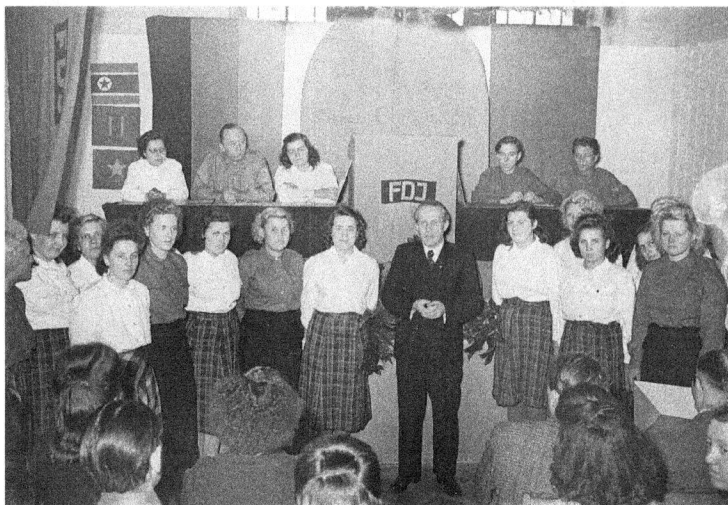

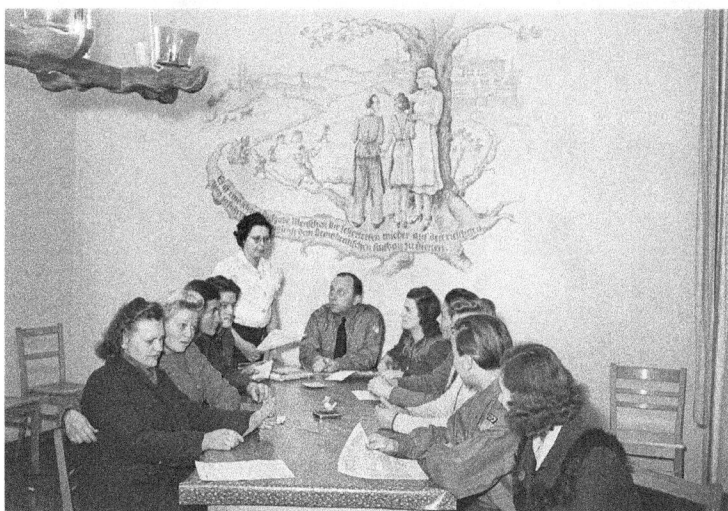

Figures 4.5a–b Two images of the political education and organisations in the *Fürsorge-heim Leuben* in December 1950

Note: (a) A meeting of the FDJ organisation with Superintendent Hofmann in the middle; (b) a political seminar, which is led by the head of the FDJ branch in the *Fürsorgeheim*. Caption of the mural in the background: "It is a great task to lead humans, who failed, back to the right way and thus serve the democratic transformation".

Source: SLUB Dresden/Deutsche Fotothek/Erich Höhne und Erich Pohl: Dresden, Leuben. Fürsorge-heim Leuben, Dezember 1950, Aufn.-Nr. df_hp_0023605_006; SLUB Dresden/Deutsche Fotothek/ Erich Höhne und Erich Pohl: Dresden, Leuben. Fürsorgeheim Leuben, Dezember 1950, Aufn.-Nr. df_hp_0023607_002.

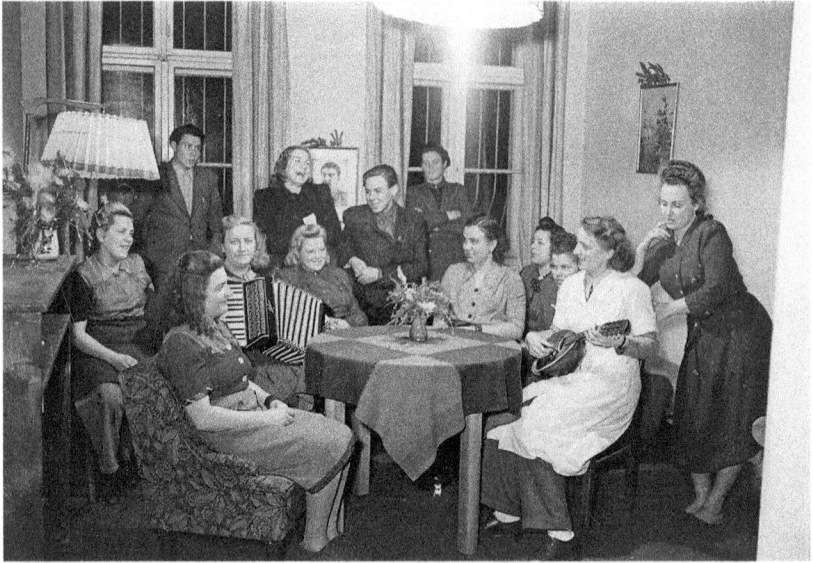

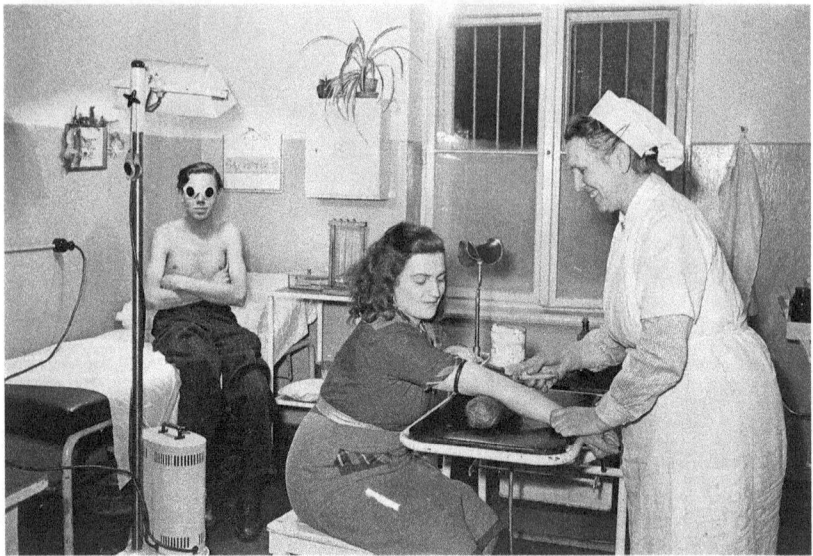

Figures 4.6a–b Two images of other activities in the *Fürsorgeheim Leuben* in December 1950

Note: (a) Both female and male inmates spend a merry evening together (visible in the background is a picture of Stalin); (b) one of the nurses' rooms in the institution, in which both female and male patients are treated.

upbringing in the form of medical memories – the report rationalised actions and the behaviour of women in the present.

They argued in another case, Rosalinde,[159] who was born in 1928, that she "was *continuously in care homes* and was *continuously arrested* and put under [medical] control as a *person suffering from STDs* [emphasis as in the original, M.W.]".[160] The language and stigmatisation inherent in this statement and the case histories, in general, show the continued existence of a biased mentality towards STDs and of medical control into the postwar era, revealed in Chapter 2. The medical memories of the medical and social constructions of these diseases in the form of concepts, diagnoses, and treatment became the medical experience of women, denounced as 'promiscuous' at the time. Both Petra and Rosalinda, as well as most of the ten other women in this file, were admitted to Leuben several times.

However, this unbroken cycle, in which many of the inmates of Leuben were trapped, not only was due to the tight medical monitoring and regulations of confinement of the officials, but also was often provoked by inmates themselves; a phenomenon, though, which was not unique for the postwar era, as this statement from January 1936 proves:

> Lately, it has been repeatedly noted here that even young people make all possible efforts to be remanded into the *Fürsorgeheim Leuben*. The reason is probably that the inmates of the *Fürsorgeheim* have to do relatively little work for good meals.[161]

Firstly, this quotation shows not only a questionable perception of parts of the youth during the Third Reich, but also that the food provision had apparently improved since the revolt in Leuben in 1929. However, it also indicates that, secondly, an institution which provided a daily routine, care, and support might have seemed attractive for the 'uprooted' youth, especially if they had lost their relatives and were displaced after the war.

The problem of the so-called *Dauer-* or *Stammgäste* [permanent and regular guests] continued into the 1950s, and they were continuously criticised for their negative influence on other inmates who were seen as 'educatable'.[162] The 'regulars' who, according to the authorities, were incapable of being re-socialised had been confined to Leuben multiple times and stayed there for a prolonged period. This fact indicates that the medical experiences of the inmates and thus their view of this institution – from the inside – was a rather positive one.

However, this finding must be qualified because their personal freedom had been restricted and they were subject to the compulsory character of the measures of social and medical control in this institution. Nonetheless, the underlying assumption is supported by Goffman, who described for 'colonisers' the tendency of 'messing up' before their planned release – a procedure which often finds support by staff to prolong the stay of inmates for social reasons.[163]

The reality in 'total institutions' generally, and in the *Fürsorgeheim Leuben* in particular, was far removed from the state narrative, the local authorities' claims, and also the staff's justifications about the aims and purpose of the workhouse. The relapse of targeted people into confinement was an inherent characteristic of this institution – it could not re-socialise or re-integrate the inmates into society.[164]

However, the reason why former inmates after their release quickly looked for a way to return to the same institution was not only that the conditions within Leuben might appear as supportive and family-like, but also that they realised "that release means moving from the top of a small world to the bottom of a large one".[165] Superintendent Hofmann was very conscious of the latter fact, as the name *Fürsorgeheim* was itself a life-long stigma which people who were confined to this institution had to live with. The re-branding of Leuben failed to have the desired effect of changing the attitudes of either staff, inmates, or the surrounding population, nor the social environment.

The unfavourable perception of the institution persisted not least because the address and the location, which were connected with the medical memories of the space and the institution itself, remained the same, maintaining an inseparable bond.[166] As a result, to be an inmate of, or referred from, *Altleuben 10* continued to be an embarrassing fact; and thus the engraved institutional medical memories became part of the individual ones, affecting her or his present life and future perspectives as shown for Petra and Rosalinde.

The stigma attached to the people often prevented their re-integration into society, which, despite all the aftercare efforts of the social welfare department in the form of providing room and work for the released Leuben inmate, supported the cycle of social and medical control. In many of the case histories mentioned earlier, the women quickly disappeared after release from their appointed job and home, and were roving around until they were arrested by the police and brought back into the *Fürsorgeheim*.[167]

In conclusion, the workhouse in Dresden constituted continuity on all four levels of the medical memories and experience concept: it remained a deterrence lesson for the outside population in its aims, procedures, name, and language, while it failed to reform and re-socialise the inmate as in the past. In Goffmanian terms, workhouses were viewed as 'storage dumps', where the "contradiction, between what the institution does and what its officials must say it does, forms the basic context of the staff's daily activity".[168]

This general limitation also applies to this analysis: due to methodological issues of obtaining material from the inside of Leuben, the reconstruction of individual medical memories and experiences occurred mostly from an outsider perspective. However, this section showed, with critically engaging Goffman's sociological analysis of 'total institutions', that the implementation of laws, criticisms, and also ideals at the local level were obstructed by the medical memories of staff, as well as inmates themselves. Many examples of reports and images point towards a very different atmosphere in Leuben that was contradictory to state officials' aims and narratives.

Therefore, this section emphasises the acknowledgement of every actor's agency in a historical context, even if confined in a 'total institution'. The medical memories and experiences of the individual determine their social conduct and actions. If inmates felt that they were unable to cope with the outside world, a renewed social and medical transgression of laws provided them with a way back into the institution. Here, they had memories of receiving care and medical treatment, of having work and, most importantly, an 'environment of equals' or even friends – they did not have to be ashamed. This finding does not belittle the deprivations which inmates experienced during their stay in the workhouse. By contrast, it is an attempt to incorporate the complexity of individual decisions and the state response.

On the outside of Leuben, the stigmatised 'promiscuous' women had – as shown in Chapter 1 – to deal with doctors who derived their medical and social concepts from their past. They often faced – as shown in Chapter 2 – medical monitoring, which heavily relied on denunciation, compulsory hospitalisation, and invasive medical treatment, often seamlessly continuing Third Reich language, medical concepts, and practices. They were quickly used as 'subjects' – as shown in Chapter 3 for the 'depraved' youth and in this chapter for the inmates of workhouses – for demarcating the 'new socialist identity' from what was 'abnormal', and for the state's narrative of the ideological struggles of the imminent Cold War. From this perspective, the *Fürsorgeheim Leuben* appeared as an alternative and last resort for the former inmate. Consequently, both the outside world's hostile attitudes towards the stigmatised as well as the apparent insular existence of Leuben ultimately supported the failure of this institution, if judged according to its aims of re-socialisation.

Notes

1 For a biography of Peter Martin Lampel, see Rolf Badenhausen, 'Lampel, Peter Martin', *Neue Deutsche Biographie*, 13 (1982), 460–1.
2 Peter Martin Lampel, *Revolte im Erziehungshaus* (Berlin: Kiepenheuer, 1929), p. 37.
3 *Revolte im Erziehungshaus* took place in a Prussian reformatory, somewhere around Berlin, and thus illustrates that these institutions were in a bad condition across the Weimar Republic, and revolts common in the late 1920s, as Leuben was not a singular case. Lars Herrmann, 'Straßen und Plätze in Leuben', *Dresdener Stadtteile* <www.dresdner-stadtteile.de/Ost/Leuben/Strassen_Leuben/strassen_leuben.html> [accessed 30 January 2019].
4 For example, a 1922 newspaper article already acknowledged the disputed results of Leuben as a reformatory. 'Ausschnitt aus dem Dresdner Anzeiger vom 21. April 1922': StA DD, Fürsorgeamt, 2.3.25, AV III Arbeitsanstalt, Rep. II: Anstaltsverwaltung, Section B: Die Organisation der Anstalt, Nr. 12, Bl. 57.
5 In the following the term 'workhouse' is used in the German and not in the Dickensian sense. While at the beginning, the workhouse in England and Germany was part of the Poor Laws system that provided accommodation and work to the poor, in Germany it increasingly developed to a place where people would be confined by penalty laws in order to 'sanitise' the industrialised cities. It was connected with the views that only those who work should receive food and support by the state and thus was part of the general socio-cultural development of the nineteenth and twentieth centuries. In contrast to this development in Germany, English workhouses became places for the infirm and elderly by the late-nineteenth century, before they were dissolved during the 1930s.
6 For further information about the history of the multifunctional character, see Wolfgang Ayaß, *Das Arbeitshaus Breitenau: Bettler, Landstreicher, Prostituierte, Zuhälter und*

Fürsorgeempfänger in der Korrektions- und Landarmenanstalt Breitenau (1874–1949) (Kassel: Verein für hessische Geschichte und Landeskunde e.V., 1992), pp. 25–34. here 29; Wolfgang Ayaß, 'Die "korrektionelle Nachhaft": Zur Geschichte der strafrechtlichen Arbeitshausunterbringung in Deutschland', *Zeitschrift für Neuere Rechtsgeschichte*, 15 (1993), 184–201; Elisabeth Elling-Ruhwinkel, *Sichern und Strafen: Das Arbeitshaus Benninghausen (1871–1945)* (Paderborn: Schöningh, 2005), pp. 17–18; Sven Korzilius, *'Asoziale' und 'Parasiten' im Recht der SBZ/DDR* (Cologne: Böhlau, 2005), p. 63.

7 Korzilius, p. 70; Doris Foitzik, '"Sittlich verwahrlost": Disziplinierung und Diskriminierung geschlechtskranker Mädchen in der Nachkriegszeit am Beispiel Hamburg', *Neunzehnhundertneunundneunzig*, 1 (1997), 68–82. Eva Gehltomholt and Sabine Hering, for example, show continuity regarding the legal, social, and medical treatment of the 'depraved girl' and in the terminology, educational programmes, personnel in and the institutions themselves after 1945. Eva Gehltomholt and Sabine Hering, *Das verwahrloste Mädchen: Diagnostik und Fürsorge in der Jugendhilfe zwischen Kriegsende und Reform (1945–1965)* (Opladen: Barbara Budrich Verlag, 2006), pp. 31–3. See also Chapter 3.

8 Ayaß, *Das Arbeitshaus Breitenau*, pp. 338–45; Ayaß, 'Die "korrektionelle Nachhaft"', pp. 199–200.

9 Ayaß, 'Die "korrektionelle Nachhaft"', pp. 200–1.

10 For Goffman's analysis of the features, which an institution needs to fulfil in order to be called a 'total' one, see Erving Goffman, *Asylums: Essays on the Social Situation of Mental Patients and Other Inmates* (London: Penguin Books, 1991), pp. 15–18.

11 For example, see the language used and the legal and social treatment proposed by Franz von Liszt, *Strafrechtliche Aufsätze und Vorträge: Erster Band, 1875 bis 1891* (Berlin: J. Guttentag, 1905), p. 165.

12 In the nineteenth and most of the twentieth century, as Ayaß and Ellis-Ruhwinkel illustrate, workhouses required state subsidies and were not able to sustain themselves through profits from manufacturing. Ayaß, *Das Arbeitshaus Breitenau*, pp. 28, 41–2; Elling-Ruhwinkel, p. 21.

13 For the history and the economic relevance of workhouses in the nineteenth and twentieth centuries, see Ayaß, *Das Arbeitshaus Breitenau*, pp. 25–34; Andrea Rudolph, *Die Kooperation von Strafrecht und Sozialhilferecht bei der Disziplinierung von Armen mittels Arbeit: Vom Arbeitshaus bis zur gemeinnützigen Arbeit* (Frankfurt a.M.: Lang, 1995), pp. 18, 157; Korzilius, pp. 61–70.

14 'Ausschnitt aus dem Dresdner Anzeiger vom 21. April 1922': StA DD, Fürsorgeamt, 2.3.25, AV III Arbeitsanstalt, Rep. II: Anstaltsverwaltung, Section B: Die Organisation der Anstalt, Nr. 12, Bl. 57. For the documents about the acquisition of this farm by the city council, see StA DD, Bauamt, 8.22, Nr. 1205, unpaginated.

15 Ayaß, *Das Arbeitshaus Breitenau*, pp. 73–4.

16 David J. Rothman, *The Discovery of the Asylum: Social Order and Disorder in the New Republic* (Boston: Little, Brown & Company, 1971), pp. 81–96; Carla Yanni, *The Architecture of Madness: Insane Asylums in the United States* (Minneapolis, MN: University of Minnesota Press, 2007), pp. 7–15. For the famous, but disputed exploration, especially of the panoptical prison, see Michel Foucault, *Descipline and Punish: The Brith of the Prison*, trans. by Robert Hurley (London: Penguin Books, 1991), pp. 195–228.

17 Ayaß, *Das Arbeitshaus Breitenau*, pp. 73–4.

18 These are the adapted features, which Goffman listed as being common to all 'total institutions'. Goffman, *Asylums*, p. 17.

19 For the problem of "disculturation" and the subsequent "civil death" of inmates, see Goffman, *Asylums*, pp. 23–5; Rothman, pp. 81–2, 95–6.

20 Goffman, *Asylums*, p. 23.

21 Ayaß, *Das Arbeitshaus Breitenau*, pp. 40–1. For the differentiation of 'general preventive' versus the 'specific preventive effect', see Rudolph, p. 158.
22 Evans shows that also the juvenile workhouses in East Germany after 1945 were in terrible conditions and the confined youth often had to face abusive staff, a lack of food and heating, and a general absence of cleanliness in these institutions. Jennifer V. Evans, *Life Among the Ruins: Cityscape and Sexuality in Cold War Berlin* (Houndmills: Palgrave Macmillan, 2011), pp. 201–2.
23 For this claim, see Ayaß, *Das Arbeitshaus Breitenau*, pp. 40–1, here 40. For the theoretical background of the deterrent effect and its impact on individual motivation and social conduct, see Franklin E. Zimring and Gordon J. Hawkins, *Deterrence: The Legal Threat in Crime Control* (Chicago: University of Chicago Press, 1973), pp. 134–6.
24 According to Goffman, anyone would be diagnosed with a mental disorder in this situation, only due to the institutional framework and the circumstances of being sent to the asylum. Goffman, *Asylums*, pp. 306–7, here 307.
25 Rothman, p. 154; Yanni, p. 11.
26 For an insightful discussion of the relation between memory and history and its use, see Aleida Assmann, 'History and Memory', *International Encyclopedia of the Social & Behavioral Sciences* (Elsevier, 2001), pp. 6822–29.
27 'Protokoll über die Sitzung der Kommission zur Prüfung der Frage der Beibehaltung des Arbeitshauses, 1. Januar 1946': BArch, DP 1/6935, unpaginated.
28 'Protokoll über die Sitzung der Kommission zur Prüfung der Frage der Beibehaltung des Arbeitshauses, 1. Januar 1946': BArch, DP 1/6935, unpaginated; For biographical information of most people who participated in this commission, see Hermann Wentker, *Justiz in der SBZ/DDR 1945–1953: Transformation und Rolle ihrer zentralen Institutionen* (Munich: Oldenbourg, 2001), pp. 42, 53–9, 65–8, 122, 203–4.
29 For more details about their life paths in the Third Reich and in the postwar era, see Wentker, pp. 53, 67, 254.
30 See Chapter 1.
31 For an official biography of Eduard Kohlrausch, see Jeanette Gonisor, 'Eduard Kohlrausch: Rektor der Friedrich-Wilhelms-Universität Zu Berlin 1932/33', *Humboldt-Universität Zu Berlin*, 2013 <www.hu-berlin.de/de/ueberblick/geschichte/rektoren/kohlrausch> [accessed 30 January 2019].
32 Korzilius, pp. 49–50.
33 Quotation taken from Korzilius, pp. 49–50, here 49.
34 Josef Wißkirchen, 'Brauweiler bei Köln: Frühes Konzentrationslager in der Provinzial-Anstalt 1933–1934', in *Konzentrationslager im Rheinland und in Westfalen 1933–1945: Zentrale Steuerung und regionale Initiative*, ed. by Jan Erik Schulte (Paderborn: Schöningh, 2005), pp. 65–86.
35 'Protokoll über die Sitzung der Kommission zur Prüfung der Frage der Beibehaltung des Arbeitshauses, 1. Januar 1946': BArch, DP 1/6935, unpaginated. For the situation in Hamburg, see Foitzik, p. 80.
36 In his recent study of chemical and biological warfare research in Porton Down, Ulf Schmidt offers an example for the politics of medical memories regarding the veterans who were exposed to different warfare agents in order to assess their impact on the human nature, and the state's denial to compensate veterans for their sufferings. Their medical memories and experiences did not fit into the overarching state narrative, which was supposed to portray the United Kingdom as a heroic nation, defeating the Prussians and the Nazis in two world wars. Ulf Schmidt, *Secret Science: A Century of Poison Warfare and Human Experiments* (Oxford: Oxford University Press, 2015), chapter 10.
37 'Protokoll über die Sitzung der Kommission zur Prüfung der Frage der Beibehaltung des Arbeitshauses, 1. Januar 1946': BArch, DP 1/6935, unpaginated.

188   *Institutionalised treatments of the past*

38 'Protokoll über die Sitzung der Kommission zur Prüfung der Frage der Beibehaltung des Arbeitshauses, 1. Januar 1946': BArch, DP 1/6935, unpaginated. For a similar argumentation of the origins and purpose to incarcerate youth for an indefinite period, see Evans, *Life Among the Ruins*, pp. 145–6.

39 For § 361 in its form, valid from 1943 until 1953, which targeted, inter alia, 'vagabonds', 'beggars', 'workshy' people, gamblers, and prostitutes, see '§ 361 StGB, [30. März 1943–1. Oktober 1953]', *Lexetius*, 2016 <http://lexetius.com/StGB/361,8> [accessed 30 January 2019].

40 'Gesetz gegen gefährliche Gewohnheitsverbrecher und Maßregeln der Sicherung und Besserung vom 24. November 1933', *ALEX: Historische Rechts- Und Gesetzestexte Online*, 2011, p. 996 <http://alex.onb.ac.at/cgi-content/alex?aid=dra&datum=1933&page=1120> [accessed 30 January 2019].

41 'Protokoll über die Sitzung der Kommission zur Prüfung der Frage der Beibehaltung des Arbeitshauses, 1. Januar 1946': BArch, DP 1/6935, unpaginated.

42 'Protokoll über die Sitzung der Kommission zur Prüfung der Frage der Beibehaltung des Arbeitshauses, 1. Januar 1946': BArch, DP 1/6935, unpaginated; 'Grundlage, Zweck, Notwendigkeit und Ausgestaltung der Einrichtung des Arbeitshauses. Referat, erstattet in der Kommission zur Prüfung der Frage der Beibehaltung des Arbeitshauses am 31. Januar 1946 durch Vortragenden Rat Fenner, DJV [DZVJ]': BArch, DP 1/6935, unpaginated.

43 'Grundlage, Zweck, Notwendigkeit und Ausgestaltung der Einrichtung des Arbeitshauses. Referat, erstattet in der Kommission zur Prüfung der Frage der Beibehaltung des Arbeitshauses am 31. Januar 1946 durch Vortragenden Rat Fenner, DJV [DZVJ]': BArch, DP 1/6935, unpaginated.

44 Korzilius, *'Asoziale' und 'Parasiten'*, 64–8. 'Bewahrungsgesetz, [1949]': BArch, DQ 1/20626, unpaginated.

45 'Gutachterliche Äußerung der Gesetzgebungsabteilung der Deutschen Justizverwaltung zur Frage der Beibehaltung des Arbeitshauses, 4. Februar 1946': BArch, DP 1/6935, unpaginated.

46 Evans also identifies that the workhouse was "[n]ot simply a throwback to Weimarera rehabilitative policy, youth penal policy inherited significant Nazi-era measures as well". Jennifer V. Evans, 'Bahnhof Boys: Policing Male Prostitution in Post-Nazi Berlin', *Journal of the History of Sexuality*, 12 (2003), 605–36.

47 'Gutachterliche Äußerung der Gesetzgebungsabteilung der Deutschen Justizverwaltung zur Frage der Beibehaltung des Arbeitshauses, 4. Februar 1946': BArch, DP 1/6935, unpaginated. For comparison with the original text from Nagler and Mezger, see the quotation used by Martin Fenner in his paper: 'Grundlage, Zweck, Notwendigkeit und Ausgestaltung der Einrichtung des Arbeitshauses. Referat, erstattet in der Kommission zur Prüfung der Frage der Beibehaltung des Arbeitshauses am 31. Januar 1946 durch Vortragenden Rat Fenner, DJV [DZVJ]': BArch, DP 1/6935, unpaginated.

48 'Parteivorstand SED an Herrn Staatssekretär Peschke, Ministerium für Arbeit und Gesundheitswesen, 7. Juli 1950': BArch, DP 1/7110, Bl. 13.

49 For a claim for gender-equality in the measures to confine people in workhouses, see 'Richtlinien für die Einweisung in die Arbeitskolonne Schönebeck, 10. Oktober 1949': BArch, DQ 1/292, unpaginated.

50 For example, see 'Vermerk über die Besprechung beim Ministerium für Arbeit am 27. März über die Neuregelung der Arbeitshausfrage, 29. März 1952': BArch, DP 1/107, Bl. 70; 'Stellungnahme zum Entwurf zur "Verordnung zur Verhütung und Bekämpfung der Geschlechtskrankheiten", 29. Juli 1958': BArch, DQ 1/20626, unpaginated.

51 As Verena Zimmermann concludes, admitting the existence of social problems in the GDR would question the system as a whole. Verena Zimmermann, *'Den neuen Menschen schaffen': Die Umerziehung von schwererziehbaren und straffälligen Jugendlichen in der DDR (1945–1990)* (Cologne: Böhlau, 2004), p. 237.

52 Erving Goffman, *Behavior in Public Places: Notes on the Social Organization of Gatherings* (New York: The Free Press, 1985), p. 248.
53 For the decision to convert Leuben back into a workhouse for 'promiscuous' women and girls on 1 July 1949, see 'Aktennotiz': BArch, DQ 1/2209, Bl. 430.
54 'Bericht über das Heim, 3. September 1952': BArch, DQ 1/20619, unpaginated.
55 'Ausschnitt aus dem Dresdner Anzeiger vom 21. April 1922': StA DD, Fürsorgeamt, 2.3.25, AV III Arbeitsanstalt, Rep. II: Anstaltsverwaltung, Section B: Die Organisation der Anstalt, Nr. 12, Bl. 57. For the documents about the acquisition of this farm by the city council and the extension and construction of new buildings, see StA DD, Bauamt, 8.22, Nr. 1205, unpaginated; StA DD, Bauamt, 8.22, Nr. 1206, unpaginated.
56 For § 361 in its form, valid from 1943 until 1953, see '§ 361 StGB, [30. März 1943–1. Oktober 1953]', p. 361.
57 Wolf Gruner, *Öffentliche Wohlfahrt und Judenverfolgung: Wechselwirkungen lokaler und zentraler Politik im NS-Staat (1933–1942)* (Munich: Oldenbourg Verlag, 2009), p. 42; Julia Hörath, *'Asoziale' und 'Berufsverbrecher' in den Konzentrationslagern 1933 bis 1938* (Göttingen: Vandenhoeck & Ruprecht, 2017), pp. 106–7; Wolfgang Ayaß, 'Pflichtarbeit und Fürsorgearbeit: Zur Geschichte der „Hilfe zur Arbeit" außerhalb von Anstalten', in *Arbeitsdienst – wieder salonfähig? Zwang zur Arbeit in Geschichte und Sozialstaat*, ed. by Frankfurter Arbeitslosenzentrum – FALZ (Frankfurt a. M.: Fachhochschulverlag, 2015), pp. 59–60. Regarding the institution in Leuben, this law was used to incarcerate especially 'endangered women', see Korzilius, p. 66.
58 'Ausschnitt aus dem Dresdner Anzeiger vom 21. April 1922': StA DD, Fürsorgeamt, 2.3.25, AV III Arbeitsanstalt, Rep. II: Anstaltsverwaltung, Section B: Die Organisation der Anstalt, Nr. 12, Bl. 57.
59 Annette Dubbers, *Leuben: Aus der Geschichte eines Dresdner Stadtteils* (Dresden: Dubbers, 2005), pp. 33–4.
60 Dubbers, pp. 33–4.
61 'Gesetz gegen gefährliche Gewohnheitsverbrecher und Maßregeln der Sicherung und Besserung vom 24. November 1933'. § 42 d specified the incarceration of reformatory institutions such as workhouses if transgressing § 361 No. 3–5, 6, 6a, and 8, and § 42 f determined the duration of the incarceration in these institutions such as the workhouse.
62 'Anordnung der Überprüfung von Leuben nach politischen Gesichtspunkten, 11. September 1935': StA DD, Fürsorgeamt, 2.3.25, Nr. 339, Bl. 68.
63 'Arbeitsdank e.V., Arbeitsgauobmann, Bericht, 26. November 1935': StA DD, Fürsorgeamt, 2.3.25, Nr. 339, Bl. 68.
64 'Antwort zum Bericht vom 26. November 1935, (Without Date)': StA DD, Fürsorgeamt, 2.3.25, Nr. 339, Bl. 74.
65 'Aufgrund des Gesetzes zur Verhütung erbkranken Nachwuchses: Änderung der Heimordnung, 7. März 1934': StA DD, Fürsorgeamt, 2.3.25, Nr. 339, Bl. 56.
66 Korzilius, *'Asoziale' und 'Parasiten'*, 69–70.
67 For example, see the report about the problematic perception of Leuben by the population and inmates, in 'Fürsorgeheim Leuben, 13. März 1933': StA DD, Fürsorgeamt, 2.3.25, Nr. 338, Bl. 53.
68 'Bericht Betr. Altersheim und Krankenhaus Leuben, 7. September 1945': StA DD, Dezernat Sozial- und Wohnungswesen, 4.1.10, Nr. 71, Bl. 1.
69 Ayaß, *Das Arbeitshaus Breitenau*, pp. 328–33; Elling-Ruhwinkel, p. 371.
70 'Bericht Betr. Altersheim und Krankenhaus Leuben, 7. September 1945': StA DD, Dezernat Sozial- und Wohnungswesen, 4.1.10, Nr. 71, Bl. 1.
71 For the use of the *Fürsorgeheim Leuben* after 1945, see 'Bericht über die Aufbauarbeit der Sozialen Fürsorge auf dem Gebiete des Anstalts- und Heimwesens der Stadt Dresden, [1951]': StA DD, Dezernat Gesundheitswesen, 4.1.12, Nr. 69, Bl. 184.

72 See Chapter 2. For a comparison with the medical and social control regarding STDs in postwar Hamburg, see Foitzik, pp. 74–80.

73 Korzilius, pp. 72–3. Korzilius also argues that due to similar Soviet laws and views regarding re-socialisation and re-education in 'total institutions', the SMAD was willing to allow the retention of the workhouse in the SBZ. Korzilius, p. 71.

74 Korzilius also argues that due to similar Soviet laws and views regarding re-socialisation and re-education, the SMAD was willing to allow the retention of the workhouse in East Germany. Korzilius, p. 71.

75 'Bericht über die Aufbauarbeit der Sozialen Fürsorge auf dem Gebiete des Anstalts- und Heimwesens der Stadt Dresden, [1951]': StA DD, Dezernat Gesundheitswesen, 4.1.12, Nr. 69, Bl. 184; 'Fürsorgeheim Leuben, 10. Februar 1947': StA DD, Dezernat Sozial- und Wohnungswesen, 4.1.10, Nr. 71, Bl. 10.

76 'Dienstvorschrift für die Fürsorgeanstalt Leuben, [mid-1946?]': StA DD, Fürsorgeamt, 2.3.25, Nr. 339, Bl. 107.

77 For the documents regarding the extension and construction of House H, the infirmary, see StA DD, Bauamt, 8.22, Nr. 1206, unpaginated.

78 Rainer Behring, 'Das Personal der kommunistischen Diktaturdurchsetzung: Parteifunktionäre und Kommunalpolitiker in Chemnitz 1945–1949', in *Von Stalingrad zur SBZ: Sachsen 1943 bis 1949*, ed. by Mike Schmeitzner, Clemens Vollnhals, and Francesca Weil (Göttingen: Vandenhoeck & Ruprecht, 2016), pp. 239–58; Sebastian Rick, 'Diktaturdurchsetzung auf dem flachen Lande am Beispiel der Landkreise Liebenwerda und Schweidnitz 1945–1949', in *Von Stalingrad zur SBZ: Sachsen 1943 bis 1949*, ed. by Mike Schmeitzner, Clemens Vollnhals, and Francesca Weil (Göttingen: Vandenhoeck & Ruprecht, 2016), pp. 259–76; Tilman Pohlmann, 'Generationen und Herrschaftsetablierung: Die 1: SED-Kreissekretäre der Nachkriegszeit', in *Von Stalingrad zur SBZ: Sachsen 1943 bis 1949*, ed. by Mike Schmeitzner, Clemens Vollnhals, and Francesca Weil (Göttingen: Vandenhoeck & Ruprecht, 2016), pp. 277–92.

79 For his biography as a disputed postwar figure in Dresden, see Jörg Osterloh, ' "Der Totenwald von Zeithain": Die Sowjetische Besatzungsmacht und die Untersuchung des Massensterbens im Stalag 204 (IV H) Zeithain', in *Von Stalingrad zur SBZ: Sachsen 1943 bis 1949*, ed. by Mike Schmeitzner, Clemens Vollnhals, and Francesca Weil (Göttingen: Vandenhoeck & Ruprecht, 2016), pp. 329–52.

80 'Fürsorgeheim Leuben, 10. Februar 1947': StA DD, Dezernat Sozial- und Wohnungswesen, 4.1.10, Nr. 71, Bl. 10. For Richter's letter to the Saxon Ministry of Labour and Social Welfare, see 'An die Landesregierung Sachsen, Ministerium für Arbeit und Sozialfürsorge, 17. Mai 1947': StA DD, Fürsorgeamt, 2.3.25, AV I, Nr. 647, Bl. 108.

81 Rothman, p. 154; Yanni, p. 11.

82 Criticisms on the outcome of workhouses or multifunctional institutions was nothing new, but existed since their creation and was often supported by pointing towards the failure to reform people, as most of the inmates would be confined several times. For criticisms of Leuben, see, for example, 'Ausschnitt aus dem Dresdner Anzeiger vom 21. April 1922': StA DD, Fürsorgeamt, 2.3.25, AV III Arbeitsanstalt, Rep. II: Anstaltsverwaltung, Section B: Die Organisation der Anstalt, Nr. 12, Bl. 57.

83 'Übersendung eines Diskussionsbeitrages, Gedanken zur Errichtung eines Arbeitshauses, Anstaltsdirektor Hofmann, 16. Juni 1949': StA DD, Dezernat Sozial- und Wohnungswesen, 4.1.10, Nr. 71, Bl. 93.

84 'Übersendung eines Diskussionsbeitrages, Gedanken zur Errichtung eines Arbeitshauses, Anstaltsdirektor Hofmann, 16. Juni 1949': StA DD, Dezernat Sozial- und Wohnungswesen, 4.1.10, Nr. 71, Bl. 93.

85 Peter Schneck, *Linser, Karl*, 2009 <www.bundesstiftung-aufarbeitung.de/wer-war-wer-in-der-ddr-%2363%3B-1424.html?ID=2117> [accessed 30 January 2019]. 'Rat der Stadt Dresden, Dezernat Gesundheitswesen an Herrn Präs. Prof. Dr. Linser, DWK, HA GW, 7. Dezember 1948': BArch, DQ 1/128, Bl. 214.

86 'Übersendung eines Diskussionsbeitrages, Gedanken zur Errichtung eines Arbeitshauses, Anstaltsdirektor Hofmann, 16. Juni 1949': StA DD, Dezernat Sozial- und
Wohnungswesen, 4.1.10, Nr. 71, Bl. 93.

87 'Bericht über die von der Landtagskommission für die Heime für soz. Betreuung am
Dienstag, dem 22. April 1952, durchgeführte Besichtigung des Heims für soziale
Betreuung in Dresden A45, Altleuben 10, 2. Mai 1952': HSA DD, Sächsischer Land-
tag 1946–1952, 11347, Nr. 136, unpaginated.

88 'Aktennotiz, 26. August 1949': DQ 1/2209, Bl. 430.

89 Leuben stood in contrast to the establishment of workhouses in former 'total insti-
tutions' such as monasteries, for example, in the case of Breitenau: Ayaß, *Das
Arbeitshaus Breitenau*, pp. 69–78. An exception to the rule is the care home in Olten,
Switzerland, which was newly built and designed for its purposes: Adolf Spring,
'Alters- Und Fürsorgeheim Ruttigerhof Bei Olten', *Schweizerische Bauzeitung*, 111
(1938), 140–2.

90 For concerns regarding the escape of inmates and the problematic security standards
of the *Fürsorgeheim Leuben*, see 'Behandlung von Untersuchungshäftlingen und
Insassen von Strafanstalten in Leuben, 2. August 1947': StA DD, Dezernat Gesundheitswesen, 4.1.12, Nr. 84, Bl. 49.

91 'Hauptabteilung III, Vermerk – Rücksprache mit der Hauptabteilung Justiz, Haupt-
referent Müller, in Dresden, über die Frage des Arbeitshauses, 29. November 1951':
Bundesarchiv (BArch), DP 1/107, Bl. 37.

92 Goffman identified the existence of dormitories or common sleeping rooms as a typical humiliating practice in the 'total institution'. Goffman, *Asylums*, p. 32.

93 StA DD, 8.22, Bauamt, Nr. 1206, unpaginated; StA DD, Bau- und Grundstücksakten,
10, Nr. 37116.

94 Ayaß, *Das Arbeitshaus Breitenau*, pp. 40–2; Elling-Ruhwinkel, pp. 17–26.

95 'Übersendung eines Diskussionsbeitrages, Gedanken zur Errichtung eines Arbeitshauses, Anstaltsdirektor Hofmann, 16. Juni 1949': StA DD, Dezernat Sozial- und
Wohnungswesen, 4.1.10, Nr. 71, Bl. 94.

96 Zimmermann, pp. 49–70. The works of Makarenko had, at least on paper, an important impetus for the educational programmes of correctional facilities throughout the
GDR in the 1950s and beyond.

97 An example represented a report from 1958, in which the author still emphasised the
punitive character of the institution. '[Without Title], 23. Oktober 1958': BArch, DQ
1/20619, unpaginated.

98 'Übersendung eines Diskussionsbeitrages, Gedanken zur Errichtung eines Arbeitshauses, Anstaltsdirektor Hofmann, 16. Juni 1949': StA DD, Dezernat Sozial- und
Wohnungswesen, 4.1.10, Nr. 71, Bl. 94.

99 For the best example for this claim, see the study of Anne Digby about the York
Retreat and its history of treating its mental patients. Anne Digby, *Madness, Morality,
and Medicine: A Study of the York Retreat, 1796–1914* (New York: Cambridge University Press, 1985). Goffman described the system of privileges and punishments
as a guideline for inmates to become "a model of conduct that is at once ideal and
staff-sponsored – a model felt by its advocates to be in the best interests of the very
persons to whom it is applied" (p. 64). Goffman, *Asylums*, pp. 51, 63–4.

100 Goffman concluded that most of the work in asylums was 'demoralising' and the
inmates plagued by boredom. Goffman, *Asylums*, p. 21.

101 Rothman, p. 154. 'Übersendung eines Diskussionsbeitrages, Gedanken zur Errichtung eines Arbeitshauses, Anstaltsdirektor Hofmann, 16. Juni 1949': StA DD, Dezernat Sozial- und Wohnungswesen, 4.1.10, Nr. 71, Bl. 95.

102 Goffman, *Asylums*, pp. 23–5, 71. 'Übersendung eines Diskussionsbeitrages,
Gedanken zur Errichtung eines Arbeitshauses, Anstaltsdirektor Hofmann, 16. Juni
1949': StA DD, Dezernat Sozial- und Wohnungswesen, 4.1.10, Nr. 71, Bl. 95.

103 'Übersendung eines Diskussionsbeitrages, Gedanken zur Errichtung eines Arbeits-hauses, Anstaltsdirektor Hofmann, 16. Juni 1949': StA DD, Dezernat Sozial- und Wohnungswesen, 4.1.10, Nr. 71, Bl. 95.

104 'Aus der Arbeit der Abteilung Sozialwesen im Jahre 1951, 17. Januar 1952': StA DD, Dezernat Gesundheitswesen, 4.1.12, Nr. 69, Bl. 75.

105 'Aktenvermerk über die Dienstreise nach Dresden, Leipzig, Freiberg, Chemnitz (Land Sachsen) in der Zeit vom 12. bis einschließlich 16. Dezember 1949': BArch, DQ 1/20626, unpaginated; 'Heim für soziale Betreuung, 3. Januar 1953': BArch, DQ 1/20626, unpaginated. Verena Zimmermann and Uta Falck claim that *Heime für soziale Betreuung* were not created before 1955, which this study could refute; both, however, also identify that the rebranding was a conscious decision to disguise the inherent tradition of the workhouse. Zimmermann, p. 227; Uta Falck, *VEB Bordell: Geschichte der Prostitution in der DDR* (Berlin: Links, 1998), p. 65.

106 'Heim für soziale Betreuung, Dresden, 3. Januar 1953': BArch, DQ 1/20619, unpaginated.

107 For example, see Cappelletto's study of an Italian village as a mnemonic commu-nity. Francesca Cappelletto, 'Introduction', in *Memory and World War II: An Ethno-graphic Approach*, ed. by Francesca Cappelletto (Oxford: Berg, 2005), pp. 4–5.

108 For the problems regarding costs incurred by Leuben, see 'Arbeitshaus, 22. Juli 1946': BArch, DP 1/106, Bl. 11; 'Offene Abteilung für Geschlechtskranke, 29. April 1947': StA DD, Fürsorgeamt, 2.3.25, AV I, Nr. 647, Bl. 109a.

109 For the split of competencies, see 'Unterbringung von etwa 40 geschlechtskranken Männern aus dem Behelfskrankenhaus Winterbergstraße im Fürsorgeheim Dresden-Leuben, 9. Februar 1948': StA DD, Fürsorgeamt, 2.3.25, AV I, Nr. 647, Bl. 133.

110 'Arbeitshaus, 22. Juli 1946': BArch, DP 1/106, Bl. 11

111 'Offene Abteilung für Geschlechtskranke, 29. April 1947': StA DD, Fürsorgeamt, 2.3.25, AV I, Nr. 647, Bl. 109a, 109b.

112 Already in the newspaper article from 1922, the author argued that the outcome and usefulness of the workhouse was highly disputed. 'Ausschnitt aus dem Dresdner Anzeiger vom 21. April 1922': StA DD, Fürsorgeamt, 2.3.25, AV III Arbeitsanstalt, Rep. II: Anstaltsverwaltung, Section B: Die Organisation der Anstalt, Nr. 12, Bl. 57.

113 For the responsibilities and overlapping competencies of this dual-leadership of the *Fürsorgeheim Leuben*, see 'Dienstvorschrift für die Fürsorgeanstalt Leuben, [1946]': StA DD, Fürsorgeamt, 2.3.25, Nr. 339, Bl. 107.

114 'An die Landesregierung Sachsen, Ministerium für Arbeit und Sozialfürsorge, 17. Mai 1947': StA DD, Fürsorgeamt, 2.3.25, AV I, Nr. 647, Bl. 108.

115 'Fürsorgeheim Leuben, 28. Mai 1947': StA DD, Fürsorgeamt, 2.3.25, AV I, Nr. 647, Bl. 109.

116 'Abschrift, Herrn Stadtrat Prof. Dr. Hübner, 5. Februar 1948': StA DD, Fürsorgeamt, 2.3.25, AV I, Nr. 647, Bl. 135.

117 'Unterbringung von etwa 40 geschlechtskranken Männern aus dem Behelfskranken-haus Winterbergstraße im Fürsorgeheim Dresden-Leuben, 9. Februar 1948': StA DD, Fürsorgeamt, 2.3.25, AV I, Nr. 647, Bl. 133.

118 'Unterbringung von etwa 40 geschlechtskranken Männern aus dem Behelfskranken-haus Winterbergstraße im Fürsorgeheim Dresden-Leuben, 9. Februar 1948': StA DD, Fürsorgeamt, 2.3.25, AV I, Nr. 647, Bl. 134.

119 'Unterbringung von etwa 40 geschlechtskranken Männern aus dem Behelfskranken-haus Winterbergstraße im Fürsorgeheim Dresden-Leuben, 9. Februar 1948': StA DD, Fürsorgeamt, 2.3.25, AV I, Nr. 647, Bl. 134.

120 'Unterbringung im Arbeitshaus Dresden-Leuben, 17. Oktober 1949': BArch, DP 1/7110, Bl. 4.

121 'Unterbringung von etwa 40 geschlechtskranken Männern aus dem Behelfskranken-haus Winterbergstraße im Fürsorgeheim Dresden-Leuben, 9. Februar 1948': StA DD, Fürsorgeamt, 2.3.25, AV I, Nr. 647, Bl. 133.

122 For a report that heavily criticised the conditions of the Homes for Social Care in Saxony in general and Leuben in particular, see 'Hauptabteilung III, Vermerk – Rücksprache mit der Hauptabteilung Justiz, Hauptreferent Müller, in Dresden, über die Frage des Arbeitshauses, 29. November 1951': BArch, DP 1/107, Bl. 36–7. For the overstretched laws to confine people in Saxony, see 'Unterbringung im Arbeitshaus Dresden-Leuben, 11. August 1949': BArch, DP 1/7110, Bl. 2; 'Deutsche Wirtschafts-kommission an die Deutsche Justizverwaltung, 6. September 1949': BArch, DP 1/7110, Bl. 1; 'Unterbringung im Arbeitshaus Leuben, 17. Oktober 1949': BArch, DP 1/7110, Bl. 3–4.

123 'Heim für soziale Betreuung, 3. Januar 1953': BArch, DQ 1/20619, unpaginated.

124 For the historiographically overstretched argument of the putative 'totalitarian' GDR, see Peter Grieder, *The East German Leadership, 1946–1973: Conflict and Crisis* (Manchester: Manchester University Press, 1999); Jürgen Kocka, 'Eine durchherr-schte Gesellschaft', in *Sozialgeschichte der DDR*, ed. by Hartmut Kaelble, Jür-gen Kocka, and Hartmut Zwahr (Stuttgart: Klett-Cotta, 1994), pp. 547–53; Klaus Schroeder, *Der SED-Staat: Geschichte und Strukturen der DDR* (Munich: Bayrische Landeszentrale für politische Bildungsarbeit, 1998).

125 Behring; Rick; Pohlmann.

126 'Heim für soziale Betreuung, 3. Januar 1953': BArch, DQ 1/20619, unpaginated. The dissolution of the *Heim für soziale Betreuung Dresden-Leuben* was accomplished during the year 1955, transforming this institution into a retirement home, which opened in 1956. 'Zentrale Einweisungsstelle für Heime für soziale Betreuung, 15. November 1955': BArch, DQ 1/20618, unpaginated; StA DD, Bau- und Grundstücks-akten, 10, Nr. 37116, unpaginated.

127 'Heim für soziale Betreuung, 3. Januar 1953': BArch, DQ 1/20619, unpaginated.

128 'Heim für soziale Betreuung, 3. Januar 1953': BArch, DQ 1/20619, unpaginated.

129 Goffman, *Asylums*, pp. 23–5, 71.

130 'Heim für soziale Betreuung, 3. Januar 1953': BArch, DQ 1/20619, unpaginated.

131 'Heim für soziale Betreuung, 3. Januar 1953': BArch, DQ 1/20619, unpaginated.

132 'Heim für soziale Betreuung, 3. Januar 1953': BArch, DQ 1/20619, unpaginated.

133 'Deutsche Wirtschaftskommission an die Deutsche Justizverwaltung, 6. Septem-ber 1949': BArch, DP 1/7110, Bl. 1.

134 For the response and rejection of the state to ease the strict regulations for sentencing people into workhouses, see 'Unterbringung im Arbeitshaus Leuben, 17. Oktober 1949': BArch, DP 1/7110, Bl. 3–4. For another example of the critic on the Saxon procedure, see 'Entwurf einer Verordnung über die Einweisungen in Heime für soziale Betreuung der Landesregierung Sachsen, 4. Januar 1950': BArch, DQ 1/20626, unpaginated.

135 'Hauptabteilung III, Vermerk – Rücksprache mit der Hauptabteilung Justiz, Haupt-referent Müller, in Dresden, über die Frage des Arbeitshauses, 29. November 1951': BArch, DP 1/107, Bl. 36.

136 'Hauptabteilung III, Vermerk – Rücksprache mit der Hauptabteilung Justiz, Haupt-referent Müller, in Dresden, über die Frage des Arbeitshauses, 29. November 1951': BArch, DP 1/107, Bl. 36.

137 'Hauptabteilung III, Vermerk – Rücksprache mit der Hauptabteilung Justiz, Haupt-referent Müller, in Dresden, über die Frage des Arbeitshauses, 29. November 1951': BArch, DP 1/107, Bl. 36.

138 'Hauptabteilung III, Vermerk – Rücksprache mit der Hauptabteilung Justiz, Haupt-referent Müller, in Dresden, über die Frage des Arbeitshauses, 29. November 1951': BArch, DP 1/107, Bl. 36–7.

139 For the legal base of the incarceration, see SMAD Commands 030 and 273 regard-ing prostitution and 'promiscuous' women, as well as SMAD Command 92/1947 regarding the social welfare measures, which replaced § 20 of the German Empire's

Social Welfare Obligation Directive [*Reichsfürsorgepflichtverordnung*] from 1924. Korzilius, pp. 70–1, Footnote 278.

140 For example, see Richter's complaint: 'Fürsorgeheim Leuben, 10. Februar 1947': StA DD, Dezernat Sozial- und Wohnungswesen, 4.1.10, Nr. 71, Bl. 10.

141 In the archival files, 20 case histories were found, of which 15 were women and five were men. Twelve women but no men had been confined to the *Fürsorgeheim Leuben* at some point in their life. '[Without title], [December 1951]': StA DD, Dezernat Gesundheitswesen, 4.1.12, Nr. 69, Bl. 64–7.

142 In the case of the *Fürsorgeheim Leuben*, they took over 120 pictures, of which this study selected ten, which appeared as the most appropriate to offer a glimpse into this institution with its inmates and staff. For more information and their biographies, see Kerstin Delang and Jens Bove, 'Höhne, Erich', *SLUB/Deutsche Fotothek*, 2006 <www.deutschefotothek.de/documents/kue/90024061> [accessed 30 January 2019]; Kerstin Delang and Jens Bove, 'Pohl, Erich', *SLUB/Deutsche Fotothek*, 2006 <www. deutschefotothek.de/documents/kue/90024062> [accessed 30 January 2019].

143 Goffman, *Asylums*, pp. 117–55, 281–336; Rothman, pp. 79–154, 206–95. For comparison, see the analysis of the establishment of the clinic as an institution of medical and social control by Michel Foucault, *The Birth of the Clinic*, trans. by Alan M. Sheridan (London: Routledge, 2003).

144 Goffman, *Asylums*, pp. 18–19. 'Dienstvorschrift für die Fürsorgeanstalt Leuben, [1946]': StA DD, Fürsorgeamt, 2.3.25, Nr. 339, Bl. 107.

145 Goffman, *Asylums*, pp. 18–19, 33, 45, 89.

146 Goffman, *Asylums*, p. 107. For example, see 'Heim für soziale Betreuung, Dresden, 3. Januar 1953': BArch, DQ 1/20619, unpaginated.

147 Goffman, *Asylums*, p. 46.

148 Goffman, *Asylums*, pp. 18–20, here 18. Ayaß also identifies this rift in the Workhouse Breitenau in West Germany after 1945. Inmates convinced US-officials that they were confined due to minor crimes and thus in this institution with no real legal basis. Subsequently, the occupation power blamed staff and German civil servants for this intolerable situation and enacted the closure of the institution in 1949. Ayaß, *Das Arbeitshaus Breitenau*, pp. 338–42.

149 'Dienstvorschrift für die Fürsorgeanstalt Leuben, [mid-1946?]': StA DD, Fürsorgeamt, 2.3.25, Nr. 339, Bl. 108.

150 For an exploration of the use of photography during the GDR, especially in the private sphere, and how it was encouraged by the postwar East German state to establish a new form of 'socialist realism', see Paul Betts, *Within Walls: Private Life in the German Democratic Republic* (Oxford: Oxford University Press, 2010), pp. 194–208.

151 'Bericht über das Heim, 3. September 1952': BArch, DQ 1/20619, unpaginated.

152 'Bericht über das Heim, 3. September 1952': BArch, DQ 1/20619, unpaginated.

153 'Bericht über das Heim, 3. September 1952': BArch, DQ 1/20619, unpaginated.

154 Goffman, *Asylums*, pp. 66, 134–5.

155 Goffman, *Asylums*, p. 142.

156 '[Without title], [December 1951]': StA DD, Dezernat Gesundheitswesen, 4.1.12, Nr. 69, Bl. 64–7.

157 The name was made anonymous due to public and archival restrictions. Therefore, the fictitious name Petra is used to enhance comprehension in the following.

158 '[Without title], [December 1951]': StA DD, Dezernat Gesundheitswesen, 4.1.12, Nr. 69, Bl. 66.

159 The name was made anonymous due to public and archival restrictions. Therefore, the fictitious name Rosalinde is used to enhance comprehension in the following.

160 '[Without title], [December 1951]': StA DD, Dezernat Gesundheitswesen, 4.1.12, Nr. 69, Bl. 65.

161 '[Without Title], 24. Januar 1936': StA DD, Fürsorgeamt, 2.3.25, Nr. 339, Bl. 69.

162 'Heim für soziale Betreuung, Dresden, 3. Januar 1953': BArch, DQ 1/20619, unpaginated.
163 Goffman, *Asylums*, pp. 55–8.
164 Goffman, *Asylums*, p. 69.
165 Goffman, *Asylums*, p. 71.
166 'Übersendung eines Diskussionsbeitrages, Gedanken zur Errichtung eines Arbeitshauses, Anstaltsdirektor Hofmann, 16. Juni 1949': StA DD, Dezernat Sozial- und Wohnungswesen, 4.1.10, Nr. 71, Bl. 95.
167 '[Without title], [December 1951]': StA DD, Dezernat Gesundheitswesen, 4.1.12, Nr. 69, Bl. 64–6.
168 Goffman, *Asylums*, p. 73.

Bibliography

Primary sources

Unpublished

BUNDESARCHIV (BARCH)

Ministry of Healthcare

BArch, DQ 1/128 – Schriftwechsel mit Landes- und Provinzialverwaltungen; Sachsen, 1945–1949
BArch, DQ 1/292 – Rechtsvorschriften, Erarbeitung und Durchsetzung, Bd. 3, 1947–1949
BArch, DQ 1/2209 – Bekämpfung der Geschlechtskrankheiten, 1948–1951
BArch, DQ 1/20618 – Heime für soziale Betreuung, Bd. 4, 1954–1961
BArch, DQ 1/20619 – Heime für soziale Betreuung, Bd. 1, 1953–1960
BArch, DQ 1/20626 – Heime für soziale Betreuung, Bd. 3, 1954–1960

Ministry of Justice

BArch, DP 1/106 – Errichtung von Arbeitshäusern, Bd. 1, 1946 – -1948
BArch, DP 1/107 – Errichtung von Arbeitshäusern, Bd. 2, 1950 – -1955
BArch, DP 1/6935 – Gemeinsame Handakten der Abteilungsleiter Dr. Ernst Melsheimer und Dr. Paul Winkelmann, Bd. 3, 1945–1947
BArch, DP 1/7110 – Vorschriften zur Bekämpfung von Geschlechtskrankheiten: Mitarbeit, Entwürfe, Durchführung, Bd. 2, 1949–1955

DRESDEN, HAUPTSTAATSARCHIV (HSA DD)

HSA DD, Sächsischer Landtag 1946–1952, 11347, Nr. 136

DRESDEN, STADTARCHIV (STA DD)

StA DD, Bauamt, 8.22, Nr. 1205
StA DD, Bauamt, 8.22, Nr. 1206
StA DD, Bau- und Grundstücksakten, 10, Nr. 37116
StA DD, Dezernat Gesundheitswesen, 4.1.12, Nr. 69
StA DD, Dezernat Gesundheitswesen, 4.1.12, Nr. 84
StA DD, Dezernat Sozial- und Wohnungswesen, 4.1.10, Nr. 71

StA DD, Fürsorgeamt, 2.3.15, AV I/Nr. 647
StA DD, Fürsorgeamt, 2.3.25, AV III Arbeitsanstalt, Rep. II: Anstaltsverwaltung, Section B: Die Organisation der Anstalt, Nr. 12
StA DD, Fürsorgeamt, 2.3.25, Nr. 338
StA DD, Fürsorgeamt, 2.3.25, Nr. 339

SÄCHSISCHE LANDESBIBLIOTHEK, STAATS- UND UNIVERSITÄTSBIBLIOTHEK
DRESDEN (SLUB) – DEUTSCHE FOTOTHEK

Collection of Erich Höhne and Erich Pohl from 1949

www.deutschefotothek.de/documents/obj/70603379
SLUB Dresden/Deutsche Fotothek/Erich Höhne und Erich Pohl: Dresden, Leuben. Fürsorgeheim Leuben, 1949, Aufn.-Nr. df_hp_0022793_007
SLUB Dresden/Deutsche Fotothek/Erich Höhne und Erich Pohl: Dresden, Leuben. Fürsorgeheim Leuben, 1949, Aufn.-Nr. df_hp_0022794_009
SLUB Dresden/Deutsche Fotothek/Erich Höhne und Erich Pohl: Dresden, Leuben. Fürsorgeheim Leuben, 1949, Aufn.-Nr. df_hp_0022795_014
SLUB Dresden/Deutsche Fotothek/Erich Höhne und Erich Pohl: Dresden, Leuben. Fürsorgeheim Leuben, 1949, Aufn.-Nr. df_hp_0022796_038
SLUB Dresden/Deutsche Fotothek/Erich Höhne und Erich Pohl: Dresden, Leuben. Fürsorgeheim Leuben, 1949, Aufn.-Nr. df_hp_0022797_001
SLUB Dresden/Deutsche Fotothek/Erich Höhne und Erich Pohl: Dresden, Leuben. Fürsorgeheim Leuben, 1949, Aufn.-Nr. df_hp_0022797_042

Collection of Erich Höhne and Erich Pohl from 1950

www.deutschefotothek.de/documents/obj/70603430
SLUB Dresden/Deutsche Fotothek/Erich Höhne und Erich Pohl: Dresden, Leuben. Fürsorgeheim Leuben, Dezember 1950, Aufn.-Nr. df_hp_0023605_006
SLUB Dresden/Deutsche Fotothek/Erich Höhne und Erich Pohl: Dresden, Leuben. Fürsorgeheim Leuben, Dezember 1950, Aufn.-Nr. df_hp_0023607_002
SLUB Dresden/Deutsche Fotothek/Erich Höhne und Erich Pohl: Dresden, Leuben. Fürsorgeheim Leuben, Dezember 1950, Aufn.-Nr. df_hp_0023608_004
SLUB Dresden/Deutsche Fotothek/Erich Höhne und Erich Pohl: Dresden, Leuben. Fürsorgeheim Leuben, Dezember 1950, Aufn.-Nr. df_hp_0023610_002

Published

'§ 361 StGB, [30. März 1943–1. Oktober 1953]', *Lexetius*, 2016 <http://lexetius.com/StGB/361,8> [accessed 30 January 2019]
'Gesetz gegen gefährliche Gewohnheitsverbrecher und Maßregeln der Sicherung und Besserung vom 24. November 1933', *ALEX: Historische Rechts- und Gesetzestexte Online*, 2011 <http://alex.onb.ac.at/cgi-content/alex?aid=dra&datum=1933&page=1120> [accessed 30 January 2019]
Spring, Adolf, 'Alters- und Fürsorgeheim Ruttigerhof bei Olten', *Schweizerische Bauzeitung*, 111 (1938), 140–2
von Liszt, Franz, *Strafrechtliche Aufsätze und Vorträge: Erster Band, 1875 bis 1891* (Berlin: J. Guttentag, 1905)

Secondary sources

Assmann, Aleida, 'History and Memory', *International Encyclopedia of the Social & Behavioral Sciences* (Elsevier, 2001), pp. 6822–29

Ayaß, Wolfgang, *Das Arbeitshaus Breitenau: Bettler, Landstreicher, Prostituierte, Zuhälter und Fürsorgeempfänger in der Korrektions- und Landarmenanstalt Breitenau (1874–1949)* (Kassel: Verein für hessische Geschichte und Landeskunde e.V., 1992)

———, 'Die "korrektionelle Nachhaft": Zur Geschichte der strafrechtlichen Arbeitshausunterbringung in Deutschland', *Zeitschrift für Neuere Rechtsgeschichte*, 15 (1993), 184–201

———, 'Pflichtarbeit und Fürsorgearbeit: Zur Geschichte der „Hilfe zur Arbeit" außerhalb von Anstalten', in *Arbeitsdienst – wieder salonfähig? Zwang zur Arbeit in Geschichte und Sozialstaat*, ed. by Frankfurter Arbeitslosenzentrum – FALZ (Frankfurt a. M.: Fachhochschulverlag, 2015)

Badenhausen, Rolf, 'Lampel, Peter Martin', *Neue Deutsche Biographie*, 13 (1982), 460–1

Behring, Rainer, 'Das Personal der kommunistischen Diktaturdurchsetzung: Parteifunktionäre und Kommunalpolitiker in Chemnitz 1945–1949', in *Von Stalingrad zur SBZ: Sachsen 1943 bis 1949*, ed. by Mike Schmeitzner, Clemens Vollnhals, and Francesca Weil (Göttingen: Vandenhoeck & Ruprecht, 2016), pp. 239–58

Betts, Paul, *Within Walls: Private Life in the German Democratic Republic* (Oxford: Oxford University Press, 2010)

Cappelletto, Francesca, 'Introduction', in *Memory and World War II: An Ethnographic Approach*, ed. by Francesca Cappelletto (Oxford: Berg, 2005)

Delang, Kerstin, and Jens Bove, 'Höhne, Erich', *SLUB/Deutsche Fotothek*, 2006 <www.deutschefotothek.de/documents/kue/90024061> [accessed 30 January 2019]

———, 'Pohl, Erich', *SLUB/Deutsche Fotothek*, 2006 <www.deutschefotothek.de/documents/kue/90024062> [accessed 30 January 2019]

Digby, Anne, *Madness, Morality, and Medicine: A Study of the York Retreat, 1796–1914* (New York: Cambridge University Press, 1985)

Dubbers, Annette, *Leuben: Aus der Geschichte eines Dresdner Stadtteils* (Dresden: Dubbers, 2005)

Elling-Ruhwinkel, Elisabeth, *Sichern und Strafen: Das Arbeitshaus Benninghausen (1871–1945)* (Paderborn: Schöningh, 2005)

Evans, Jennifer V., 'Bahnhof Boys: Policing Male Prostitution in Post-Nazi Berlin', *Journal of the History of Sexuality*, 12 (2003), 605–36

———, *Life Among the Ruins: Cityscape and Sexuality in Cold War Berlin* (Houndmills: Palgrave Macmillan, 2011)

Falck, Uta, *VEB Bordell: Geschichte der Prostitution in der DDR* (Berlin: Links, 1998)

Foitzik, Doris, ' "Sittlich verwahrlost": Disziplinierung und Diskriminierung geschlechtskranker Mädchen in der Nachkriegszeit am Beispiel Hamburg', *Neunzehnhundertneunundneunzig*, 1 (1997), 68–82

Foucault, Michel, *Discipline and Punish: The Brith of the Prison*, trans. by Robert Hurley (London: Penguin Books, 1991)

———, *The Birth of the Clinic*, trans. by Alan M. Sheridan (London: Routledge, 2003)

Gehltomholt, Eva, and Sabine Hering, *Das verwahrloste Mädchen: Diagnostik und Fürsorge in der Jugendhilfe zwischen Kriegsende und Reform (1945–1965)* (Opladen: Barbara Budrich Verlag, 2006)

Goffman, Erving, *Asylums: Essays on the Social Situation of Mental Patients and Other Inmates* (London: Penguin Books, 1991)

————, *Behavior in Public Places: Notes on the Social Organization of Gatherings* (New York: The Free Press, 1985)

Gonisor, Jeanette, 'Eduard Kohlrausch: Rektor der Friedrich-Wilhelms-Universität Zu Berlin 1932/33', *Humboldt-Universität Zu Berlin*, 2013 <www.hu-berlin.de/de/ueberblick/geschichte/rektoren/kohlrausch> [accessed 30 January 2019]

Grieder, Peter, *The East German Leadership, 1946–1973: Conflict and Crisis* (Manchester: Manchester University Press, 1999)

Gruner, Wolf, *Öffentliche Wohlfahrt und Judenverfolgung: Wechselwirkungen lokaler und zentraler Politik im NS-Staat (1933–1942)* (Munich: Oldenbourg Verlag, 2009)

Herrmann, Lars, 'Straßen und Plätze in Leuben', *Dresdener Stadtteile* <www.dresdner-stadtteile.de/Ost/Leuben/Strassen_Leuben/strassen_leuben.html> [accessed 30 January 2019]

Hörath, Julia, *'Asoziale' und 'Berufsverbrecher' in den Konzentrationslagern 1933 bis 1938* (Göttingen: Vandenhoeck & Ruprecht, 2017)

Kocka, Jürgen, 'Eine durchherrschte Gesellschaft', in *Sozialgeschichte der DDR*, ed. by Hartmut Kaelble, Jürgen Kocka, and Hartmut Zwahr (Stuttgart: Klett-Cotta, 1994), pp. 547–53

Korzilius, Sven, *'Asoziale' und 'Parasiten' im Recht der SBZ/DDR* (Cologne: Böhlau, 2005)

Lampel, Peter Martin, *Revolte im Erziehungshaus* (Berlin: Kiepenheuer, 1929)

Osterloh, Jörg, ' "Der Totenwald von Zeithain": Die Sowjetische Besatzungsmacht und die Untersuchung des Massensterbens im Stalag 204 (IV H) Zeithain', in *Von Stalingrad zur SBZ: Sachsen 1943 bis 1949*, ed. by Mike Schmeitzner, Clemens Vollnhals, and Francesca Weil (Göttingen: Vandenhoeck & Ruprecht, 2016), pp. 329–52

Pohlmann, Tilman, 'Generationen und Herrschaftsetablierung: Die 1: SED-Kreissekretäre der Nachkriegszeit', in *Von Stalingrad zur SBZ: Sachsen 1943 bis 1949*, ed. by Mike Schmeitzner, Clemens Vollnhals, and Francesca Weil (Göttingen: Vandenhoeck & Ruprecht, 2016), pp. 277–92

Rick, Sebastian, 'Diktaturdurchsetzung auf dem flachen Lande am Beispiel der Landkreise Liebenwerda und Schweidnitz 1945–1949', in *Von Stalingrad zur SBZ: Sachsen 1943 bis 1949*, ed. by Mike Schmeitzner, Clemens Vollnhals, and Francesca Weil (Göttingen: Vandenhoeck & Ruprecht, 2016), pp. 259–76

Rothman, David J., *The Discovery of the Asylum: Social Order and Disorder in the New Republic* (Boston: Little, Brown & Company, 1971)

Rudolph, Andrea, *Die Kooperation von Strafrecht und Sozialhilferecht bei der Disziplinierung von Armen mittels Arbeit: Vom Arbeitshaus bis zur gemeinnützigen Arbeit* (Frankfurt a.M.: Lang, 1995)

Schmidt, Ulf, *Secret Science: A Century of Poison Warfare and Human Experiments* (Oxford: Oxford University Press, 2015)

Schneck, Peter, *Linser, Karl*, 2009 <www.bundesstiftung-aufarbeitung.de/wer-war-wer-in-der-ddr-%2363%3B-1424.html?ID=2117> [accessed 30 January 2019]

Schroeder, Klaus, *Der SED-Staat: Geschichte und Strukturen der DDR* (Munich: Bayrische Landeszentrale für politische Bildungsarbeit, 1998)

Wentker, Hermann, *Justiz in der SBZ/DDR 1945–1953: Transformation und Rolle ihrer zentralen Institutionen* (Munich: Oldenbourg, 2001)

Wißkirchen, Josef, 'Brauweiler bei Köln: Frühes Konzentrationslager in der Provinzial-Anstalt 1933–1934', in *Konzentrationslager im Rheinland und in Westfalen 1933–1945: Zentrale Steuerung und regionale Initiative*, ed. by Jan Erik Schulte (Paderborn: Schöningh, 2005), pp. 65–86

Yanni, Carla, *The Architecture of Madness: Insane Asylums in the United States* (Minneapolis, MN: University of Minnesota Press, 2007)

Zimmermann, Verena, *'Den neuen Menschen schaffen': Die Umerziehung von schwererziehbaren und straffälligen Jugendlichen in der DDR (1945–1990)* (Cologne: Böhlau, 2004)

Zimring, Franklin E., and Gordon J. Hawkins, *Deterrence: The Legal Threat in Crime Control* (Chicago: University of Chicago Press, 1973)

Epilogue

"I am fed up with this", replied Walter Korinek at 8 am on 27 September 1950 when questioned by his colleagues as to why he had packed his suitcase and left work before even starting. He explained to them that at 4 am that morning the police had stopped him in his car and led him in handcuffs to the police station, only because he forgot his identity documents. For him, this treatment was unbearable because, as a reputable doctor, he felt he had not been paid due respect.[1] Korinek's extraordinary fraud case has persisted throughout this book, demonstrating that while this statement is far from the truth it fits into Korinek's narrative as a known doctor from Dresden. Despite never finishing his medical studies he was able to use the chaotic postwar years and his medical skills acquired during the Second World War to his advantage, and in doing so developed the self-confidence necessary to perpetuate his masquerade.

In the epilogue that follows, I will summarise the findings of this book and discuss the analytical tool of medical memories and experiences on a conceptual level before pointing towards potential avenues for future research. Medical memories and experiences are a tool that connects to the methodology of socio-cultural history, the history of everyday life, and memory studies. It investigates human behaviour by incorporating the memories and experiences from the past that determined the present and future of an individual's life; and Korinek has been a vivid demonstration of this concept.

Upon his leaving work, colleagues and the *Betriebsgewerkschaftsleitung* [The Direction of the Company Union, the official representatives of the GDR trade union on site] visited Korinek at home and tried to convince him to come back; he refused. Only after Dresden's City officials threatened him with immediate dismissal did he give in, and he returned to work the following day.[2] The archival files suggest that this was a persistent pattern: Dresden's authorities were openly frustrated with Korinek and wanted to sack him, but his chief doctor always protected him due to his apparent medical skill and the persistent lack of specialists.[3]

This struggle between the ideal version of medical personnel in Socialism and the urgent need for specialists regardless of background and political predisposition was true for many doctors analysed in the first chapter. It investigated the different ways in which physicians *treated their past* to establish an identity that was compatible with the political framework of postwar East Germany and in doing so secured their social and professional position. Furthermore, the study exposed the fact that the primary socialisation for each age cohort, their medical memories, and their involvement in former political systems shaped their adaptation strategies in the GDR – such as their willingness to become a party member or socially active again after 1945. In this way, the analysis aligned itself with Fulbrook and others but offers a more nuanced picture of the transition of individuals of different ages from war to postwar in East Germany.

The first chapter went beyond Fulbrook, arguing that the ability of a physician to continue his or her medical practice after the Second World War was a highly individualised negotiation between the person, the local community and authorities, as well as the state. Here, doctors were able to continue their practice often only thanks to the medical predicaments of the postwar era, the protection of influential people, the difficulties of obtaining information about doctors, or the lack of medical specialists that necessitated a pragmatic de-Nazification process among the medical profession by occupation and local authorities. These conditions ultimately allowed incriminated physicians, former Nazi party members, and fraudulent doctors like Korinek to evade East Germany's de-Nazification and certification systems.

In the following decades, the selecting, sanitising, and silencing of these medical memories and experiences by the doctor and the state were embedded in the Cold War struggle with the FRG. It became part of legitimisation and international recognition strategies of both German states, as well as in the GDR's ideological claim of having established an 'anti-Fascist state'. Therefore, a Nazi doctor who carried out sterilisations or 'euthanasia' had no place in this narrative. In some cases, East German authorities decided to prosecute physicians, especially if they were not involved in the political system, if they were judged as dispensable, or, moreover, were labelled 'stubborn' private practitioners. Nonetheless, the political situation and the established life and state narratives ultimately prevented the GDR from achieving a clear break with the past of the medical profession, as well as creating a 'socialist medical intelligentsia'.

Korinek was also not a 'socialist' doctor, apart from his membership in the SED. For the Dresden City officials and local branches of the party, the described behaviour of Korinek had nothing to do with their idealised visions and rather became a nuisance. Already in a letter from June 1950, one of the directors of Dresden's Health Department justified the disapproval of rewarding Korinek with a performance bonus due to the following issues:

1 Immediate stop to work at the outpatient clinic for orthopaedics [. . .] due to financial reasons,
2 Termination outside of the period of notice with the reason that if he is not put in the next higher salary group with the same performance level immediately,
3 Unmedical behaviour, which should have been disciplined (regarding his behaviour with his Gonorrhoea infection, documents are available at the Department of the Interior),
4 Awful brawl with another doctor in the hospital.[4]

However, this behaviour never had real consequences for him. Instead, despite all his legal transgressions following the end of the Second World War, which included fraud, illegal abortions, and trade with narcotics, it took 22 years, until 1967, before he was completely prohibited from working in the medical field.[5]

This continuity of medical personnel paved the way for the continued existence of medical and social *treatments from the past*, which the second chapter has revealed for patients who suffered from STDs. Within these long-standing mentalities that shaped the medical treatment and resultant medical experiences of infected people, it was the persistent gender bias that stood out in the analysis of postwar East German health policies.

The analysis has used Moser and Harsch's approach, describing East Germany's main health paradigm as 'medicalised social hygiene', but has specified this for patients with STDs. In this process, this study has revealed that the concept has limitations: it might describe the state level, but fails to capture the diversity of mentalities, as well as the medical and social concepts of these diseases at the local level. In this way, this chapter has been able to broaden the understanding of the societal mechanics in cities like Dresden regarding the curbing of STDs, as well as refute the claim that the centralisation of the SBZ overruled the agency of local authorities.

Despite state attempts to 'de-gender' STD prevention and treatment, the local attitudes of doctors and the general public prevented their realisation. Staff at the specialised STD health clinics mostly targeted female parties to sexual intercourse and used their position to employ medicine as deterrent for supposed 'promiscuous' women. Moreover, ambiguous categories like a 'person with frequent promiscuous behaviour' fostered a system of denunciation within communities in which females accused other females, neighbours accused neighbours, men accused women, state officials accused local officials, and so forth. Such a system was welcomed by the state. It was recognised that even false denunciations served as deterrence and thus supported the efforts against diseases to the detriment of personal rights. In this way, many women experienced medical and social control that was akin to the previous political systems.[6]

Additionally, the continuity of medical memories in the form of mentalities towards STDs was identified in health campaigns and exhibitions in postwar East Germany. Inherently biased street posters drew attention to the woman seducing the man as being the site of the 'immoral' sexual conduct, thus making her responsible for the spread of venereal diseases. In summary, this chapter demonstrated that authorities, doctors, and the general public used old medical and social treatments for denounced 'fallen' women not only to treat but also to deter and educate them – an ethically questionable application of medicine.

Alongside women, East Germany's 'war youth' were also confronted with persistent medical concepts, moral judgments, and mentalities that pre-dated 1945. The third chapter has clarified that the past of 'war children' was not treated medically, but used to legitimise the future of the East German state. By pathologising the social conduct of young people – emphasising the negative connotation and medical description of behaviour as a disease – authorities established a narrative that cast the Nazis as the cause for the uprooted and morally corrupted children as another tool to demarcate the new state from the Third Reich.

This postwar narrative neglected the complex war experiences of hunger, loss, violence, and diseases that influenced the behaviour of the youth, but more so it denied their agency, such as the search for adventure and survival. As a result, state authorities excused the 'war children' from any involvement in the Third Reich and the Second World War, and placed all their hope upon this generation to become the future of the new, socialist society. However, this definition incorporated the condemnation of any 'socially deviant behaviour', meaning that stigmatised children were trapped in a perpetual social hygienic cycle of transfers between social institutions and care homes for re-socialisation purposes, such as the *Fürsorgeheim Leuben*.

In this pathologising of social conduct, a 'para-medicalised' terminology evolved that was derived from the medical memories and experiences of 'war children' and social hygienic and eugenic concepts of the past, which where in turn employed by the state to legitimise its interventions into 'asocial' families. The third chapter has questioned this political strategy and the supposed 'scientific' medical terms, such as 'trauma', that were used to narrate and correct social phenomena – not least given that elderly 'war youth' today depict themselves as a 'traumatised and forgotten generation' who initiated a discussion of 'victimhood' that critics view as a trivialisation of Holocaust survivors' sufferings.[7] Therefore, the analysis has contributed to the current public debate in Germany by differentiating the war experiences and their use by the East German state, as well as by the self-ascribed, and retrospectively constructed, 'war youth generation' today – the latter has established themselves as a mnemonic community with strong social ties and political weight.

Even if illegitimately, Korinek too became part of a strong mnemonic community: that of the medical profession. His membership in this community allowed many of his legal transgressions to be overlooked, and as such the outcome of the event detailed earlier was unsurprising. After he came back to work on 28 September 1950, Korinek was again arrested that same day, this time because of 'resistance against state authority', and was subsequently sentenced to five months in prison.[8] The sources suggest that he was a *Stammkunde* [regular] in local pubs and drank alcohol excessively. His alcoholism caused these conflicts with the state organs and, in the end, his dismissal from his position in a Dresden hospital as well as his expulsion from the SED.[9] However, after a couple years of probation in the countryside as a doctor in a refugee camp and as a *Betriebsarzt* [company physician], Korinek was able to get another job as senior consultant of orthopaedics in Dresden in May 1954. Despite the seniority of this new position, Korinek never provided the requested certifications, yet was able to continue his practice until his arrest by the MfS during Christmas 1959.[10]

Korinek's example encapsulates the purpose of this book, which has been to expose inherent patterns of continuity and discontinuity after 1945 that were common to all three groups analysed throughout: incriminated doctors, stigmatised women, and 'delinquent' children. It has illustrated that a physician, for example, who was trained during the Weimar Republic and practised his profession in the Third Reich would have developed a mentality towards sexually transmitted diseases and uprooted adolescents that could not be altered overnight and would instead shape his medical and social conduct during the postwar era.

This form of transition was possible even after a potentially deep caesura such as the end of a war. In a similar vein, institutions survived the Second World War not only in their structural substance – in their 'being' and spatial capacity if they were not destroyed through bombing or battle – but also in their conceptions and medical or social views projected onto them by the population, inmates, medical personnel, and authorities alike. This continuity that transgressed the proclaimed *Stunde Null* [Zero Hour or Year Zero] in 1945 in the particular form of medical memories and experiences was part of every chapter in this study, questioning this historically and politically constructed watershed.[11]

Medical memories and experiences capture this interdependency between the past, present, and future as well as between the state, institutions, mnemonic communities, and the individual. The final chapter was both a summary of all three main chapters and a case study illustrating the application of medical memories and experiences as a methodological approach. In the discussion of whether the workhouse should be part of postwar East Germany's future, this study has identified that behind the established state narrative, people with individual medical memories and experiences were able to shape the outcome of this political-motivated issue.

Consequently, whether in the upper echelons or local levels of society, influential or not, it is always people with their individual medical memories and experiences who shape state narratives, mnemonic communities, medical concepts, or stigmatisations of 'socially deviant' groups. From their views and specific interpretations of the past they draw conclusions for their contemporary context and justify corresponding actions in the future.

Future studies could continue to investigate the complex interdependencies between the medical memories of influential societal agents, local communities, and the state to achieve legitimisation of actions and stigmatisations as well as medical diagnoses and treatments. For example, how did the treatment of prostitutes correspond to the changing state narratives over time? Why were most of the doctors unaware of the social construction of many of the medical diagnoses that they applied in their everyday routine? What ethical ramification did this ignorance have on the doctor–patient relationship? These are only a few questions that could be investigated with the help of the concept of medical memories and experiences.

As shown, a few people can generate a state narrative that can then be imposed on the citizens if it offers enough leeway to integrate individual narratives among the majority of the population – or if it is heralded and propagated in such a way to ultimately replace individual memories with the desired one. One example is the establishment of socially accepted 'scapegoats' that can then always be used by the state. Therefore, it was important to explore the *Fürsorgeheim Leuben*, even with limited means, in order to clarify the concept of medical memories and experiences. This exploration has revealed that the STD diagnosis that brought the majority of the inmates into this institution not only had a deep-rooted social impact on people's lives, but was also intentionally imposed by the state to deter the wider population from becoming 'promiscuous' while simultaneously locking away the 'medicalised' 'social deviant'.

However, the implementation of the state's decision and the subsequent policies were often limited by the local communities, conditions, and buildings, such as the layout of the *Fürsorgeheim Leuben*. This institution carried 'memories' engraved in its walls that shaped the inmates' or staff's experience of the place and space and the local population's and authorities' perception of the address *Altleuben 10*. As a result, people in charge at the local level, such as Superintendent Hofmann, tried to introduce their visions of society into this institution, derived from their medical memories of, and experiences with, reformatories in the past – a fact that reveals their agency in the postwar period in a supposedly centralised state construct.

Within the proposed concept of medical memories and experiences, the level of the institution determines both the survival of buildings as well as the concepts projected onto them by authorities, doctors, inmates, and the general public. By moving away from an exterior perspective of appearance and layout, the concept encompasses the interior of the buildings, the design, the utilisation, and the subsequent experiences of individuals working and living in them. Consequently, architecture, often connected with medical and social concepts regarding the function of an institution, plays a major role in the analysis; the walls – in a metaphorical sense – carry the memory of contemporary attitudes towards disease and 'social deviance', as well as their interrelationship.

Therefore, the question could be raised whether the design of an institution reflects the deprivation of privacy, especially for declared 'promiscuous' women.[12] Is it possible to identify legacies of medical memories in the retention of institutions, their functions, and their layouts? Additionally, the focus of interest could be shifted towards the furniture and medical equipment used inside medical facilities. For example, did the medical profession withhold or delay the introduction of new equipment or easier methods of treatment into the workhouse in order to make the deterrence more empathic for inmates? The second chapter identified that some doctors in the GDR saw their roles not only from a medical but also from a social perspective and thus differentiated how they treated 'normal' and 'promiscuous' people with STDs.

In the case of the *Fürsorgeheim Leuben*, different mnemonic communities in the form of Dresden's Health, Justice, Police, and Social Welfare Departments established their individual narratives of the workhouse's purpose and utilisation as a place for 'socially deviant' child or 'promiscuous' woman. Despite its questionable past, every profession judged the institution's existence as a necessity, but none wanted to take over sole responsibility, leading to constant conflicts and changes to the workhouse in Dresden-Leuben. The blurred responsibility distributed among local authorities shaped inmates' and staff's medical experiences inside the *Fürsorgeheim* and also opened limited opportunities for the agency of the individual.

Future research could continue to reveal the role of local agency in stigmatisation practices, as well as the medical and social control of minorities defined according to the medical memories and experiences of specific mnemonic communities. These local perceptions of 'social deviance' often differ from the state narrative and have to be explored at the local rather than the national level.

This claim is also true for the level of the individual within the concept of medical memories and experiences. This analysis has revealed that life in the Care Home Leuben was removed from the state and local narratives. This finding proved the assumption that the latter were purely justifications of the workhouse's existence rather than a reflection of their actual contribution to society. As Goffman concluded, asylums and 'total institutions' like Leuben often just locked away, instead of reformed, those deemed to be 'socially deviant'.[13]

In this way, the individual level can investigate a patient's medical history and its impact on her or his actions and behaviour. For example, a past adverse experience with the healthcare system could mean that the patient avoids medical treatment in the future. However, it also offers an insight into the other side of this relationship, for example, the motivations of the individual doctor to deny treatment with Penicillin to women whom he has identified as being 'promiscuous'.

Moreover, every person, patient, nurse, or doctor is part of many overlapping mnemonic communities that have an influence on individual medical memories and vice versa. A doctor, for example, is part of the medical profession – a mnemonic community in regard to its social bond derived from its shared medical memories – and simultaneously is part of the medical community of his institution, his local environment, and his family, which are all mnemonic communities in and of themselves. Future research into different historical settings and time periods would reveal the interdependency of the individual and the state narrative, the institutional memories, and the mnemonic communities.

In summary, all four levels of the proposed concept – the state narrative, the mnemonic community, the institution, and the individual – are intertwined, and every level consists of individuals, either alone or in groups, whose medical memories and experiences shaped their social conduct, self-perception, and life-narration. Therefore, this book, in particular the fourth chapter, has contributed a case study of an institution to the ever-growing body of research in medicine and space, as well as microcosm studies, revealing in the context of postwar East Germany continuity and change on the local level, often removed from the state level.

In his book *Asylums*, Goffman identified that an "apolitical medicine" does not exist and, instead, is always connected with moral judgements that are an essential part of societies.[14] This study has identified the persistence of this fictional narrative of a 'neutral science' or the 'apolitical doctor' throughout its analysis. It was a strategy employed by physicians to justify themselves after the medical crimes carried out throughout the Third Reich, and to preserve their societal position in postwar East Germany. Nevertheless, the claim of an 'apolitical position' was also the long-standing narrative of their mnemonic community, the medical profession, since the nineteenth century, a tradition that gave credence to the individual doctor's perception of being 'foreign to politics'.

Furthermore, the 'para-medicalised' terminology that East German authorities applied to describe 'socially deviant behaviour' is another example of how assumed 'objective' scientific terms and theories were used to provide a scientific legitimacy to public discourses. However, disease concepts are often ambiguous in the medical realm as well, and rely on social definitions and indications such as the social environment of a patient. The failure to acknowledge the social construction of and the moral judgment implied by diagnoses from the medical profession led to the misconception of authorities and the public that they integrated a 'scientific' terminology into their language explaining social phenomena, thereby shaping the medical experience and social treatment of patients with STDs.

This book has embedded postwar East Germany in the overall developments in medicine and society during the twentieth century. It challenged the historical watershed of 1945 by exposing continuity and discontinuities in local communities and individuals who used their given agency and shaped their present and future with their knowledge of the past – their medical memories and experiences – and sought to achieve their goals within the possibilities of the given situation.

Notes

1 'Niederschrift, 27. September 1950': StA DD, Dezernat Gesundheitswesen, 4.1.12, Nr. 21, Bl. 48.
2 'Niederschrift, 27. September 1950': StA DD, Dezernat Gesundheitswesen, 4.1.12, Nr. 21, Bl. 48.
3 For example, the correspondence between city officials and the chief doctor of Korinek from 2 May 1950 in BArch, DQ 1/12052, unpaginated.
4 'Ablehnung der Prämierung von Walter Korinek, 17. Juni 1950': BArch, DQ 1/12052, unpaginated.
5 'Sachstandsbericht, 7. Januar 1960': BStU, MfS, AU 43/60, Bl. 95, 99–100; 'MfG – Recht – an HO-Gaststätten- und Hotelbetrieb Dresden, Betr.: Walter Korinek, geb. 19.4.1914, 7. Februar 1967': BArch, DQ 1/12052, unpaginated; 'Schreiben der HO-Gaststätten- und Hotelbetrieb Dresden an das MfG – Recht –, 14. Februar 1967': BArch, DQ 1/12052, unpaginated.
6 Annette F. Timm, 'Sex with a Purpose: Prostitution, Venereal Disease, and Militarized Masculinity in the Third Reich', *Journal of the History of Sexuality*, 11 (2002), 223–55. For the similar situation in West Germany in the postwar period, see Doris Foitzik, ' "Sittlich verwahrlost": Disziplinierung und Diskriminierung geschlechtskranker Mädchen in der Nachkriegszeit am Beispiel Hamburg', *neunzehnhundertneunundneunzig*, 1 (1997), 68–82.
7 For a critical analysis about the current debates, see Michael Heinlein, 'Das Trauma der deutschen Kriegskinder zwischen nationaler und europäischer Erinnerung: Kritische Anmerkungen zum gegenwärtigen Wandel der Erinnerungskultur', in *Narratives of Trauma: Discourses of German Wartime Suffering in National and International Perspective*, ed. by Helmut Schmitz and Annette Seidel-Arpacı (Amsterdam: Rodopi, 2011), pp. 111–28.

8 'Schreiben von Korinek, 30. Oktober 1950': BArch, DQ 1/12052, unpaginated.
9 'Einschätzung zu Operativ-Vorgang "Spinne", 15. Dezember 1959': BStU, MfS, BV Dresden, AU 43/60, Bl. 19.
10 'Sachstandsbericht, 7. Januar 1960': BStU, MfS, AU 43/60, Bl. 95.
11 Richard Bessel, *Germany 1945: From War to Peace* (London: Simon & Schuster, 2009); Christoph Kleßmann, *1945 – welthistorische Zäsur und 'Stunde Null'*, 2010 <http://docupedia.de/zg/klessmann_1945_v1_de_2010> [accessed 2 February 2017].
12 Goffman identified that the deprivation and constant penetration of an inmate's private sphere were the key features that separate a 'total institution' from any other forms. Erving Goffman, *Asylums: Essays on the Social Situation of Mental Patients and Other Inmates* (London: Penguin Books, 1991), pp. 18, 36.
13 Goffman, pp. 69, 73.
14 Goffman, p. 318.

Bibliography

Primary sources

Unpublished

BUNDESARCHIV (BARCH)

Ministry of Healthcare

BArch, DQ 1/12052 – Personalakte Walter Korinek, 1948–1967

ARCHIV DES BUNDESBEAUFTRAGTEN FÜR DIE UNTERLAGEN DES
STAATSSICHERHEITSDIENSTES DER EHEMALIGEN DEUTSCHEN DEMOKRATISCHEN
REPUBLIK (BSTU)

BStU, MfS, BV Dresden, AU 43/60

DRESDEN, STADTARCHIV (STA DD)

StA DD, Dezernat Gesundheitswesen, 4.1.12, Nr. 21

Secondary sources

Bessel, Richard, *Germany 1945: From War to Peace* (London: Simon & Schuster, 2009)
Foitzik, Doris, ' "Sittlich verwahrlost": Disziplinierung und Diskriminierung geschlechts-kranker Mädchen in der Nachkriegszeit am Beispiel Hamburg', *Neunzehnhundertneu-nundneunzig*, 1 (1997), 68–82
Goffman, Erving, *Asylums: Essays on the Social Situation of Mental Patients and Other Inmates* (London: Penguin Books, 1991)
Heinlein, Michael, 'Das Trauma der deutschen Kriegskinder zwischen nationaler und europäischer Erinnerung: Kritische Anmerkungen zum gegenwärtigen Wandel der Erin-nerungskultur', in *Narratives of Trauma: Discourses of German Wartime Suffering in National and International Perspective*, ed. by Helmut Schmitz and Annette Seidel-Arpacı (Amsterdam: Rodopi, 2011), pp. 111–28

Kleßmann, Christoph, *1945 – welthistorische Zäsur und 'Stunde Null'*, 2010 <http://docupedia.de/zg/klessmann_1945_v1_de_2010> [accessed 2 February 2017]

Timm, Annette F., 'Sex with a Purpose: Prostitution, Venereal Disease, and Militarized Masculinity in the Third Reich', *Journal of the History of Sexuality*, 11 (2002), 223–55

Appendix

Excerpt of the database[1]

Overview of the total numbers (N = 128)

Totals		Members in GDR organisations	Not politically involved after 1945
	128	82	46
Members in NS organisations	89	52	37
KPD members	9	9	0
Not politically involved before 1945	30	21	9

Detailed overview of membership (multiple affiliations included), overlap, and transition between the Third Reich and the GDR

Totals		SED	FDJ	FDGB	DSF	CDU	LDPD	NDPD	Not politically involved after 1945
	128	38	2	52	18	5	5	9	46
NSDAP	81	17	0	26	7	5	3	7	34
HJ	11	4	0	2	2	1	1	1	4
SA	32	6	0	14	4	0	1	5	13
SS	13	2	0	3	1	0	0	1	8
NSÄB	21	8	0	12	6	1	1	0	5
NSV	16	4	0	8	2	1	0	0	5
DAF	3	2	0	3	2	0	1	0	0
KPD	9	9	0	8	4	0	0	0	0
Not politically involved before 1945	30	10	2	15	6	0	2	0	9

Cohort A (1886–1895): the World War One Generation

Last name	Name	DOB	Politically involved before 1945 in					Politically involved after 1945 in					Main reference
			NSDAP	NSÄB	SA	SS	Other	SED	FDGB	FDJ	DSF	Other	
Brekenfeld	Friedrich	13/09/1887	Yes	No	No	No	N/A	No	No	No	No	N/A	BStU, MfS, HA XX, 5749, Bl. 135.
Carriere	Reinhard	09/04/1891	Yes	Yes	No	No	N/A	No	No	No	No	CDU	BStU, MfS, HA XX, 5749, Bl. 164.
Claus	Martin	28/09/1888	Yes	Yes	Yes	Yes	N/A	No	No	No	No	N/A	BStU, MfS, HA IX/11, RHE 57/79 DDR, Bl. 12–16.
Hämel	Josef	18/11/1894	Yes	Yes	Yes	No	N/A	No	Yes	No	No	N/A	BStU, MfS, HA XX, 5750, Bl. 133.
Katsch	Gerhard	14/05/1887	Yes	No	Yes	No	N/A	No	No	No	No	N/A	BStU, MfS, HA XX, 5751, Bl. 17–18.
Konitzer	Paul	01/02/1894	No	No	No	No	N/A	Yes	No	No	No	N/A	Schneck, Peter, *Wer war wer in der DDR?* (2009)
Krostitz	Alfred	17/12/1893	Yes	No	No	No	N/A	No	Yes	No	No	N/A	BStU, MfS, BV Leipzig, AOP 143/55, Bd. 7, Bl. 32.
Lammert	Hette	15/01/1895	No	No	No	No	KPD	Yes	Yes	No	Yes	N/A	BStU, MfS, HA IX/11, AV 4/74, Bd. 10, Bl. 5–8.
Linser	Karl	10/05/1895	No	No	Yes	No	N/A	Yes	No	No	No	N/A	Schneck, Peter, *Wer war wer in der DDR?* (2009)
Neumann	Paul	04/07/1888	Yes	No	No	No	N/A	No	Yes	No	No	N/A	BStU, MfS, HA IX/11, RHE 1/66 VRP, Bl. 93–95.
Rupp	Johannes	06/04/1891	Yes	No	No	No	N/A	No	Yes	No	No	LDP	BStU, MfS, BV Leipzig, AOP 143/55, Bd. 9, Bl. 185.
Schenk	Johann	15/02/1895	Yes	Yes	No	No	N/A	No	No	No	No	N/A	BStU, MfS, HA XX, 5755, Bl. 357.
Schnurrer	Josef	21/06/1890	Yes	No	Yes	No	N/A	No	No	No	No	NDP	BStU, MfS, HA XX, 5752, Bl. 94–95.
Schwarz	Egbert	22/06/1890	Yes	Yes	No	Yes	N/A	No	No	No	No	N/A	BStU, MfS, HA XX, 5752, Bl. 130–32.
Waßmund	Wilhelm	19/03/1894	No	No	No	No	N/A	No	Yes	No	No	LDP	BStU, MfS, BV Leipzig, AOP 143/55, Bd. 5, Bl. 21.
Wedig	August	07/10/1891	Yes	No	No	No	N/A	No	No	No	No	N/A	BStU, MfS, AU 131/60, Bd. 1.

Cohort B (1896–1905): the Weimar Generation

Last name	Name	DOB	Politically involved before 1945 in					Politically involved after 1945 in					Main reference
			NSDAP	NSDÄB	SA	SS	Other	SED	FDGB	FDJ	DSF	Other	
Amon	Franz	04/06/1896	Yes	No	Yes	No	N/A	No	No	No	No	N/A	BStU, MfS, HA XX, 5749, Bl. 27.
Barthel	Karl	13/08/1905	Yes	No	Yes	No	N/A	No	No	No	No	NDPD	BStU, MfS, HA XX, 5749, Bl. 42.
Becker	Herbert	01/02/1900	Yes	No	No	No	N/A	No	No	No	No	N/A	BStU, MfS, HA XX, 5755, Bl. 41.
Dietz	Hans	13/04/1899	Yes	No	No	No	N/A	Yes	No	No	No	N/A	BStU, MfS, BV Leipzig, AOP 143/55, Bd. 1, Bl. 61.
Gelbke	Carl	09/07/1899	No	No	No	No	KPD	Yes	No	No	No	N/A	StA Lpz, Stadtverwaltung und Rat, Nr. 1611.
Hebold	Otto	27/07/1896	Yes	No	Yes	No	N/A	No	Yes	No	No	NDPD	BStU, MfS, HA XX, 5755, Bl. 40.
Heißmeyer	Kurt	26/12/1905	Yes	No	No	No	N/A	No	No	No	No	N/A	BStU, MfS, HA XX, 16974, Bl. 1–70.
Henneberg	Hermann	31/08/1904	Yes	Yes	No	Yes	N/A	Yes	Yes	No	Yes	N/A	BStU, MfS, HA XX, 5750, Bl. 203–09.
Hielscher	Mar-garete	12/09/1899	Yes	Yes	No	No	N/A	Yes	No	No	Yes	N/A	BStU, MfS, HA XX, 5755, Bl. 343.
Hoffgaard	Willy	27/08/1898	Yes	No	No	No	N/A	No	No	No	No	N/A	BStU, MfS, HA XX, 5755, Bl. 39.
Kraatz	Helmut	06/08/1902	Yes	No	Yes	No	N/A	No	Yes	No	No	Kulturbund	BStU, MfS, HA XX, 5755, Bl. 43.
Kuniß	Johannes	25/10/1904	Yes	Yes	Yes	No	N/A	Yes	Yes	No	Yes	N/A	BStU, MfS, AP 6338/77, Bl. 15–17.
Lemm	Karl	10/10/1900	No	No	No	No	N/A	No	Yes	No	No	N/A	BStU, MfS, BV Leipzig, AOP 143/55, Bd. 1, Bl. 23.
Lochner	Herbert	29/06/1901	Yes	No	Yes	No	N/A	No	No	No	No	N/A	BStU, MfS, HA IX/11, AK 1453/75-1454/75, Bl. 4.
Marcusson	Erwin	11/06/1899	No	No	No	No	KPD	Yes	Yes	No	Yes	N/A	BStU, MfS, HA IX/11, AV 4/74, Bd. 11, Bl. 137–40.
Marquardt	Karl	24/01/1897	No	No	No	No	N/A	No	No	No	No	N/A	BStU, MfS, BV Leipzig, AOP 143/55, Bd. 1, Bl. 36–37.
Meyer	Wilhelm	30/04/1902	Yes	No	No	No	N/A	No	Yes	No	No	N/A	BStU, MfS, HA IX/11, ZA I 7414, Akte 31, Bl. 2-3.

													Source
Nauwald	Karl	08/01/1904	Yes	No	Yes	No	N/A	No	No	No	No	N/A	BStU, MfS, HA IX/11, AV 8/84, Bl. 126–29.
Neumann	Rudolf	13/11/1899	No	No	No	No	N/A	Yes	Yes	No	Yes	N/A	BStU, MfS, HA IX/11, AV 4/74, Bd. 14, Bl. 7.
Osselmann	Herbert	25/08/1904	Yes	Yes	No	Yes	N/A	No	Yes	No	No	N/A	BStU, MfS, HA XX, 5751, Bl. 323–24.
Pietzuch	Arthur	10/09/1898	No	No	No	No	N/A	No	No	No	No	N/A	BStU, MfS, GH, 19/59, Bl. 1.
Pusch	Frie-derike	20/06/1905	Yes	No	No	No	N/A	No	Yes	No	No	N/A	BStU, MfS, HA IX/11, RHE-West 178/2, Bl. 121.
Reichen-bach	Erwin	01/08/1897	Yes	Yes	Yes	No	N/A	Yes	Yes	No	No	N/A	BStU, MfS, HA XX, 5755, Bl. 32.
Schneider	Johannes	09/02/1896	Yes	No	No	No	N/A	No	No	No	No	N/A	BStU, MfS, BV Leipzig, AOP 746/66, Bl. 185.
Schröder	Kurt	23/07/1902	Yes	No	No	No	N/A	No	No	No	No	N/A	BStU, MfS, HA XX, 5755, Bl. 44.
Schulte	Johannes	06/01/1905	Yes	Yes	Yes	No	N/A	No	Yes	No	Yes	LDP	BStU, MfS, HA XX, 5752, Bl. 117–18.
Steidle	Luitpcld	12/03/1898	Yes	No	No	No	N/A	No	No	No	No	CDU	BStU, MfS, HA XX, 5752, Bl. 158–61.
Stolze	Martin	03/08/1900	Yes	No	Yes	No	N/A	No	Yes	No	No	N/A	BStU, MfS, HA IX/11, ZA VI 654, Akte 24, Bl. 19–22.
Uebermuth	Herbert	18/01/1901	Yes	Yes	No	No	N/A	No	Yes	Yes	Yes	NDPD	BStU, MfS, HA XX, 5752, Bl. 225–26.
Velhagen	Karl	22/09/1897	Yes	Yes	Yes	No	NSFK	No	Yes	Yes	Yes	N/A	BStU, MfS, HA XX, 5752, Bl. 237–39.
von Kraus	Karl	12/09/1905	Yes	No	No	Yes	N/A	No	No	No	No	N/A	BStU, MfS, HA XX, 5751, Bl. 122–23.
Wand	Aloys	23/07/1905	Yes	No	No	No	N/A	No	No	No	No	N/A	BStU, MfS, HA XX, 5755, Bl. 41.
Welcker	Ernst-Rulo	11/12/1904	Yes	Yes	Yes	No	N/A	Yes	No	No	No	N/A	BStU, MfS, HA XX, 5755, Bl. 171.
Zwingen-berger	Marianne	19/01/1896	No	No	No	No	N/A	No	No	No	No	N/A	StA DD, Dezernat Gesundheitswesen, 4.1.12, Nr. 22.

Cohort C (1906–1915): the Generation of Depression and Upheaval

Last name	Name	DOB	Politically involved before 1945 in					Politically involved after 1945 in					Main reference
			NSDAP	NSÄB	SA	SS	Other	SED	FDGB	FDJ	DSF	Other	
Albrecht	Rosemarie	19/03/1915	No	No	No	No	N/A	No	No	No	No	N/A	BStU, MfS, HA XX, 5755, Bl. 333.
Anxxxxx	Axxxxx	xx/09/1912	No	No	No	No	N/A	No	No	No	No	N/A	BStU, MfS, HA IX/11, RHE-West 203, Bl. 1–3.
Bexxxxx	Exxxxx	xx/02/1908	Yes	No	Yes	No	N/A	No	Yes	No	No	N/A	BStU, MfS, HA IX/11, ZB II 4553, Akte 2, Bl. 2–3.
Bexxxxx	Cxxxxx	xx/05/1908	Yes	Yes	No	No	N/A	No	Yes	No	No	N/A	BStU, MfS, HA IX/11, ZA I, Akte 145, Bl. 1–20.
Blxxxxx	Fxxxxx	xx/09/1909	No	No	No	No	N/A	No	No	No	No	N/A	BStU, MfS, HA IX/11, RHE-West 178/2, Bl. 18–20.
Boxxxxx	Uxxxxx	xx/12/1908	Yes	No	No	No	N/A	No	No	No	No	CDU	BStU, MfS, HA XX, 5749, Bl. 115.
Dixxxxx	Kxxxxx	xx/04/1911	Yes	No	No	No	N/A	No	No	No	No	N/A	BStU, MfS, HA IX/11, ZB II 4553, Akte 1, Bl. 2–3.
Döxxxxx	Exxxxx	xx/10/1908	Yes	No	Yes	No	N/A	Yes	Yes	No	Yes	N/A	BStU, MfS, HA II/10, 1037.
Emxxxxxx	Rxxxxx	xx/08/1910	Yes	No	Yes	No	N/A	No	No	No	No	N/A	BStU, MfS, HA XX, 5749, Bl. 242–45.
Eßxxxxx	Hxxxxx	xx/03/1909	Yes	Yes	No	No	N/A	No	No	No	No	N/A	BStU, MfS, HA XX, 5749, Bl. 249.
Faxxxxx	Gxxxxx	xx/06/1913	Yes	No	No	No	N/A	Yes	No	No	No	N/A	BStU, MfS, HA XX, 5749, Bl. 266.
Fexxxxx	Pxxxxx	xx/09/1908	No	No	Yes	No	N/A	No	Yes	No	No	N/A	BStU, MfS, HA IX/11, ZA I 7413, Akte 1, Bl. 2–3.
Fischer	Horst	31/12/1912	Yes	No	No	Yes	N/A	No	No	No	No	N/A	BStU, MfS, HA XX, 5755, Bl. 337.
Fuxxxxx	Hxxxxx	xx/05/1911	Yes	No	No	Yes	N/A	Yes	No	No	No	N/A	BStU, MfS, HA XX, 5749, Bl. 311–14.
Gäxxxxxx	Jxxxxx	xx/03/1915	No	No	No	No	N/A	Yes	Yes	Yes	Yes	N/A	BStU, MfS, BV Dresden, AIM 1272/82, Bl. 21.
Gexxxxx	Hxxxxx	xx/03/1913	Yes	Yes	No	No	N/A	No	Yes	No	No	N/A	BStU, MfS, HA IX/11, ZA 11858, Objekt 13, Bl. 4.
Grxxxxx	Fxxxxx	xx/12/1907	No	No	No	No	N/A	No	Yes	No	No	N/A	BStU, MfS, BV Dresden, KD Sebnitz, 4409, Teil 2, Bl. 292.
Grxxxxx	Hxxxxx	xx/05/1908	No	No	Yes	No	N/A	No	Yes	No	No	NDPD	BStU, MfS, HA IX/11, ZUV 49, Bd. 1, Bl. 11–17.

Surname	First name	DOB											Source
Grxxxxx	Hxxxxxx	xx/08/1910	Yes	No	Yes	No	N/A	No	Yes	No	No	N/A	BStU, MfS, HA IX/11, ZB II 5842, Akte 1, Bl. 12–13.
Grxxxxx	Exxxxxx	xx/08/1907	Yes	No	No	No	N/A	Yes	No	No	No	N/A	BStU, MfS, HA XX, 5755, Bl. 341.
Guxxxxx	Hxxxxxx	xx/08/1908	Yes	No	No	No	N/A	Yes	No	No	No	N/A	BStU, MfS, HA XX, 5750, Bl. 110–14.
Güxxxxx	Hxxxxxx	xx/03/1912	Yes	Yes	Yes	No	N/A	Yes	Yes	No	No	N/A	BStU, MfS, HA XX, 5750, Bl. 104–05.
Güxxxxx	Hxxxxxx	xx/03/1912	Yes	No	Yes	No	N/A	No	Yes	No	No	N/A	BStU, MfS, HA XX, 5750, Bl. 109.
Haxxxxx	Hxxxxxx	xx/06/1911	Yes	No	Yes	No	N/A	No	Yes	No	No	N/A	BStU, MfS, HA XX, 5755, Bl. 32.
Häxxxxx	Axxxxxx	xx/10/1913	No	No	No	Yes	NSFK	Yes	No	No	Yes	N/A	BStU, MfS, HA IX/11, ZA 12.212/55, Objekt 12, Bl. 4–7.
Haxxxxx	Wxxxxxx	xx/12/1909	No	No	No	No	N/A	No	Yes	No	No	N/A	BStU, MfS, BV Leipzig, AOP 143/55, Bd. 1, Bl. 22.
Hexxxxx	Kxxxxxx	xx/12/1908	Yes	No	No	No	N/A	Yes	Yes	No	No	N/A	BStU, MfS, BV Leipzig, AOP 143/55, Bd. 1, Bl. 143.
Hempel	Hans-Christoph	15/08/1912	No	No	No	No	N/A	No	No	No	No	N/A	BStU, MfS, HA XX, 5628, Bl. 16–22.
Hoxxxxx	Hxxxxxx	xx/03/1910	No	No	Yes	No	N/A	No	No	No	No	N/A	BStU, MfS, HA XX, 5755, Bl. 343.
Höxxxxx	Gxxxxxx	xx/02/1914	Yes	No	No	Yes	N/A	No	No	No	No	N/A	BStU, MfS, BV Leipzig, AOP 143/55, Bd. 1, Bl. 55.
Ilxxxxx	Gxxxxxx	xx/12/1910	Yes	No	Yes	No	N/A	No	No	No	No	N/A	BStU, MfS, HA XX, 5755, Bl. 338.
Kaxxxxx	Axxxxxx	xx/05/1915	No	No	No	No	KPD	Yes	Yes	No	Yes	N/A	BStU, MfS, HA IX/11, AV 4/74, Bd. 11, Bl. 12–13.
Korinek	Walter	19/04/1914	No	Yes	No	No	N/A	Yes	No	No	No	N/A	BStU, MfS, BV Dresden, AU 43/60, Bd. 1, Bl. 17–19.
Krxxxxx	Hxxxxxx	xx/05/1909	No	No	No	No	N/A	No	Yes	No	No	N/A	BStU, MfS, HA XX, 4244.
Lexxxxx	Gxxxxxx	xx/06/1911	No	No	No	No	N/A	No	No	No	No	N/A	BStU, MfS, HA XX, 5755, Bl. 348.
Loxxxxx	Axxxxxx	xx/04/1909	Yes	No	No	No	N/A	Yes	No	No	No	N/A	BStU, MfS, HA XX, 5751, Bl. 201.
Marcusson	Hildegard	14/01/1910	No	No	No	No	N/A	Yes	Yes	No	Yes	N/A	BStU, MfS, HA IX/11, AV 4/74, Bd. 11, Bl. 137–40.
Mexxxxxx	Gxxxxxx	xx/09/1908	Yes	No	Yes	No	N/A	No	No	No	No	N/A	BStU, MfS, HA XX, 5751, Bl. 240.
Mexxxxxx	Gxxxxxx	xx/07/1913	Yes	No	No	No	N/A	No	No	No	No	CDU	BStU, MfS, HA XX, 5751, Bl. 247.

(Continued)

Last name	Name	DOB	Politically involved before 1945 in					Politically involved after 1945 in					Main reference
			NSDAP	NSÄB	SA	SS	Other	SED	FDGB	FDJ	DSF	Other	
Mexxxxx	Hxxxxx	xx/09/1912	No	No	No	No	SAJ	Yes	Yes	No	Yes	N/A	BStU, MfS, HA IX/11, AV 4/74, Bd. 12, Bl. 6–9.
Mixxxxx	Rxxxxx	xx/08/1914	No	No	No	Yes	N/A	No	No	No	No	N/A	BStU, MfS, HA XX, 5755, Bl. 41.
Mixxxxx	Hxxxxx	xx/05/1910	No	No	No	No	N/A	No	No	No	No	N/A	BStU, MfS, BV Dresden, KD Sebnitz, 4409, Teil 2, Bl. 279.
Munkwitz	Günther	13/03/1912	Yes	Yes	No	No	N/A	Yes	Yes	No	No	N/A	BStU, MfS, HA XX, 3828, Bl. 30–34.
Mustafa	Konstantin	05/08/1911	Yes	No	No	No	N/A	No	Yes	No	No	N/A	BStU, MfS, BV Dresden, KD Sebnitz, 4409, Teil 2, Bl. 279.
Nexxxxx	Wxxxxx	xx/05/1911	Yes	No	No	No	N/A	No	No	No	No	N/A	BStU, MfS, HA XX, 5751, Bl. 287.
Nixxxxx	Kxxxxx	xx/02/1908	Yes	No	Yes	No	N/A	No	No	No	No	N/A	BStU, MfS, HA XX, 5751, Bl. 294
Ochsen-farth	Elfriede	28/06/1914	No	No	No	No	N/A	Yes	No	No	No	N/A	BStU, MfS, BV Leipzig, AOP 746/66, Bl. 147–48.
Pexxxxx	Hxxxxx	xx/06/1910	No	No	No	No	KPD	Yes	Yes	No	No	N/A	BStU, MfS, HA IX/11, AV 4/74, Bd. 14, Bl. 10–12.
Rexxxxx	Wxxxxx	xx/08/1907	Yes	Yes	No	No	N/A	Yes	No	No	No	N/A	BStU, MfS, HA XX, 5751, Bl. 397–98.
Reckzeh	Paul	04/11/1913	Yes	No	No	No	N/A	No	No	No	No	N/A	BStU, MfS, HA XX, 5751, Bl. 399–401.
Rixxxxx	Kxxxxx	xx/03/1914	Yes	No	No	No	N/A	No	No	No	No	N/A	BStU, MfS, BV Leipzig, AOP 143/55, Bd. 1, Bl. 160.
Rixxxxx	Fxxxxx	xx/10/1915	Yes	No	No	No	N/A	No	No	No	No	NDPD	BStU, MfS, HA XX, 5751, Bl. 446–47.
Rißmann	Eitel-Friedrich	07/03/1906	Yes	No	No	No	N/A	No	No	No	No	N/A	BStU, MfS, HA XX, 5755, Bl. 355.
Roxxxxx	Wxxxxx	xx/10/1908	No	No	No	No	KPD	Yes	Yes	No	No	N/A	BStU, MfS, HA IX/11, AV 4/74, Bd. 17, Bl. 6–13.
Rühle	Otto	10/02/1914	Yes	No	No	No	N/A	No	No	No	No	NDPD	BStU, MfS, HA XX, 5755, Bl. 47.
Scxxxxx	Kxxxxx	xx/04/1913	No	No	No	Yes	N/A	No	No	No	No	NDPD	BStU, MfS, HA XX, 5755, Bl. 357.
Scxxxxx	Fxxxxx	xx/01/1915	Yes	No	Yes	No	N/A	No	No	No	No	N/A	BStU, MfS, HA XX, 5755, Bl. 39.
Scxxxxx	Jxxxxx	xx/05/1911	No	No	No	No	N/A	Yes	Yes	No	Yes	N/A	StA DD, Dezernat Gesundheitswesen, 4.1.12, Nr. 22, Bl. 100.
Sixxxxx	Exxxxx	xx/04/1915	No	No	No	No	N/A	No	Yes	No	No	LDP	BStU, MfS, BV Leipzig, AOP 143/55, Bd. 2, Bl. 5

Stxxxxx	Rxxxxxx	xx/10/1909	No	No	No	No	KPD	Yes	Yes	No	No	N/A	BStU, MfS, HA IX/11, AV 4/74, Bd. 18, Bl. 7–8.
Stxxxxx	Axxxxxx	xx/09/1910	Yes	No	No	Yes	N/A	No	Yes	No	No	N/A	BStU, MfS, BV Leipzig, AOP 143/55, Bd. 2, Bl. 56.
von Cxxxxx	Hxxxxxx	xx/08/1911	Yes	No	No	No	N/A	No	No	No	No	N/A	BStU, MfS, HA XX, 5755, Bl. 335.
Winter	Kurt	11/05/1910	No	No	No	No	KPD	Yes	Yes	No	No	N/A	BStU, MfS, HA IX/11, AV 4/74, Bd. 19, Bl. 7.
Zexxxxx	Wxxxxxx	xx/01/1907	Yes	No	No	Yes	N/A	No	No	No	No	N/A	BStU, MfS, HA XX, 5755, Bl. 381.

Cohort D (1916–1926): the National Socialist Generation

Last name	Name	DOB	Politically involved before 1945 in					Politically involved after 1945 in					Main reference
			NSDAP	NSÄB	SA	SS	Other	SED	FDGB	FDJ	DSF	Other	
Adxxxxx	Jxxxxx	xx/09/1923	No	No	No	Yes	N/A	No	No	No	No	N/A	BStU, MfS, HA XX, 5755, Bl. 333.
Bergmann	Charlotte	30/11/1920	Yes	No	No	No	N/A	No	No	No	No	LDP	BStU, MfS, HA XX, 5749, Bl. 75.
Fixxxxx	Gxxxxx	xx/03/1920	Yes	No	No	No	N/A	No	No	No	No	CDU	BStU, MfS, HA XX, 5749, Bl. 279–80.
Garten	Johannes	20/08/1920	Yes	No	No	No	DJV	No	No	No	No	N/A	BStU, MfS, HA IX/11, ZA 7294, Objekt 13, Bl. 5–9, 21.
Hexxxxx	Fxxxxx	xx/07/1920	No	No	No	No	N/A	No	Yes	No	Yes	N/A	BStU, MfS, BV Dresden, KD Sebnitz, 4409, Teil 2, Bl. 291.
Hexxxxx	Wxxxxx	xx/12/1918	No	No	No	No	N/A	No	Yes	No	No	N/A	BStU, MfS, HA IX/11, AV 8/84, Bl. 126–29.
Hoxxxxx	Kxxxxx	xx/09/1919	No	No	No	No	N/A	No	Yes	No	No	N/A	BStU, MfS, BV Dresden, KD Sebnitz, 4409, Teil 2, Bl. 327.
Kexxxxx	Kxxxxx	xx/09/1923	No	No	No	No	N/A	Yes	No	No	No	N/A	BStU, HA VII, 2125, Bl. 31–33.
Matthies	Hans-Jürgen	06/03/1925	Yes	No	No	No	N/A	Yes	No	No	No	N/A	BStU, MfS, HA XX, 5755, Bl. 228.
Mecklinger	Ludwig	14/11/1919	No	No	No	No	N/A	Yes	No	Yes	No	N/A	BStU, MfS, HA XX, 527, Bl. 354–57.
Ocxxxxx	Mxxxxx	xx/01/1920	No	No	No	No	N/A	Yes	No	No	No	N/A	BStU, MfS, HA XX, 3364, Bl. 47–48.
Schwarz-lose	Erich	28/08/1918	Yes	No	No	No	N/A	No	No	No	No	NDPD	BStU, MfS, HA XX, 5755, Bl. 144–58.
Voxxxxx	Kxxxxx	xx/07/1917	No	No	No	No	N/A	No	Yes	No	Yes	N/A	BStU, MfS, BV Leipzig, KD Leipzig-Land, 3738, Bl. 2–5.
Wixxxxx	Gxxxxx	xx/02/1919	No	No	No	No	N/A	No	Yes	No	No	N/A	BStU, MfS, AS 2453/67, Bl. 18.

Note

1 Some names were made anonymous due to public and archival restrictions, especially for people not in any political or public offices born 1907 and later. Therefore, only the first two letters of the last name, the first letter of the first name, and the birth month and year are provided in the following in order to comply with the German Data Protection Law of the archives, i.e. BStU and BArch (restrictions until 110 years after birth, if the DOD is unknown).

Index

For Product Safety Concerns and Information please contact our EU
representative GPSR@taylorandfrancis.com
Taylor & Francis Verlag GmbH, Kaufingerstraße 24, 80331 München, Germany

www.ingramcontent.com/pod-product-compliance
Lightning Source LLC
Chambersburg PA
CBHW060406220326
41598CB00023B/3035